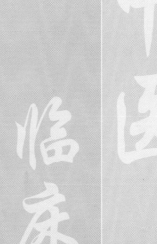

中医
临
床

The herb shown on the cover is **Ài Yè**艾叶 *(Folium Artemisiae Argyi), commonly known as mugwort. Its therapeutic actions include warming the channels, stopping bleeding, dissipating cold, regulating menstruation, and calming a restless fetus. In Chinese medical gynecology, mugwort is commonly used in the treatment of uterine bleeding, amenorrhea and infertility.*

Project Editor: Liu Shui, Jiang Qian & Zeng Chun
Book Designer: Li Xi
Cover Designer: Li Xi
Typesetter: Wei Hong-bo

The Clinical Practice of Chinese Medicine

Menstrual Disorders I:
Dysfunctional Uterine Bleeding & Amenorrhea

中医
临床

The Clinical Practice of Chinese Medicine

Menstrual Disorders I:
Dysfunctional Uterine Bleeding & Amenorrhea

by **Si-tu Yi**
*Professor of Chinese Medical Gynecology,
the Second Teaching Hospital of Guangzhou
University of CM, Guangzhou, China*

Wang Xiao-yun
*Professor of Chinese Medical Gynecology,
Director of Department of Gynecology,
the Second Teaching Hospital of Guangzhou
University of CM, Guangzhou, China*

Contributors
Lu Hua, Ph.D. TCM   **Yang Hong-yan**, Ph.D. TCM   **Liu Ge**, Ph.D. TCM
Ran Qing-zhen, Ph.D. TCM   **Wen Ming-hua**, M.S. TCM

Translated by
Yang Guang-ning, M.S. TCM & **Liu Lu**, M.S. TCM

Edited by
Harry F. Lardner, R.Ac.

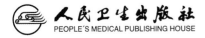
人民卫生出版社
PEOPLE'S MEDICAL PUBLISHING HOUSE

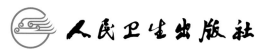

PMPH PEOPLE´S MEDICAL PUBLISHING HOUSE

Website: http://www.pmph.com

Book Title: The Clinical Practice of Chinese Medicine:
Menstrual Disorders I: Dysfunctional Uterine Bleeding & Amenorrhea
中医临床实用系列：月经病I：功能失调性子宫出血与闭经

Contact address: Bldg 3, 3 Qu, Fang Qun Yuan, Fang Zhuang, Beijing 100078, P. R. China, Phone/fax: 86 10 6761 7315, E-mail: pmph@pmph.com

---

Disclaimer

This book is for educational and reference purposes only. In view of the possibility of human error or changes in medical science, neither the author, editor nor the publisher nor any other party who has been involved in the preparation or publication of this work guarantees that the information contained herein is in every respect accurate or complete. The medicinal therapy and treatment techniques presented in this book are provided for the purpose of reference only. If readers wish to attempt any of the techniques or utilize any of the medicinal therapies contained in this book, the publisher assumes no responsibility for any such actions.

It is the responsibility of the readers to understand and adhere to local laws and regulations concerning the practice of these techniques and methods. The authors, editors and publishers disclaim all responsibility for any liability, loss, injury, or damage incurred as a consequence, directly or indirectly, of the use and application of any of the contents of this book.

First published: 2007
ISBN: 978-7-117-08820-6/R · 8821

Cataloguing in Publication Data:
A catalog record for this book is available from the
CIP - Database China.

Printed in P.R. China

ISBN 978-7-117-08820-6

9 787117 088206 >

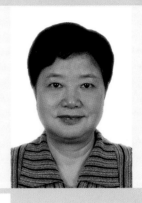

司徒仪 教授

Professor **Si-tu Yi** was born in May 1945. She is a professor & Ph.D. supervisor & postdoctoral cooperative supervisor at the Second Teaching Hospital of Guangzhou University of Chinese Medicine (also known as Guangdong Provincial Hospital of Chinese Medicine). She is also the instructor of "Guangzhou Municipal Outstanding Clinical Talent Research Project", and chief physician. In addition, she serves as the key special subject leader of the State Administration of Traditional Chinese Medicine on the "10th Five-Years Key Programs for Science and Technology Development of China", the vice chairman of the Gynecology Committee of China Association of Chinese Medicine, the member of the Chinese Association of the Integration of Traditional and Western Medicine - the Third Gynecology Committee, the councilor of the Guangdong Association of the Integration of Traditional and Western Medicine – Gynecology Committee, the member of Guangdong Technical Appraisal for the Medical Negligence Committee, and the member of the Chinese Medical Appraisal Committee for Science and Technology Award & Chinese Medical Youth Prize of the Chinese Medical Association.

She is in charge of the vice president and executive director of the First Gynecology Specialty Committee of World Federation of Chinese Medicine Societies, the director of the Guangdong Association of the Integration of Traditional and Western Medicine, the deputy director of the Editorial Board of the *Chinese Journal of Chinese Medicine Gynecology*, and the editorial member of *Chinese Journal of Modern Integrative Medicine*. She is the chief editor of four monographs and the editorial member of another four monographs, including *Integrative Medicine Gynecology and Geared to the 21st Century Medical College Teaching Materials*. Endometriosis is her main direction. She has compiled the book *Integrative Medical Treatment on Endometriosis* published by People's Medical Publishing House, which is popular in the majority of professionals and patients. In 2001, she won the "Outstanding Award" of Kanglaite-Cup National Chinese Medicine Outstanding Academic Book Award for editing the book *Clinical Chinese Medical Diagnosis and Treatment on Gynecological Diseases*.

So far, she has published more than 60 articles on the provincial-level magazines, taken charge of or participated in totally 20 research projects at all levels, and accomplished more than 10 scientific research achievements, including 3 ministerial-level achievements.

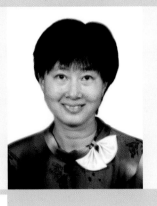

王小云 教授

Professor **Wang Xiao-yun** serves as a professor and Ph.D. supervisor of Chinese medical gynecology at the Second Teaching Hospital of the Guangzhou University of Chinese Medicine (also known as Guangdong Provincial Hospital of Chinese Medicine). She engages in the clinic, scientific research and teaching work of the integrative medical diagnosis and treatment of gynecological diseases, specializes in clinical diagnosis and treatment and mechanism researches on gynecological endocrine diseases and tumors, especially does well in menopause syndrome, depression, insomnia, infertility and gynecological tumors.

Professor Wang was awarded the honorary title "Bethune-Medical Worker" by the Department of Health of Guangdong Province in 1996, and was rated the honorary title "Guangdong Nanyue Outstanding Teacher" in 2003. She is the member of the Gynecology Committee of China Association of Chinese Medicine, the member of the Gynecology Specialty Committee of World Federation of Chinese Medicine Societies, the director of the Chinese Medical Council of Guangdong Province, the vice chairman of the Gynecology Committee of Guangdong Provincial Association of Chinese Medicine.

Inheriting the classical theories of Chinese medicine, Professor Wang is good at the treatment of emergent and stubborn gynecological diseases with classical formulas. She holds that fully taking advantage of the combined therapy of Chinese medicine will gain a satisfactory result in the clinic. Due to her achievements, she enjoys a relatively high reputation among patients in USA, Canada, Australia, Singapore, Hong Kong, Macao and other areas around the country.

During the period of learning evidence-based medicine in Newcastle Northumbria University in Britain, she treated a paralysis patient with acupuncture for only three times. After the treatment, the patient, who had suffered movement disturbance for 3 years, can walk freely again. Therefore, she was eulogized as "magical needle"acupucturist. With upright academy style and noble professional quality, Professor Wang cultivates and encourages students without selfishness. Now, she has trained 23 masters and 6 doctors in total.

Foreword

Chinese medicine is a broad and profound art of healing. It is a well-established and comprehensive system of medicine with an ancient origin and a long rich history. Throughout the ages, it has made a significant contribution to the prosperity of the Chinese civilization. The system of pattern differentiation and treatment fully reflects the Chinese medical view of health and disease as a holistic concept, the emphasis on the body's ability to regulate itself and adapt to the environment, and the need for individualized treatment. The integration of diseases and syndromes is the consummation of treatment based on pattern differentiation; it fully displays the superior characteristic of this discipline, and has an extensive influence on the development of the art of Chinese medicine.

The intention of this series of books is to introduce accurate Chinese medical diagnosis and treatment of various diseases to overseas readers.

The Chinese edition of *The Clinical Practice of Chinese Medicine* was edited by the Second Teaching Hospital of Guangzhou University of CM (also known as Guangdong Provincial Hospital of TCM), and published by People's Medical Publishing House. When the series was published in 2000, it was widely accepted in clinical practice due to its originality, distinguishing features, richness in content, completeness, accuracy, and outstanding emphases. This series has become a trademark of standard in the eyes of Chinese and integrative medical practitioners. During the second printing of this series of books, Professor Deng Tie-tao praised, "For a series to be printed a multiple number of times, shows that it is highly regarded and has received excellent reviews." In order to keep up with the constant development of medical science, this series was revised and re-published in 2004 by People's Medical Publishing House. Due to its popularity, it has been reprinted numerous times since.

The English edition of this series of books includes 20 volumes:
- ✧ *COPD & Asthma*
- ✧ *Coronary Artery Disease & Hyperlipidemia*
- ✧ *Stroke & Parkinson's Disease*
- ✧ *Chronic Gastritis & Irritable Bowel Syndrome*
- ✧ *Diabetes & Obesity*
- ✧ *Gout & Rheumatoid Arthritis*
- ✧ *Menstrual Disorders I: Dysfunctional Uterine Bleeding & Amenorrhea*
- ✧ *Menstrual Disorders II: Premenstrual Syndrome, Dysmenorrhea & Perimenopause*
- ✧ *Endometriosis & Uterine Fibroids*
- ✧ *Pelvic Inflammatory Disease & Miscarriage*
- ✧ *Postpartum Hypogalactia & Breast Hyperplasia*
- ✧ *Male & Female Infertility*
- ✧ *Urticaria*
- ✧ *Eczema & Atopic Dermatitis*
- ✧ *Lupus Erythematosus*
- ✧ *Scleroderma & Dermatomyositis*
- ✧ *Diseases of the Accessory Organs of the Skin*
- ✧ *Psoriasis & Cutaneous Pruritis*
- ✧ *Herpes Zoster & Fungal Skin Infections*

❖ *Pigmentary Disorders of the Skin*

Clinical application varies by individual and by location; when this is combined with the rapid development of medical science, the treatment methods and medicinal dosages may also vary accordingly. When using these books as a reference guide, overseas readers should confirm the formulas and dosages of medicinals according to the individual health condition of the patient, as well as take into account the origin of the Chinese medicinals.

The quotes in these books were taken from various medical literature during the compilation process. We have deleted some of the contents of the original texts for the purpose of uniformity and ease in readability. We ask for the reader's forgiveness and express our respect and gratitude toward the original authors.

Due to the complicated nature of the diagnoses and treatments covered in these books, and the wide range of topics they touch upon, it is inevitable that one may encounter errors while reading through them. We respectively welcome constructive criticism and corrections from our readers.

The clinical practice of medicine changes with the constant development of medical science. The books in this series will be revised regularly to continuously adapt to the development of traditional Chinese medicine.

Editorial Board for the English edition of
The Clinical Practice of Chinese Medicine **series**
September, 2006

Wu Xian-zhong

Specialist of Integrative Medicine, Academician of Chinese Academy of Engineering, Professor, Tianjin Medical University, Chairman of Tianjin Institute of Acute Abdomen Research on Integrative Medicine

Wang Yong-yan

Specialist of Chinese Internal Medicine, Academician of Chinese Academy of Engineering, Professor and former President of Beijing University of CM, and Honorary President of China Academy of Chinese Medical Science

Chen Ke-ji

Specialist of Cardiovascular & Aging Diseases, Academician of Chinese Academy of Science, Professor of Medicine, Xiyuan Hospital, and Institute of Aging Medicine, China Academy of Chinese Medical Science, Consultant on Traditional Medicine, WHO

General Coordinator

Lü Yu-bo

Professor & Vice President, Guangzhou University of CM, President, the Second Teaching Hospital of Guangzhou University of CM

Editors-in-Chief

Luo Yun-jian

Guangdong Province Entitled Famous Chinese Medicine Physician, Professor of Chinese Internal Medicine, & former Vice President of the Second Teaching Hospital of Guangzhou University of CM

Liu Mao-cai

Guangdong Province Entitled Famous Chinese Medicine Physician, Professor of Chinese Internal Medicine, & former Vice President of the Second Teaching Hospital of Guangzhou University of CM, Former Chairman of Institute for Aging Cerebral Diseases, Guangzhou University of CM

Members (Listed alphabetically by name)

Deng Zhao-zhi

Professor of Chinese Internal Medicine, Guangzhou University of CM

Fan Guan-jie

Professor of Chinese Internal Medicine, Director of Department of Education, the Second Teaching Hospital of Guangzhou University of CM

Fan Rui-qiang

Professor of Chinese External Medicine, Director of Department of Dermatology, the Second Teaching Hospital of Guangzhou University of CM

Huang Jian-ling

Professor of Chinese Medicine Gynecology, Director of the First Department of Gynecology, the Second Teaching Hospital of Guangzhou University of CM

Huang Pei-xin

Professor of Chinese Internal Medicine, the Second Teaching Hospital of Guangzhou University of CM, Head of the Research Project of Cerebral Disease Treatment on Chinese Internal Medicine, Sponsored by SATCM China

Huang Sui-ping

Professor of Chinese Internal Medicine, Director of Department of Digestion, the Second Teaching Hospital of Guangzhou University of CM

Li Li-yun

Guangdong Province Entitled Famous Chinese Medicine Physician, Professor of Chinese Medicine Gynecology, the Second Teaching Hospital of Guangzhou University of CM

Liang Xue-fang

Professor of Chinese Medicine Gynecology, Director of the Third Department of Gynecology, the Second Teaching Hospital of Guangzhou University of CM

Lin Lin

Professor of Chinese Internal Medicine, Director of Department of Respiratory, the Second Teaching Hospital of Guangzhou University of CM

Lin Yi

Professor of Mastopathy in Chinese Medicine , the Second Teaching Hospital of Guangzhou University of CM, Head of the National Key Subject – Mastopathy in Chinese Medicine

Liu Wei-sheng

Master of the National Master and Apprentice Education Program, Professor of Chinese Internal Medicine, the Second Teaching Hospital of Guangzhou University of CM

Si-tu Yi

Professor of Chinese Medicine Gynecology, the Second Teaching Hospital of Guangzhou University of CM, Head of the National Key Subject-Chinese Medicine Gynecology

Wang Xiao-yun

Professor of Chinese Medicine Gynecology, Director of Department of Gynecology, Head of Teaching Division of Gynecology, the Second Teaching Hospital of Guangzhou University of CM

Sponsored by

The Second Teaching Hospital of Guangzhou University of CM, also known as **Guangdong Provincial Hospital of TCM**

Preface

Chinese medicine is proved to be significantly effective in the treatment of menstrual diseases, which highlights its characteristics and advantages in clinical practice. Along with the development of gynecology, researches on menstrual diseases have already been standardized and systemized. This book is intended to provide effective formulas, medicinals, and multiple-route therapies for Chinese medical professionals, practitioners and students at home and abroad. Also, it provides a therapeutic tool for biomedical doctors of gynecology in the treatment of stubborn gynecological diseases.

Dysfunctional uterine bleeding and amenorrhea discussed in this book are commonly and frequently seen in the gynecology, which may severely influence female health and quality of life and is always emphasized by doctors since ancient times. Chinese medical doctors of every dynasty have accumulated rich experience in practice. Based on the holism, in order to regulate endocrine and restore normal menstruation they balance Kidney yin and Kidney yang, promote the Kidney function, and re-establish yin-yang equilibrium of the Kidney-Heart-Uterus Axis, combining the periodic variation of the ovaries. Our editorial board made a refined summarization of Chinese medical clinical diagnosis and treatment, according to long-time clinical observation and current research results. Indeed, the book is considered as a gospel of medical treatment for patients.

This book is edited by clinical experts and professors of rich knowledge and experience of clinical practices. They are engaged in integrative medical diagnosis and treatment of dysfunctional uterine bleeding and amenorrhea for a long time. Taken professional opinions from the editorial board and experts of related subjects into account, its content includes detailed introduction of traditional pattern differentiation, diagnosis and treatment, quotation of classics such as *"The Yellow Emperor's Inner Classic"* and *"Classic on Medical Problems"*, experience of clinical treatment, clinical practice essence of contemporary famous domestic scholars, updated progressions of current researches. This compilation places much emphasis on the thinking and refinement of the key points and challenges of diseases. Under the guidance of Chinese medicine theories, each disease introduction is clearly and concisely expounded as etiology & pathomechanism, treatment principle, formula, medicinals, while empirical cases and perspectives of many elderly renowned TCM doctors are involved in this book as clinical evidences.

Besides, combining the advantages of Chinese medicine and the appropriate timing and modalities of biomedicine, it provides for foreign readers clear ideas of thinking in the integrative medical treatment. In addition, it also analyzes and discusses current domestic and international research results. The part **modern research** that appends to each disease provides informative reference for readers as detailedly as possible.

This book extensively collects medical classics and research information of current magazines, which is a comprehensive clinical book of gynecology. Including the rich experience of clinical specialists, it covers refined classical medical treatises, relatively new scientific developments and practical experience in the clinic.

Its clear and concise statements as well as the expression style that simplify profound ideas make it more systematic and complete, and therefore is more applicable to those clinical medical students and gynecologist of all levels at home and abroad.

In this series of books, readers will find an organized and thorough presentation of each disease, including a brief overview, etiology, pathomechanism, Chinese medical treatment using various treatment modalities, prognosis, preventive healthcare practices, case studies, comments from famous physicians, integrative treatment approaches, quotes from classical texts, and modern research.

The **brief overview** offers a general introduction to the biomedical view of the disease.

Discussions of etiology, pathomechanism, and Chinese medical treatment are from the angle of Chinese medicine, and reflect upon the onset, diagnosis, pattern differentiation, and treatment of the disease.

Cases and comments from many famous physicians are collected in the section of clinical experience of renowned physicians.

The chapter on **integrative treatment approaches** emphasizes the advantages of Chinese medical treatments, as well as discussing the proper time for the intervention of biomedicine. To the Western reader, this section presents a clear mode of thinking in terms of the integration of Chinese medicine and biomedicine.

Quotes from classical texts and modern research provide abundant references on these diseases.

This series of books presents a clear description of each disease as well as the key points for diagnosis and treatment using Chinese medicine. These books discuss, in detail, the clinical experience of ancient and modern-day renowned physicians, thereby enabling the practitioner to become more adept at using Chinese medicine in the diagnosis and treatment of common diseases.

As objective readers of this book, foreign teachers and students of Chinese medical college or acupuncture college, practitioners engaged in Chinese medicine and acupuncture, biomedical doctors who are interested in Chinese medicine, and all of those involved in the field of Chinese medicine can read it for study reference in the clinical diagnosis and treatment.

The book has referred to a great number of literatures, and cited some contents of various medical books, journals, and magazines. In the process of compilation, it has undergone repeatedly careful modifications and much consideration for its accuracy. However, due to the nature of clinical medicine, we apologize for any out-dated or incorrect information that may appear in these books. We hope that readers will not hesitate to offer their comments and suggestions on how to improve the content of this material. Meanwhile, we express our heartfelt thanks to those experts for their enlightenments and help. Salute the originators for their diligence and great efforts.

This book is designed to collect the whole Chinese medical diagnosis and treatment of the two diseases mentioned above, correct the errors, gather the scattered parts and sort out the information, and is expected to spread around the world for a little contribution to the inheritance and development of traditional Chinese medicine.

Si-tu Yi & Wang Xiao-yun
Guangzhou China
March 2007

Contents

Amenorrhea 223

Dysfunctional Uterine Bleeding

by **Si-tu Yi**, Professor of Chinese Medical Gynecology

Wang Xiao-yun, Professor of Chinese Medical Gynecology

Lu Hua, Ph. D. TCM

Yang Hong-yan, Ph. D. TCM

Liu Ge, Ph. D. TCM

OVERVIEW

Dysfunctional uterine bleeding (DUB) is abnormal genital tract bleeding that is not due to any organic or structural cause. After all other causes of abnormal uterine bleeding are ruled out, DUB is caused by an imbalance of the neuroendocrine which is related to ovulation. Being the most commonly encountered disease in gynecology, DUB may occur at any time during a woman's reproductive life. The main clinical symptoms are menstruation that vary in cycle, duration, and volume. Bleeding patterns range from scant menses to profuse vaginal hemorrhage. Clinically, DUB can be classified as ovulatory and anovulatory types.

Approximately 80% DUB cases belong to anovulatory type, 90% of which occur during adolescence and premenopause. The incidence in premenopause is higher than in adolescence.The main characteristics of anovulatory DUB are irregular cycles with excessive bleeding, or intermenstrual bleeding lasting from 10 days to several months. Ovulatory type may present shortened cycle, excessively increased menstrual bleeding, and prolonged duration that can spontaneously stop.

In Chinese medicine, dysfunctional uterine bleeding (DUB) refers to clinical conditions such as flooding and spotting, early menstruation, profuse menstruation, prolonged menstruation and ovulatory bleeding. Both ovulatory and anovulatory DUB may lead to infertility.

CHINESE MEDICAL ETIOLOGY AND PATHOMECHANISM

The Chinese medicine etiology of DUB can be understood in three aspects. Heat, stasis and deficiency are regarded as three main causes responsible for this disease. Each of them attacks human body individually or in combination. Furthermore, there may be mutual causation among these three causes. All eventually lead to an impairment of the penetrating and conception vessels, resulting in uncontrolled bleeding.

1. Heat Disturbing the Penetrating and Conception Vessels, Restlessness of the Sea of Blood

(1) Deficienct Heat

This pattern is associated with an underlying yin deficiency that may result from a variety of factors. Causes include longstanding diseases, congenital deficiency, sudden or chronic damage to yin-blood, yin essence decline during menopause, sexual intemperance, or excessive childbirth. Yin deficiency often leads to internal heat. Heat injures the vessels and the blood may not be contained, resulting in yin-blood deficiency. As yin-blood becomes more deficient, the heat condition progresses. Yin deficiency and blood-heat conditions often tangle with each other, leading to a rapid exacerbation of the patient's condition.

(2) Excessive Heat

Heat conditions may originate from either external or internal causes. The internal causes are listed as follows.

➢ Liver fire resulting from a constitutional condition of excessive yang.

➢ Severe or sudden anger.

➢ Liver qi constraint associated with emotional depression, leading to fire.

➢ Excessive consumption of foods that are acrid, dry or yang-assisting in nature, leading to fire or pathogenic heat accumulating in the penetrating and conception vessels.

➢ Improper diet and taxation may impair the Spleen which may fail to transform and transport, resulting in turbid dampness pouring downward and transforming into heat.

➢ When damp-heat invades the uterus and uterine collaterals, the penetrating and conception vessels become damaged due to heat disturbance and dampness obstruction. This often occurs during the menstrual period, or following childbirth and surgery.

Heat patterns may also develop as a result of contracting an external pathogen. Pathogenic heat or damp-heat may be contracted unexpectedly during any season. Internal heat then forces the blood to move frenetically, leading to a depletion of yin-blood, resulting in a deficient heat condition. Therefore, excess heat conditions must be addressed as they often lead to deficiency patterns that may further severely damage yin-blood.

2. DEFICIENCY AND INSECURITY OF THE PENETRATING AND CONCEPTION VESSELS

(1) Deficiency of the Internal Organs

Deficiencies of the viscera mainly involve the Kidney, Liver and Spleen. As both the root of congenital constitution and the source of *Tian Gui*, the Kidney is responsible for storing essence and also absorbing qi. Abundant Kidney qi is fundamental to normal menstrual function. Chronic Kidney deficiency may be associated with congenital conditions or a lack of abundant Kidney qi during adolescence. During the reproductive period, intemperate sexual activity and excessive childbirth also lead to deficiency. Kidney qi naturally declines during menopause, and may also be depleted as a result of any severe or longstanding disease. As the source of menses, Kidney deficiency also leads to disorders of storage.

Loss of blood also damages the Liver, disrupting its function of storage and discharge. Since the Liver and Kidney share the same source, disordered menstruation may result.

The Spleen governs both the transformation and management of blood. Spleen qi deficiency may result from a congenital weakness of the Stomach and Spleen, insufficiency of the middle qi, overwork, over-thinking, or improper nutrition. The impairment of Spleen qi may cause lack of the origin, leading to the dysfunction of the Spleen.

(2) Qi and Blood Deficiency

Qi is the commander of blood, and blood is the mother of qi. Due to this relationship, qi and blood originate from the same source and engender each other. Qi deficiency may result in blood deficiency, and vice versa.

Blood deficiency results in an insufficient source of nourishment for the penetrating and conception vessels. Qi and blood may be deficient as a result of congenital factors, or they may become deficient due to any chronic disease, including DUB.

Qi deficiency impairs the Spleen's function of containment, and also affects the penetrating and conception vessels, leading to frenetic movement of blood. The condition of the penetrating and conception vessels is closely related to the sufficiency of qi and blood, so these patterns often lead to one another.

In addition, congenital yang deficiency may also generate conditions of internal cold. Eating too many cold or raw foods or taking medicinals of a cold nature may impair yang qi or deplete the life gate fire. As a result, the viscera are unable to warm and transform, leading to further qi and blood deficiency. Finally, the penetrating and conception vessels are unable to manage the blood, leading to DUB.

3. STASIS IN THE PENETRATING AND CONCEPTION VESSELS, BLOOD NOT CONTAINED IN THE VESSELS

(1) Excessive Blood Stasis

Blood stasis may occur as a result of excess conditions such as Liver qi stagnation, heat consuming the fluids, external cold evil, congealing cold or damp-heat accumulation impairing free flow, or long-time bleeding leads to stagnation in the uterus. Eating too much cold and raw food or living in cold and damp areas may exacerbate stasis conditions.

(2) Deficient Blood Stasis

Deficienct blood stasis may result from deficient qi unable to promote the free flow of blood. The uterus and its vessels may also be damaged after surgery, leading to disordered movement of qi and blood. Stasis conditions often result from incomplete curettage. All of this leads to an impairment of the free flow in the penetrating and conception vessels, where fresh blood is prevented from circulating. As blood stasis and excessive bleeding lead to each other, these conditions tend to repeatedly occur.

4. COMPLEX PATTERNS INVOLVING DEFICIENCY, HEAT AND STASIS

The most commonly seen combinations involve:

➤ Yin deficiency with blood-heat.
➤ Qi deficiency with blood-heat.
➤ Kidney deficiency with blood-heat.
➤ Kidney deficiency with Liver qi stagnation.
➤ Spleen deficiency with Liver qi stagnation.
➤ Blood deficiency and stasis.
➤ Qi and yin deficiency with stasis.
➤ Stasis combined with heat.

➢ Yang deficiency with blood stasis.

CHINESE MEDICAL TREATMENT

The treatment of dysfunctional uterine bleeding (DUB) should be determined based on the severity and duration of condition, as well as the age and physical condition of the patient.

There are several approaches that we may consider. We may treat differently according to the presence of bleeding and non-bleeding phases. Another approach is to consider the age and reproductive health of the patient. Adolescent, childbearing and menopausal women all require specific treatment plans.

In the case of severe bleeding treating the symptom is primary, but if the condition is not acute, we may rather focus on the underlying cause. It is important to stop bleeding immediately in unusually severe cases. During non-bleeding phases the main approach is to regulate menstruation and secure the penetrating vessel.

In adolescents, we should address abnormal bleeding with an objective of establishing regular menstruation. Treatment should continue until two normal ovulatory cycles have been established.

In childbearing women, we should also determine the cause by ruling out both structural and systemic disease.

The treatment approach for menopausal women is to first stanch bleeding, after which our objective is to assist the patient throughout the transition by strengthening the Spleen and nourishing blood.

Pattern Differentiation and Treatment

1. KEY POINTS IN PATTERN DIFFERENTIATION

Pattern differentiation for abnormal bleeding is based on the quantity, color and quality of the blood, as well as the other presenting signs and symptoms. We must differentiate the main patterns of deficiency, heat, or stasis, and also the presence of more complex presentations.

(1) Deficiency Pattern Differentiation

Symptoms such as profuse bleeding with spotting, thin and light-colored menses, lassitude, and a pale tongue are generally associated with Spleen qi deficiency.

Symptoms such as weakness of the legs and lumbus, frequent urination, depressed mood, a pale tongue and a deep or weak and forceless pulse indicate an insecurity of Kidney qi.

Thin and light-colored menses, a pale complexion, cold abdominal pain that is relieved by warmth and pressure, and a pale, swollen tongue with indentations at the edges point to a debilitation of yang qi.

Symptoms and signs of qi and blood deficiency include shortness of breath, spontaneous sweating, dizziness and blurry vision, a sallow complexion, a pale tongue, and a thready or weak pulse.

(2) Heat Pattern Differentiation

Scant bleeding appearing bright red, tidal fever and night sweating, vexing heat in the chest, palms and soles, a red tongue with little coating, and a thready, rapid pulse are all signs of yin deficiency.

Damp-heat patterns may manifest as profuse bleeding of bright red or very dark-colored menses that is both viscous and foul-smelling. We may also see slight fever, taxation, distending pain of the lower abdomen, a red tongue with a greasy coating, and a slippery or rapid pulse.

(3) Blood Stasis Pattern Differentiation

Symptoms of qi stagnation and blood stasis include profuse or scant bleeding of dark color with clotting, distention and oppression of the chest and hypochondrium, distending pain of the lower abdomen that is aggravated by pressure, a bitter taste and dry throat, a red tongue, and a wiry or slippery pulse.

Excess heat with blood stasis may present profuse bleeding with clotting that is bright red in color and also foul-smelling. Other symptoms may be fever, agitation, a dry mouth, a red tongue, and a slippery or rapid pulse.

Congealing cold often presents scant bleeding with dark clots, coldness of the trunk and limbs, cold pain of the lower abdomen, a dark-colored tongue with stasis spots, and a deep, thready or weak pulse.

Blood stasis due to trauma often occurs in patients reporting a history of abortion or surgery. Signs include profuse or scant bleeding, irregular cycles with clotting and pain in the lower abdomen which is relieved upon discharge, normal tongue color with possible stasis spots, and a wiry pulse.

2. THREE APPROACHES TO THE TREATMENT OF FLOODING

These three approaches may be applied individually or together.

(1) Se Liu (Stanch Bleeding)

Bleeding of this type may be treated with upbearing and astringent medicinals. When sudden and severe flooding occurs, bleeding must be stopped or qi may become exhausted, creating a possibly life-threatening condition. In these cases, stopping bleeding to prevent exhaustion is paramount. Qi is the commander of blood and blood is the mother of qi, as both are mutually engendering and interdependent. Any excessive loss of blood inevitably creates a deficiency of qi. Deficiency may cause the origin qi to fall, and combined with a failure to contain blood in the vessels, blood loss will continue. Due to this relationship of qi and blood, sudden flooding may lead to an exhaustion of both qi and blood. So it is important while arresting bleeding to simultaneously tonify qi. The treatment principles are to secure qi to contain blood, and astringe to stanch bleeding.

(2) Cheng Yuan (Treat the Root)

This method emphasizes treating the root cause. Patterns must be differentiated based on their etiology, and treatment that follows must be clearly based on the presenting pattern. After the bleeding pattern has decreased or ceased, new treatment principles and medicinals should be selected according to the presenting etiologies and pathomechanisms. This is an important consideration in the proper treatment of DUB.

(3) Fu Jiu (Establish and Regulate Menses)

This method refers to the establishment and regulation of normal menstrual cycles. The treatment principles are to tonify the Kidney, regulate the Liver, and strengthen the Spleen. In clinic, we must consider the timing, volume, and quality of the menses as well as the specific pattern associated with the disorder. So the principle objective is to restore normal cycles while also preventing the possibility of recurrence.

The Kidney which stores the essence is the source of menses and responsible for reproduction. The Liver stores the blood and is responsible for promoting the free flow of qi and blood. It also regulates the functions of the sea of blood. The smooth flow of Liver qi ensures the timely filling of the sea of blood, which is essential for the production of regular menstrual cycles. The Spleen is responsible for the transformation and transportation of qi and blood. The Spleen also manages the blood by both generating blood and containing it within the vessels. So the Kidney, Liver and Spleen must be coordinated with the functions of the penetrating and conception vessels and the uterus. Only then can healthy menstrual cycles occur.

(4) Stanch Bleeding and Treat the Root

The proper strategy may often be to combine individual treatment principles such as tonifying deficiency while arresting bleeding, or clearing heat while also dispelling blood stasis. Multiple approaches may be indicated, with the appropriate presenting patterns. Merely astringing in order to stop bleeding may not sufficiently invigorate blood or dispel stasis. As a result, abnormal bleeding could recur. So the combination of these methods may both effectively stop bleeding while also preventing further stagnation and blood stasis.

(5) Treat the Root, Establish and Regulate Menses

The combination of these methods may shorten the course of treatment, and also benefit menstruation after the cessation of the abnormal bleeding patterns.

3. Pattern Differentiation and Treatment in the Bleeding Stage

(1) Yin Deficiency and Blood-heat

【Syndrome Characteristics】
Advanced menstruation with sudden bleeding, profuse and urgent menstruation or scant with spotting, thick red menses, tidal facial flushing, vexation, fever of the palms and soles, scant yellow urine, constipation, a red tongue with little coating, and a thready or rapid pulse.

【Treatment Principle】
Nourish yin and clear heat, stanch bleeding and regulate menstruation.

【Commonly Used Medicinals】
Commonly used medicinals are *huáng qín* (Radix Scutellariae), *huáng*

bǎi (Cortex Phellodendri Chinensis), *shēng dì huáng* (Radix Rehmanniae), *zhī mǔ* (Rhizoma Anemarrhenae), *dì gǔ pí* (Cortex Lycii), *bái sháo* (Radix Paeoniae Alba), *bái wēi* (Radix et Rhizoma Cynanchi Atrati), *hàn lián cǎo* (Herba Ecliptae), *qiàn cǎo* (Radix Rubiae), *dān pí* (Cotex Moutan), *qīng hāo* (Herba Artemisiae Annuae), *shā shēn* (Radix Adenophorae seu Glehniae), *mài dōng* (Radix Ophiopogonis), *huáng jīng* (Rhizoma Polygonati), *nǔ zhēn zǐ* (Fructus Ligustri Lucidi), *guī bǎn* (Testudinis Plastrum), *biē jiǎ* (Carapax Trionycis), and *ē jiāo* (Colla Corii Asini).

【Representative Formula】

Bǎo Yīn Jiān (保阴煎) with *Èr Zhì Wán* (二至丸) plus *yì mǔ cǎo* (Herba Leonuri), *hé shǒu wū* (Radix Polygoni Multiflori), and *ē jiāo* (Colla Corii Asini).

【Ingredients】

生地黄	shēng dì huáng	12g	Radix Rehmanniae
熟地黄	shú dì huáng	12g	Radix Rehmanniae Praeparata
白芍	bái sháo	12g	Radix Paeoniae Alba
山药	shān yào	15g	Rhizoma Dioscoreae
续断	xù duàn	12g	Radix Dipsaci
黄芩	huáng qín	12g	Radix Scutellariae
黄柏	huáng bǎi	9g	Cortex Phellodendri Chinensis
女贞子	nǔ zhēn zǐ	20g	Fructus Ligustri Lucidi
旱莲草	hàn lián cǎo	24g	Herba Ecliptae
沙参	shā shēn	12g	Radix Adenophorae seu Glehniae
麦冬	mài dōng	12g	Radix Ophiopogonis
五味子	wǔ wèi zǐ	9g	Fructus Schisandrae
甘草	gān cǎo	4g	Radix et Rhizoma Glycyrrhizae

Decoct in 500ml of water until 100ml of liquid remains. Take half warm, twice daily.

【Formula Analysis】

In this formula, *huáng qín* (Radix Scutellariae), *huáng bǎi* (Cortex

Phellodendri Chinensis) and *shēng dì huáng* (Radix Rehmanniae) clear heat and cool blood; *shú dì huáng* (Radix Rehmanniae Praeparata) and *bái sháo* (Radix Paeoniae Alba) nourish blood and astringe yin; *shān yào* (Rhizoma Dioscoreae) and *xù duàn* (Radix Dipsaci) tonify the Kidney and secure the penetrating vessel; *hé shǒu wū* (Radix Polygoni Multiflori) and *ē jiāo* (Colla Corii Asini) nourish blood and arrest bleeding; *nǚ zhēn zǐ* (Fructus Ligustri Lucidi) and *hàn lián cǎo* (Herba Ecliptae) nourish the Liver and Kidney to stanch bleeding; *shā shēn* (Radix Adenophorae seu Glehniae), *mài dōng* (Radix Ophiopogonis) and *wǔ wèi zǐ* (Fructus Schisandrae) nourish yin; *yì mǔ cǎo* (Herba Leonuri) dispels stasis to arrest bleeding; and *gān cǎo* (Radix et Rhizoma Glycyrrhizae) harmonizes the formula.

【Modifications】

➢ For flooding, add *xiān hè cǎo* (Herba Agrimoniae) 30g, and *wū zéi gǔ* (Sepium) 12g, to cool blood and astringe.

➢ For spotting, add *shēng pú huáng* (Pollen Typhae Crudum) 12g (wrap-boiled), and *shēng sān qī fěn* (Raw Radix Notoginseng Powder) 3g, to eliminate blood stasis and stanch bleeding.

➢ For dizziness and blurry vision with taxation, add *dǎng shēn* (Radix Codonopsis) 20g, *huáng qí* (Radix Astragali) 20g, *bái zhú* (Rhizoma Atractylodis Macrocephalae) 12g, and *gǒu qǐ* (Fructus Lycii) 12g, to tonify qi and blood.

(2) Qi and Yin Deficiency

【Syndrome Characteristics】

Unexpected menstruation or advanced menstruation with sudden bleeding, or profuse and urgent bleeding followed by spotting, thick red or light clear menses, lassitude with sleepiness, insomnia or dream-disturbed sleep, tidal fever with sweating, scant yellow urine, constipation, a red or pale red tongue, a thin yellow or white tongue coating, and a thready, weak and rapid pulse.

【Treatment Principle】

Nourish qi and yin, purge heat and cool blood to stanch bleeding.

【Commonly Used Medicinals】

Select *huáng qí* (Radix Astragali), *dǎng shēn* (Radix Codonopsis), *xī yáng shēn* (Radix Panacis Quinquefolii), *tài zǐ shēn* (Radix Pseudostellariae), *bái zhú* (Rhizoma Atractylodis Macrocephalae), *shān yào* (Rhizoma Dioscoreae), *gān cǎo* (Radix et Rhizoma Glycyrrhizae), *mài dōng* (Radix Ophiopogonis), *wǔ wèi zǐ* (Fructus Schisandrae), *shēng dì huáng* (Radix Rehmanniae), *huáng qín* (Radix Scutellariae), *bái sháo* (Radix Paeoniae Alba), *bái wēi* (Radix et Rhizoma Cynanchi Atrati), *hàn lián cǎo* (Herba Ecliptae), *qīng hāo* (Herba Artemisiae Annuae), *shā shēn* (Radix Adenophorae seu Glehniae), *huáng jīng* (Rhizoma Polygonati), *nǚ zhēn zǐ* (Fructus Ligustri Lucidi), and *ē jiāo* (Colla Corii Asini).

【Representative Formula】

Bǎo Yīn Jiān (保阴煎) with *Shēng Mài Yǐn* (生脉饮) plus added *huáng qí* (Radix Astragali).

【Ingredients】

黄芪	huáng qí	20g	Radix Astragali
太子参	tài zǐ shēn	15g	Radix Pseudostellariae
黄芩	huáng qín	12g	Radix Scutellariae
黄柏	huáng bǎi	9g	Cortex Phellodendri Chinensis
生地黄	shēng dì huáng	12g	Radix Rehmanniae
熟地黄	shú dì huáng	12g	Radix Rehmanniae Praeparata
山药	shān yào	20g	Rhizoma Dioscoreae
川断	chuān xù duàn	12g	Radix Dipsaci
白芍	bái sháo	12g	Radix Paeoniae Alba
麦冬	mài dōng	12g	Radix Ophiopogonis
五味子	wǔ wèi zǐ	9g	Fructus Schisandrae
甘草	gān cǎo	4g	Radix et Rhizoma Glycyrrhizae

Decoct in 500ml of water until 100ml of liquid remains. Take half warm, twice daily.

【Formula Analysis】

In this formula, *huáng qín* (Radix Scutellariae), *huáng bǎi* (Cortex Phellodendri Chinensis) and *shēng dì huáng* (Radix Rehmanniae) clear heat and cool blood. *Shú dì huáng* (Radix Rehmanniae Praeparata) and *bái sháo* (Radix Paeoniae Alba) nourish blood and astringe yin; *shān yào* (Rhizoma Dioscoreae) and *xù duàn* (Radix Dipsaci) tonify the Kidney and secure the penetrating vessel; and *gān cǎo* (Radix et Rhizoma Glycyrrhizae) harmonizes the formula. *Huáng qí* (Radix Astragali) and *rén shēn* (Radix et Rhizoma Ginseng) tonify qi and nourish blood, while *mài dōng* (Radix Ophiopogonis) nourishes yin, and *wǔ wèi zǐ* (Fructus Schisandrae) with its a sour flavor astringes.

【Modifications】

➢ For vexation and insomnia, add *bǎi zǐ rén* (Semen Platycladi) 10g and *suān zǎo rén* (Semen Ziziphi Spinosae) 12g, *yè jiāo téng*（Caulis Polygoni Multiflori）30g, or *guī bǎn* (Testudinis Plastrum) 12g, *shēng mǔ lì* (Concha Ostreae Cruda)12g and *shēng lóng gǔ* (Fossilia Ossis Mastodi Cruda) 12g. These nourish yin and blood as well as pacifying the Heart and calming the spirit.

➢ For profuse bleeding, add *jīng jiè tàn* (Herba Schizonepetae Carbonisatum) 15g, *cè bǎi tàn* (Carbonized Cacumen Platycladi) 12g, and *pú huáng tàn* (Carbonized Pollen Typhae) 12g to clear heat and astringe.

(3) Yang Excess and Blood-heat

【Syndrome Characteristics】

Irregular or advanced menstruation, flooding and spotting, thick and dark red menses, thirst and vexation, fever, or during the summer-heat season, yellow urine or constipation, a red tongue with a yellow or

功能失调性子宫出血

greasy yellow coating, and a surging or rapid pulse.

【Treatment Principle】

Purge heat and cool blood, stanch bleeding and regulate menstruation.

【Commonly Used Medicinals】

Select *huáng qín* (Radix Scutellariae), *huáng lián* (Rhizoma Coptidis), *huáng bǎi* (Cortex Phellodendri Chinensis), *zhī zǐ* (Fructus Gardeniae), *dàn zhú yè* (Herba Lophatheri), *shēng dì huáng* (Radix Rehmanniae), *chì sháo* (Radix Paeoniae Rubra), *lián qiào* (Fructus Forsythiae), *yín huā* (Flos Lonicerae), *bài jiàng cǎo* (Herba Patriniae), *qīng hāo* (Herba Artemisiae Annuae), *dà huáng* (Radix et Rhizoma Rhei), *bái huā shé shé cǎo* (Herba Hedyotis Diffusae), and *xià kū cǎo* (Spica Prunellae).

【Representative Formula】

Qīng Rè Gù Jīng Tāng (清热固经汤) plus added *shā shēn* (Radix Adenophorae seu Glehniae).

【Ingredients】

黄芩	huáng qín	12g	Radix Scutellariae
焦栀子	jiāo zhī zǐ	12g	Fructus Gardeniae (scorch-fried)
生地黄	shēng dì huáng	12g	Radix Rehmanniae
地骨皮	dì gǔ pí	12g	Cortex Lycii
地榆	dì yú	12g	Radix Sanguisorbae
阿胶（烊化）	ē jiāo	12g	Colla Corii Asini (dissolved)
生藕节	shēng ǒu jié	20g	Nodus Nelumbinis Rhizomatis (raw)
陈棕炭	chén zōng tàn	20g	Petiolus Trachycarpi (carbonized)
炙龟板	zhì guī bǎn	12g	Testudinis Plastrum (fried with liquid)
牡蛎粉	mǔ lì fěn	12g	Concha Ostreae Powder
沙参	shā shēn	9g	Radix Adenophorae seu Glehniae
生甘草	shēng gān cǎo	4g	Radix et Rhizoma Glycyrrhizae (raw)

Decoct in 500ml of water until 100ml of liquid remains. Take half warm, twice daily.

【Formula Analysis】

In this formula, *huáng qín* (Radix Scutellariae), *jiāo zhī zǐ* (Scorch-fried Fructus Gardeniae), *dì gǔ pí* (Cortex Lycii), *dì yú* (Radix Sanguisorbae) and *ǒu jié* (Nodus Nelumbinis Rhizomatis) purge heat to stop bleeding; *shā shēn* (Radix Adenophorae seu Glehniae) benefits qi. Both *shā shēn* (Radix Adenophorae seu Glehniae) and *shēng dì huáng* (Radix Rehmanniae) nourish yin and blood. *Ē jiāo* (Colla Corii Asini) nourishes blood; *guī bǎn* (Testudinis Plastrum) and *mǔ lì* (Concha Ostreae) nourish yin and astringe blood; *chén zōng tàn* (Carbonized Petiolus Trachycarpi) astringes and stanches bleeding. This formula arrests bleeding by purging heat, cooling blood, and nourishing yin.

【Modifications】

➢ For heat with blood stasis causing abdominal pain with clotting, remove *chén zōng tàn* (Carbonized Petiolus Trachycarpi) and *mǔ lì fěn* (Concha Ostreae Powder). Add *yì mǔ cǎo* (Herba Leonuri) 30g, *zhǐ qiào* (Fructus Aurantii) 12g, *shēng sān qī fěn* (Raw Radix Notoginseng Powder) 3g, and *xià kū cǎo* (Spica Prunellae) 20g, to invigorate blood and dispel stasis.

(4) Liver Constraint with Blood-heat

【Syndrome Characteristics】

Advanced or irregular menstruation, irregular menstrual flow, purplish or red clotting, distending lower abdominal pain, oppression of the chest and hypochondrium, painful distended breasts, agitation and vexation, a bitter taste and dry throat, a red tongue with a thin yellow coating, and a rapid and wiry pulse.

【Treatment Principle】

Course the Liver and resolve constraint, arrest bleeding and regulate menses.

【Commonly Used Medicinals】

Select *chái hú* (Radix Bupleuri), *zhī zǐ* (Fructus Gardeniae), *yù jīn* (Radix Curcumae), *xiāng fù* (Rhizoma Cyperi), *chuān liàn zǐ* (Fructus Toosendan), *zhǐ qiào* (Fructus Aurantii), *bái sháo* (Radix Paeoniae Alba), *huáng qín* (Radix Scutellariae) and *xià kū cǎo* (Spica Prunellae).

【Representative Formula】

Dān Zhī Xiāo Yáo Sǎn (丹栀逍遥散) with added *xià kū cǎo* (Spica Prunellae), *zhè bèi mǔ* (Bulbus Fritillariae Thunbergii), and *yù jīn* (Radix Curcumae).

【Ingredients】

牡丹皮	mǔ dān pí	12g	Cortex Moutan
炒栀子	chǎo zhī zǐ	12g	Fructus Garderniae (scorch-fried)
当归	dāng guī	9g	Radix Angelicae Sinensis
芍药	sháo yào	12g	Paeonia
柴胡	chái hú	10g	Radix Bupleuri
白术	bái zhú	12g	Rhizoma Atractylodis Macrocephalae
茯苓	fú líng	12g	Poria
炙甘草	zhì gān cǎo	4g	Radix et Rhizoma Glycyrrhizae Praeparata cum Melle
夏枯草	xià kū cǎo	20g	Spica Prunellae
浙贝母	zhè bèi mǔ	15g	Bulbus Fritillariae Thunbergii
郁金	yù jīn	10g	Radix Curcumae

Decoct in 500ml of water until 100ml of liquid remains. Take half warm, twice daily.

【Formula Analysis】

In this formula, *chái hú* (Radix Bupleuri), *zhī zǐ* (Fructus Gardeniae), *xià kū cǎo* (Spica Prunellae), *mǔ dān pí* (Cortex Moutan) and *yù jīn* (Radix Curcumae) course the Liver and resolve constraint. *Dāng guī* (Radix Angelicae Sinensis) and *bái sháo* (Radix Paeoniae Alba) nourish blood and emolliate the Liver; *zhè bèi mǔ* (Bulbus Fritillariae Thunbergii) astringes qi and blood; *bái zhú* (Rhizoma Atractylodis Macrocephalae), *fú líng* (Poria) and *gān cǎo* (Radix et Rhizoma Glycyrrhizae) strengthens the Spleen and harmonizes the middle jiao. The main function of this formula is to course the Liver and resolve constraint, cool blood, and regulate menstruation.

【Modifications】

➢ For profuse bleeding, add *dì yú* (Radix Sanguisorbae) 12g, and *guàn zhòng* (Cyrtomii Rhizoma) 18g, to cool blood and arrest bleeding.

(5) Qi Stagnation and Blood Stasis

【Syndrome Characteristics】

Sudden flooding or spotting, purplish black clotting, lower abdominal distention and pain that is aggravated by pressure yet relieved after discharge, breast distention with hypochondriac pain, a dark purple tongue with stasis spots on the right side of the tongue tip, and a deep and choppy or wiry and tight pulse.

【Treatment Principle】

Invigorate blood and dispel stasis, arrest bleeding and regulate menses.

【Commonly Used Medicinals】

Select *chuān xiōng* (Rhizoma Chuanxiong), *yì mǔ cǎo* (Herba Leonuri), *pú huáng* (Pollen Typhae), *wǔ líng zhī* (Faeces Trogopterori), *é zhú* (Rhizoma Curcumae), *chuān niú xī* (Radix Cyathulae), *yù jīn* (Radix Curcumae), *dān shēn* (Radix Salviae Miltiorrhizae), *hóng huā* (Flos Carthami), *jī xuè téng* (Caulis Spatholobi), *táo rén* (Semen Persicae), *yuè jì huā* (Flos Rosae Chinensis), *zhǐ qiào* (Fructus Aurantii), *xiāng fù* (Rhizoma Cyperi), *tái wū* (Radix Linderae) and *chái hú* (Radix Bupleuri).

【Representative Formula】

Sì Wù Tāng (四物汤) and *Shī Xiào Sǎn* (失笑散) with added *sān qī fěn* (Radix Notoginseng Powder), *qiàn cǎo tàn* (Carbonized Radix Rubiae), and *wū zéi gǔ* (Endoconcha Sepiae).

【Ingredients】

熟地黄	shú dì huáng	12g	Radix Rehmanniae Praeparata
当归	dāng guī	12g	Radix Angelicae Sinensis
川芎	chuān xiōng	9g	Rhizoma Chuanxiong
白芍	bái sháo	12g	Radix Paeoniae Alba
炒蒲黄	chǎo pú huáng	12g	Pollen Typhae (dry-fried)
五灵脂	wǔ líng zhī	12g	Faeces Trogopterori
茜草炭	qiàn cǎo tàn	12g	Radix Rubiae (carbonized)
乌贼骨	wū zéi gǔ	12g	Endoconcha Sepiae
生三七粉	shēng sān qī fěn	1.5-3g	Radix Notoginseng Powder (raw)

Decoct in 500ml of water until 100ml of liquid remains. Take half warm, twice daily.

【Formula Analysis】

In this formula, *Sì Wù Tāng* (四物汤) nourishes and regulates the blood to regulate menstruation; *Shī Xiào Sǎn* (失笑散) invigorates blood and dispels stasis; *sān qī fěn* (Radix Notoginseng Powder) and *qiàn cǎo tàn* (Carbonized Radix Rubiae) dispel stasis to arrest bleeding; *wū zéi gǔ* (Endoconcha Sepiae) astringes blood without causing stagnation. The main function of this formula is to invigorate blood, dispel stasis and regulate menstruation.

【Modifications】

➢ For longstanding blood stasis transforming into heat with a dry mouth, a bitter taste, and profuse red menses, add *huáng qín* (Radix Scutellariae) 12g, *xiān hè cǎo* (Herba Agrimoniae) 30g, *dì yú* (Radix Sanguisorbae) 12g and *xià kū cǎo* (Spica Prunellae) 20g to clear heat, regulate qi, cool blood and arrest bleeding.

(6) Kidney Deficiency with Blood-heat

【Syndrome Characteristics】

Irregular menstruation, advanced or prolonged menses, flooding or spotting, bright red menses, fever of the palms and soles, weakness of the legs or lumbar pain, a red tongue with little coating, and a thready or rapid pulse.

【Treatment Principle】

Tonify the Kidney, nourish yin, stanch bleeding and secure the penctrating vessel.

【Commonly Used Medicinals】

Select *nǚ zhēn zǐ* (Fructus Ligustri Lucidi), *hàn lián cǎo* (Herba Ecliptae), *dì huáng* (Radix Rehmanniae), *hé shǒu wū* (Radix Polygoni Multiflori), *sāng jì shēng* (Herba Taxilli), *bǔ gǔ zhī* (Fructus Psoraleae), *xù duàn* (Radix Dipsaci), *shān yào* (Rhizoma Dioscoreae), *tù sī zǐ* (Semen Cuscutae), *yín yáng huò* (Herba Epimedii), *bā jǐ tiān* (Radix Morindae Officinalis), *lù jiǎo jiāo* (Colla Cornus Cervi), *bái sháo* (Radix Paeoniae Alba), *zhī mǔ* (Rhizoma Anemarrhenae), *qīng hāo* (Herba Artemisiae Annuae), *mǔ dān pí* (Cortex Moutan), *huáng qín* (Radix Scutellariae) and *huáng bǎi* (Cortex Phellodendri Chinensis).

【Representative Formula】

Modified *Zhī Bǎi Dì Huáng Tāng* (知柏地黄汤).

【Ingredients】

生地黄	shēng dì huáng	20g	Radix Rehmanniae
熟地黄	shú dì huáng	20g	Radix Rehmanniae Praeparata
山药	shān yào	20g	Rhizoma Dioscoreae
何首乌	hé shǒu wū	15g	Radix Polygoni Multiflori
川断	chuān xù duàn	12g	Radix Dipsaci
桑寄生	sāng jì shēng	15g	Herba Taxilli
泽泻	zé xiè	10g	Rhizoma Alismatis
山萸肉	shān yú ròu	12g	Fructus Corni
茯苓	fú líng	12g	Poria
牡丹皮	mǔ dān pí	10g	Cortex Moutan

茜草	qiàn cǎo	12g	Radix Rubiae
血余炭	xuè yú tàn	12g	Crinis Carbonisatus
知母	zhī mǔ	12g	Rhizoma Anemarrhenae
黄柏	huáng bǎi	12g	Cortex Phellodendri Chinensis

Decoct in 500ml of water until 100ml of liquid remains. Take half warm, twice daily.

【Formula Analysis】

In this formula, *shú dì huáng* (Radix Rehmanniae Praeparata) nourishes Kidney yin and tonifies essence, while *shān yú ròu* (Fructus Corni) nourishes the Kidney and Liver with its sour flavor and warm nature. *Shān yào* (Rhizoma Dioscoreae) nourishes the Kidney and tonifies Spleen; *zé xiè* (Rhizoma Alismatis) with *shú dì huáng* (Radix Rehmanniae Praeparata) drain the Kidney and descend turbidity; *mǔ dān pí* (Cortex Moutan) with *shān yú ròu* (Fructus Corni) clear Liver fire; *zhī mǔ* (Rhizoma Anemarrhenae) with *huáng bǎi* (Cortex Phellodendri Chinensis) clear heat. *Fú líng* (Poria) with *shān yào* (Rhizoma Dioscoreae) percolate Spleen dampness. The main function of this formula is to tonify the Kidney and Liver by tonifying both the congenital and the acquired.

【Modifications】

➢ For blood stasis with lower abdominal pain, inhibited menstruation, and dark-colored menses with clotting, add *shēng sān qī fěn* (Raw Radix Notoginseng Powder) 3g, *yì mǔ cǎo* (Herba Leonuri) 30g, *chǎo pú huáng* (Dry-fried Pollen Typhae) 12g, *chǎo líng zhī* (Dry-fried Faeces Trogopterori) 12g, *dān shēn* (Radix Salviae Miltiorrhizae) 15g, and *chì sháo* (Radix Paeoniae Rubra) 15g to invigorate blood, dispel stasis and arrest bleeding.

➢ For profuse bleeding, add *tài zǐ shēn* (Radix Pseudostellariae) 30g, and *huáng qí* (Radix Astragali) 20g, to tonify and upbear qi and arrest bleeding.

(7) Liver and Kidney Yin Deficiency

【Syndrome Characteristics】

Advanced or irregular menstruation, dark red menses, spotting, dry throat, flushed face, vexation and tidal fever, and weakness of the legs with lumbar soreness. The tongue may be red and peeled or with little coating, and the pulse is both deep and thready, or weak.

【Treatment Principle】

Tonify the Liver and Kidney, regulate menstruation and arrest bleeding.

【Commonly Used Medicinals】

Select *shēng dì huáng* (Radix Rehmanniae), *shú dì huáng* (Radix Rehmanniae Praeparata), *nǚ zhēn zǐ* (Fructus Ligustri Lucidi), *hàn lián cǎo* (Herba Ecliptae), *gǒu qǐ zǐ* (Fructus Lycii), *hé shǒu wū* (Radix Polygoni Multiflori), *zhī mǔ* (Rhizoma Anemarrhenae), *guī bǎn* (Testudinis Plastrum), *ē jiāo* (Colla Corii Asini), *bái sháo* (Radix Paeoniae Alba), *wǔ wèi zǐ* (Fructus Schisandrae) and *shān zhū yú* (Fructus Corni).

【Representative Formula】

Zuǒ Guī Yǐn (左归饮) and *Èr Zhì Wán* (二至丸) with added *huáng qín* (Radix Scutellariae), *xià kū cǎo* (Spica Prunellae), *xiān hè cǎo* (Herba Agrimoniae), and *zhì shǒu wū* (Radix Polygoni Multiflori Praeparata cum Succo Glycines Sotae).

【Ingredients】

黄芩	huáng qín	12g	Radix Scutellariae
熟地黄	shú dì huáng	10g	Radix Rehmanniae Praeparata
山萸肉	shān zhū yú	10g	Fructus Corni
山药	shān yào	10g	Rhizoma Dioscoreae
茯苓	fú líng	10g	Poria
枸杞子	gǒu qǐ zǐ	10g	Fructus Lycii

仙鹤草	xiān hè cǎo	30g	Herba Agrimoniae
女贞子	nǚ zhēn zǐ	10g	Fructus Ligustri Lucidi
旱莲草	hàn lián cǎo	10g	Herba Ecliptae
制首乌	zhì shǒu wū	12g	Radix Polygoni Multiflori Praeparata cum Succo Glycines Sotae
夏枯草	xià kū cǎo	20g	Spica Prunellae
炙甘草	zhì gān cǎo	4g	Radix et Rhizoma Glycyrrhizae Praeparata cum Melle

Decoct in 500ml of water until 100ml of liquid remains. Take half warm, twice daily.

【Formula Analysis】

In this formula, *shú dì huáng* (Radix Rehmanniae Praeparata) nourishes yin and blood; *guī jiāo* (Colla Carapax et Plastrum Testudinis), tonifies yin and subdues yang to astringe blood; *gǒu qǐ* (Fructus Lycii), *shān yú ròu* (Fructus Corni), *tù sī zǐ* (Semen Cuscutae), *niú xī* (Radix Acanthopanacis Bidentatae) and *shān yào* (Rhizoma Dioscoreae) tonify the Liver and Kidney and nourish the penetrating and conception vessels; *lù jiǎo jiāo* (Rhizoma Dioscoreae) warms and nourishes essence and blood; *nǚ zhēn zǐ* (Fructus Ligustri Lucidi) and *hàn lián cǎo* (Herba Ecliptae) nourish the Liver and Kidney to arrest bleeding.

【Modifications】

➤ For profuse red bleeding without clotting, remove *fú líng* (Poria) and *shú dì huáng* (Radix Rehmanniae Praeparata), and add *shēng dì huáng* (Radix Rehmanniae), *huáng qí* (Radix Astragali) 15g, *shēng dì yú* (Raw Radix Sanguisorbae) 10g, *zhì jūn tàn* (Prepared Radix et Rhizoma Rhei) 10g, and *zhù má gēn* (Radix Boehmeriae) 20g, to tonify qi and cool blood.

(8) Damp-heat

【Syndrome Characteristics】

Advanced or irregular menstruation, flooding or spotting, dark purplish blood with clotting or mucus, distending pain of the lower abdomen that is aggravated by pressure, fever, taxation and heaviness of the limbs, thirst with no desire to drink, a red tongue with a yellow greasy coating, and a soggy or rapid pulse.

【Treatment Principle】

Purge heat and eliminate dampness, arrest bleeding and regulate menses.

【Commonly Used Medicinals】

Select *huáng qín* (Radix Scutellariae), *zhú rú* (Caulis Bambusae in Taenia), *bàn xià* (Rhizoma Pinelliae), *hòu pò* (Cortex Magnoliae Officinalis), *yīn chén* (Herba Artemisiae Scopariae), *cāng zhú* (Rhizoma Atracylodis), *fú líng* (Poria), *bái zhú* (Rhizoma Atractylodis Macrocephalae), *zé xiè* (Rhizoma Alismatis), *zhǐ qiào* (Fructus Aurantii), *shā rén* (Fructus Amomi), *pèi lán* (Herba Eupatorii), *huò xiāng* (Herba Agastachis), *lián qiào* (Fructus Forsythiae) and *pú gōng yīng* (Herba Taraxaci).

【Representative Formula】

Modified *Wǔ Wèi Xiāo Dú Yǐn* (五味消毒饮) .

【Ingredients】

泡参	pào shēn	15g	Radix Adenophorae
银花	yín huā	12g	Flos Lonicerae
野菊花	yě jú huā	12g	Flos Chrysanthemi Indici
蒲公英	pú gōng yīng	12g	Herba Taraxaci
紫花地丁	zǐ huā dì dīng	12g	Herba Violae
天葵子	tiān kuí zǐ	12g	Radix Semiaquilegiae
仙鹤草	xiān hè cǎo	30g	Herba Agrimoniae
茵陈	yīn chén	12g	Herba Artemisiae Scopariae
夏枯草	xià kū cǎo	20g	Spica Prunellae
枳壳	zhǐ qiào	12g	Fructus Aurantii

| 香附 | xiāng fù | 12g | Rhizoma Cyperi |
| 益母草 | yì mǔ cǎo | 30g | Herba Leonuri |

Decoct in 500ml of water until 100ml of liquid remains. Take half warm, twice daily.

【Formula Analysis】

In this formula *Wǔ Wèi Xiāo Dú Yǐn* (五味消毒饮) combines *yín huā* (Flos Lonicerae), *yě jú huā* (Flos Chrysanthemi Indici), *dì dīng* (Herba Violae), *pú gōng yīng* (Herba Taraxaci) and *tiān kuí zǐ* (Radix Semiaquilegiae) to clear heat and both detoxify and cool the blood. *Xiān hè cǎo* (Herba Agrimoniae) astringes to arrest bleeding, while *yīn chén* (Herba Artemisiae Scopariae), *xià kū cǎo* (Spica Prunellae), *zhǐ qiào* (Fructus Aurantii) and *xiāng fù* (Rhizoma Cyperi) regulate qi, invigorate blood, and dispel blood stasis.

【Modifications】

➢ For excessive dampness, remove *tiān kuí zǐ* (Radix Semiaquilegiae) and add *yì yǐ rén* (Semen Coicis) 24g, *fǎ xià* (Rhizoma Pinelliae) 12g to percolate dampness and disinhibit water.

➢ For excessive heat, add *huáng qín* (Radix Scutellariae) 12g, *dà jì* (Herba Cirsii Japonici) 10g, *xiǎo jì* (Herba Cirsii) 10g and *chūn gēn pí* (Cortex Ailanthi) 12g, which purge heat and cool blood to arrest bleeding.

(9) Kidney Yang Deficiency

【Syndrome Characteristics】

Advanced or irregular menstruation, profuse menses, spotting, pale menses, a sallow complexion, coldness of the lower abdomen and back, aversion to cold, lumbar pain, frequent urination at night, clear and profuse urine. Tongue appears pale and swollen with indentations, and the pulse is deep and thready.

【Treatment Principle】

Warm the Kidney and secure the penetrating vessel, arrest bleeding and regulate menses.

【Commonly Used Medicinals】

Select *lù jiǎo piàn* (Sliced Cornu Cervi), *bā jǐ tiān* (Radix Morindae Officinalis), *sāng jì shēng* (Herba Taxilli), *ròu cōng róng* (Herba Cistanches), *yín yáng huò* (Herba Epimedii), *xù duàn* (Radix Dipsaci), *zǐ hé chē* (Placenta Hominis), *tù sī zǐ* (Semen Cuscutae), *huáng qí* (Radix Astragali), *ròu guì* (Cortex Cinnamomi) and *fù zǐ* (Radix Aconiti Lateralis Preparata).

【Representative Formula】

Shèn Qì Wán (肾气丸) minus *mǔ dān pí* (Cortex Moutan) and *zé xiè* (Rhizoma Alismatis), plus added *huáng qí* (Radix Astragali), *fù pén zǐ* (Fructus Rubi) and *chì shí zhī* (Halloysitum Rubrum).

【Ingredients】

熟地黄	shú dì huáng	20g	Radix Rehmanniae Praeparata
山萸肉	shān zhū yú	12g	Fructus Corni
茯苓	fú líng	12g	Poria
赤石脂	chì shí zhī	12g	Halloysitum Rubrum
黄芪	huáng qí	15g	Radix Astragali
附子	fù zǐ	5g	Radix Aconiti Lateralis
肉桂	ròu guì	10g	Cortex Cinnamomi
山药	shān yào	20g	Rhizoma Dioscoreae

Decoct in 500ml of water until 100ml of liquid remains. Take half warm, twice daily.

【Formula Analysis】

In this formula, *fù zǐ* (Radix Aconiti Lateralis Praeparata) and *ròu guì* (Cortex Cinnamomi) warm and tonify Kidney yang; *shú dì huáng* (Radix Rehmanniae Praeparata), *shān zhū yú* (Fructus Corni) and *shān yào* (Rhizoma Dioscoreae) nourish Kidney yin to contain yang. *Fú líng* (Poria) promotes urination and drains heat; *huáng qí* (Radix Astragali) tonifies qi and nourishes blood; *fù pén zǐ* (Fructus Rubi) and *chì shí zhī* (Halloysitum

Rubrum) both astringe to stanch bleeding.

【Modifications】

➢ For profuse light-colored bleeding without clotting, remove *fú líng* (Poria). Add *xiān hè cǎo* (Herba Agrimoniae) 18g, *duàn lóng gǔ* (Calcined Fossilia Ossis Mastodi) 15g, *duàn mǔ lì* (Calcined Concha Ostreae) 15g, *wū zéi gǔ* (Endoconcha Sepiae) 15g, *ē jiāo* (Colla Corii Asini), *tù sī zǐ* (Semen Cuscutae), and *bái zhú* (Rhizoma Atractylodis Macrocephalae) to astringe and nourish blood, tonify the Kidney, and stanch bleeding.

(10) Qi Deficiency

【Syndrome Characteristics】

Advanced or irregular menstruation, profuse pale menses, lassitude, lower abdominal discomfort with an empty or downbearing sensation, poor appetite and loose stools, a pale tongue, and a thready or weak pulse.

【Treatment Principle】

Tonify the Spleen and Kidney, contain blood and regulate menses.

【Commonly Used Medicinals】

Select *huáng qí* (Radix Astragali), *rén shēn* (Radix et Rhizoma Ginseng), *dǎng shēn* (Radix Codonopsis), *gān cǎo* (Radix et Rhizoma Glycyrrhizae), *bái zhú* (Rhizoma Atractylodis Macrocephalae), *sāng jì shēng* (Herba Taxilli), *shān yào* (Rhizoma Dioscoreae) and *shēng má* (Rhizoma Cimicifugae).

【Representative Formula】

Bǔ Zhōng Yì Qì Tāng (补中益气汤) minus *dāng guī* (Radix Angelicae Sinensis) and *chái hú* (Radix Bupleuri), plus added *nǚ zhēn zǐ* (Fructus Ligustri Lucidi), *gǒu qǐ* (Fructus Lycii), *shān yào* (Rhizoma Dioscoreae) and *bǔ gǔ zhī* (Fructus Psoraleae).

【Ingredients】

党参	dǎng shēn	12g	Radix Codonopsis
黄芪	huáng qí	20g	Radix Astragali
陈皮	chén pí	9g	Pericarpium Citri Reticulatae
升麻	shēng má	9g	Rhizoma Cimicifugae
白术	bái zhú	12g	Rhizoma Atractylodis Macrocephalae
女贞子	nǚ zhēn zǐ	20g	Fructus Ligustri Lucidi
川断	chuān xù duàn	12g	Radix Dipsaci
山药	shān yào	18g	Rhizoma Dioscoreae
艾叶	ài yè	6g	Folium Artemisiae Argyi
炙甘草	zhì gān cǎo	4g	Radix et Rhizoma Glycyrrhizae Praeparata cum Melle

Decoct in 500ml of water until 100ml of liquid remains. Take half warm, twice daily.

【Formula Analysis】

In this formula, *huáng qí* (Radix Astragali) tonifies the middle qi and upbears the clear yang; *rén shēn* (Radix et Rhizoma Ginseng) and *gān cǎo* (Radix et Rhizoma Glycyrrhizae) tonify the Spleen and benefit qi; *bái zhú* (Rhizoma Atractylodis Macrocephalae) dries dampness and strengthens the Spleen while assisting *huáng qí* (Radix Astragali) to tonify the middle qi; *chén pí* (Pericarpium Citri Reticulatae) regulates qi; *shēng má* (Rhizoma Cimicifugae) upbears and tonifies the middle qi. *Nǚ zhēn zǐ* (Fructus Ligustri Lucidi), *gǒu qǐ* (Fructus Lycii), *shān yào* (Rhizoma Dioscoreae) and *bǔ gǔ zhī* (Fructus Psoraleae) tonify the Kidney, replenish essence, and nourish blood.

【Modifications】

➢ For qi deficiency and blood stasis with clotting, add *yì mǔ cǎo* (Herba Leonuri) 30g and *shān cí gū* (Pseudobulbus Cremastrae seu Pleiones) 20g, to invigorate blood and dispel stasis.

➢ For profuse bleeding, add *lóng gǔ* (Fossilia Ossis Mastodi) 15g and *mǔ lì* (Concha Ostreae) 15g to astringe.

➢ For blood-heat, add *huáng qín* (Radix Scutellariae) 15g.

➤ For yin deficiency, add *dān pí* (Cortex Moutan) 12g and *hàn lián cǎo* (Herba Ecliptae) 12g, to nourish yin and cool blood.

(11) Qi and Blood Deficiency

【Syndrome Characteristics】

Flooding or spotting of pale menses, a lusterless complexion, shortness of breath with no desire to speak, poor appetite, loose stools, a pale tongue with a thin white or moist coating, and a thready and weak pulse.

【Treatment Principle】

Tonify the Spleen to contain blood, conduct blood back to the vessels.

【Commonly Used Medicinals】

Select *huáng qí* (Radix Astragali), *rén shēn* (Radix et Rhizoma Ginseng), *dǎng shēn* (Radix Codonopsis), *gān cǎo* (Radix et Rhizoma Glycyrrhizae), *bái zhú* (Rhizoma Atractylodis Macrocephalae), *sāng jì shēng* (Herba Taxilli), *shān yào* (Rhizoma Dioscoreae), *shēng má* (Rhizoma Cimicifugae), *shú dì huáng* (Radix Rehmanniae Praeparata), *hé shǒu wū* (Radix Polygoni Multiflori), *ē jiāo* (Colla Corii Asini), *bái sháo* (Radix Paeoniae Alba), *nǚ zhēn zǐ* (Fructus Ligustri Lucidi), *hàn lián cǎo* (Herba Ecliptae), *yè jiāo téng* (Caulis Polygoni Multiflori) and *wǔ wèi zǐ* (Fructus Schisandrae).

【Representative Formula】

Guī Pí Tāng (归脾汤) minus *dāng guī* (Radix Angelicae Sinensis), *fú líng* (Poria) and *yuǎn zhì* (Radix Polygalae), plus added *dǎng shēn* (Radix Codonopsis), *qiàn cǎo* (Radix Rubiae), *wū zéi gǔ* (Endoconcha Sepiae) and *xiān hè cǎo* (Herba Agrimoniae).

【Ingredients】

黄芪	huáng qí	20g	Radix Astragali
党参	dǎng shēn	15g	Radix Codonopsis

酸枣仁	suān zǎo rén	15g	Semen Ziziphi Spinosae
木香	mù xiāng	10g	Radix Aucklandiae
白术	bái zhú	15g	Rhizoma Atractylodis Macrocephalae
龙眼肉	lóng yǎn ròu	15g	Arillus Longan
仙鹤草	xiān hè cǎo	15g	Herba Agrimoniae
白芍	bái sháo	12g	Radix Paeoniae Alba
茜草	qiàn cǎo	15g	Radix Rubiae
甘草	gān cǎo	4g	Radix et Rhizoma Glycyrrhizae
乌贼骨	wū zéi gǔ	15g	Endoconcha Sepiae

Decoct in 500ml of water until 100ml of liquid remains. Take half warm, twice daily.

【Formula Analysis】

In this formula, *huáng qí* (Radix Astragali) and *dǎng shēn* (Radix Codonopsis) invigorate the Spleen and tonify qi; *suān zǎo rén* (Semen Ziziphi Spinosae) and *lóng yǎn ròu* (Arillus Longan) tonify blood, nourish blood and calm the spirit; *mù xiāng* (Radix Aucklandiae) regulates qi and awakens the Spleen as well as tonifying without cloying. *Qiàn cǎo* (Radix Rubiae) dispels stasis to arrest bleeding, while *wū zéi gǔ* (Endoconcha Sepiae) and *xiān hè cǎo* (Herba Agrimoniae) astringe to arrest bleeding. The main function of this formula is to tonify the Spleen and contain blood.

【Modifications】

➢ For continuous spotting, add *shēng pú huáng* (Pollen Typhae Crudum) 12g, *wǔ líng zhī* (Faeces Trogopterori) 12g, and *shēng sān qī fěn* (Raw Radix Notoginseng Powder) 3g (infused) to dispel stasis, invigorate blood, and stanch bleeding.

(12) Spleen and Kidney Yang Deficiency

【Syndrome Characteristics】

Advanced, prolonged, or irregular menstruation, pale and profuse menses, a white complexion, lassitude, aversion to cold, cold limbs, soreness of the knees and lumbus, poor appetite, loose stools. Tongue is pale and swollen with teeth marks, and the deficient pulse is often deep and slow.

【Treatment Principle】

Warm and tonify the Spleen and Kidney, stanch bleeding and secure the penetrating vessel.

【Commonly Used Medicinals】

Select *huáng qí* (Radix Astragali), *rén shēn* (Radix et Rhizoma Ginseng), *dǎng shēn* (Radix Codonopsis), *bái zhú* (Rhizoma Atractylodis Macrocephalae), *shān yào* (Rhizoma Dioscoreae), *shēng má* (Rhizoma Cimicifugae), *lù jiǎo piàn* (Sliced Cornu Cervi), *bā jǐ tiān* (Radix Morindae Officinalis), *sāng jì shēng* (Herba Taxilli), *ròu cōng róng* (Herba Cistanches), *yín yáng huò* (Herba Epimedii), *xù duàn* (Radix Dipsaci), *zǐ hé chē* (Placenta Hominis), *tù sī zǐ* (Semen Cuscutae), *ròu guì* (Cortex Cinnamomi) and *fù zǐ* (Radix Aconiti Lateralis Praeparata).

【Representative Formula】

Modified *Yòu Guī Yǐn* (右归饮) with *Jǔ Yuán Jiān* (举元煎).

【Ingredients】

黄芪	huáng qí	15g	Radix Astragali
太子参	tài zǐ shēn	15g	Radix Pseudostellariae
白术	bái zhú	12g	Rhizoma Atractylodis Macrocephalae
熟地黄	shú dì huáng	12g	Radix Rehmanniae Praeparata
山萸肉	shān zhū yú	10g	Fructus Corni
山药	shān yào	20g	Rhizoma Dioscoreae
杜仲	dù zhòng	10g	Cortex Eucommiae
枸杞子	gǒu qǐ zǐ	10g	Fructus Lycii
煅牡蛎	duàn mǔ lì	30g	Concha Ostreae (calcined)
升麻	shēng má	10g	Rhizoma Cimicifugae

| 菟丝子 | tù sī zǐ | 12g | Semen Cuscutae |
| 鹿角胶(烊化) | lù jiǎo jiāo | 10g | Colla Cornus Cervi (dissolved) |

Decoct in 500ml of water until 100ml of liquid remains. Take half warm, twice daily.

【**Formula Analysis**】

In this formula, *tài zǐ shēn* (Radix Pseudostellariae), *huáng qí* (Radix Astragali) and *bái zhú* (Rhizoma Atractylodis Macrocephalae) supplement the middle jiao and tonify qi; *shēng má* (Rhizoma Cimicifugae) upbears yang and lifts the fallen. Upbearing of the qi also treats the blood, so this formula both astringes and secures the penetrating vessel without treating the blood directly. *Shú dì huáng* (Radix Rehmanniae Praeparata), *shān zhū yú* (Fructus Corni) and *gǒu qǐ zǐ* (Fructus Lycii) nourish Kidney yin and replenish both essence and blood; *shān yào* (Rhizoma Dioscoreae) and *tù sī zǐ* (Semen Cuscutae) tonify Kidney yang to nourish essence and qi. When yang is generated, the yin is increased as well. *Lù jiǎo jiāo* (Colla Cornus Cervi) nourishes yin and blood to arrest bleeding, and *duàn mǔ lì* (calcined Concha Ostreae) astringes to stanch bleeding.

【**Modifications**】

➤ For profuse and pale menses without clotting, add *bǔ gǔ zhī* (Fructus Psoraleae) 15g, *chì shí zhī* (Halloysitum Rubrum) 15g, and *xiān hè cǎo* (Herba Agrimoniae) 30g to secure the penetrating vessel and astringe to stanch bleeding.

➤ For blood stasis, add *dān shēn* (Radix Salviae Miltiorrhizae) 12g and *hóng huā* (Flos Carthami) 5g, to invigorate blood and dispel blood stasis.

4. PATTERN DIFFERENTIATION AND TREATMENT IN THE NON-BLEEDING STAGE

(1) Kidney Deficiency

【Syndrome Characteristics】

Insufficiency of Kidney qi during adolescence, or exhaustion of *Tian Gui* during menopause, chronic profuse bleeding or spotting, dizziness and tinnitus, soreness of the lumbus and legs, a pale or red tongue with a white or thin coating, and a deep and thready or thready and rapid pulse.

【Treatment Principle】

Tonify the Kidney, secure the penetrating vessel, and regulate menses.

【Commonly Used Medicinals】

Select *shēng dì huáng* (Radix Rehmanniae), *shú dì huáng* (Radix Rehmanniae Praeparata), *nǚ zhēn zǐ* (Fructus Ligustri Lucidi), *hàn lián cǎo* (Herba Ecliptae), *gǒu qǐ zǐ* (Fructus Lycii), *hé shǒu wū* (Radix Polygoni Multiflori), *zhī mǔ* (Rhizoma Anemarrhenae), *guī bǎn* (Testudinis Plastrum), *ē jiāo* (Testudinis Plastrum), *bái sháo* (Radix Paeoniae Alba), *shān zhū yú* (Fructus Corni), *zǐ hé chē* (Placenta Hominis), *huáng qí* (Radix Astragali), *dǎng shēn* (Radix Codonopsis), *gān cǎo* (Radix et Rhizoma Glycyrrhizae), *bái zhú* (Rhizoma Atractylodis Macrocephalae), *sāng jì shēng* (Herba Taxilli), *shān yào* (Rhizoma Dioscoreae), *shēng má* (Rhizoma Cimicifugae), *yè jiāo téng* (Caulis Polygoni Multiflori) and *wǔ wèi zǐ* (Fructus Schisandrae).

【Representative Formula】

Qǐ Jú Dì Huáng Tāng (杞菊地黄汤) plus *zǐ hé chē* (Placenta Hominis)

【Ingredients】

枸杞	gǒu qǐ	12g	Fructus Lycii

熟地黄	shú dì huáng	12g	Radix Rehmanniae Praeparata
生地黄	shēng dì huáng	12g	Radix Rehmanniae
茯苓	fú líng	12g	Poria
山茱萸	shān zhū yú	12g	Fructus Corni
牡丹皮	mǔ dān pí	10g	Cortex Moutan
泽泻	zé xiè	10g	Rhizoma Alismatis
山药	shān yào	20g	Rhizoma Dioscoreae
菊花	jú huā	12g	Flos Chrysanthemi
紫河车粉（冲服）	zǐ hé chē	3g	Placenta Hominis Powder (infused)

Decoct in 500ml of water until 100ml of liquid remains. Take half warm, twice daily.

【**Formula Analysis**】

In this formula, *shú dì huáng* (Radix Rehmanniae Praeparata) nourishes Kidney yin and replenishes essence; *shān zhū yú* (Fructus Corni) nourishes the Kidney and Liver with its sour flavor and warm nature; *shān yào* (Rhizoma Dioscoreae) nourishes the Kidney and Spleen; *zé xiè* (Rhizoma Alismatis) with *shú dì huáng* (Radix Rehmanniae Praeparata) drain the Kidney and descend the turbid; *mǔ dān pí* (Cortex Moutan) with *shān zhū yú* (Fructus Corni) clear Liver fire; *gǒu qǐ zǐ* (Fructus Lycii) and *jú huā* (Flos Chrysanthemi) nourish Kidney and Liver yin; *zǐ hé chē* (Placenta Hominis) tonifies blood with its particular affinity to flesh and blood. Both *fú líng* (Poria) and *shān yào* (Rhizoma Dioscoreae) drain Spleen dampness.

【**Modifications**】

➢ For Kidney yin deficiency with symptoms such as vexing heat in the chest, palms and sores, tidal fever and sweating, add *nǚ zhēn zǐ* (Fructus Ligustri Lucidi) 15g, *hàn lián cǎo* (Herba Ecliptae) 15g, *tù sī zǐ* (Semen Cuscutae) 10g, *fù pén zǐ* (Fructus Rubi) 10g, *dù zhòng* (Cortex Eucommiae) 10g, *ròu cōng róng* (Herba Cistanches) 10g, and *chǎo bái zhú* (Dry-fried Rhizoma Atractylodis Macrocephalae) 10g.

> For Kidney yang deficiency with symptoms such as aversion to cold, cold limbs, a sallow complexion, clear and profuse urine, remove *mǔ dān pí* (Cortex Moutan), *shēng dì huáng* (Radix Rehmanniae), *zé xiè* (Rhizoma Alismatis) and *jú huā* (Flos Chrysanthemi). Add *bǔ gǔ zhī* (Fructus Psoraleae) 20g, *tù sī zǐ* (Semen Cuscutae), *chuān xù duàn* (Radix Dipsaci), *huáng qí* (Radix Astragali), *lù dǎng shēn* (Radix Codonopsis), *xiān líng pí* (Herba Epimedii), *chǎo bái zhú* (Dry-fried Rhizoma Atractylodis Macrocephalae), *bā jǐ tiān* (Radix Morindae Officinalis), and *jiāo ài* (Scorch-fried Folium Artemisiae Argyi), 10g each.

> For Kidney essence deficiency without obvious yin or yang symptoms, add *xiān líng pí* (Herba Epimedii), *bā jǐ tiān* (Radix Morindae Officinalis), *chuān xù duàn* (Radix Dipsaci), *bǔ gǔ zhī* (Fructus Psoraleae), *jiāo shān yào* (Scorch-fried Rhizoma Dioscoreae), *tù sī zǐ* (Semen Cuscutae), *gǒu qǐ zǐ* (Fructus Lycii) and *nǔ zhēn zǐ* (Fructus Ligustri Lucidi), 15g each.

> For Heart yin deficiency with symptoms such as vexation and insomnia, add *wǔ wèi zǐ* (Fructus Schisandrae) 12g and *yè jiāo téng* (Caulis Polygoni Multiflori) 30g, to nourish Heart blood and calm the spirit.

> For phlegm-damp, obesity, heaviness of the head and body, or profuse leucorrhea, add *cāng zhú* (Rhizoma Atracylodis) 9g, *bái zhú* (Rhizoma Atractylodis Macrocephalae) 12g, *fǎ xià* (Rhizoma Pinelliae Praeparatum) 12g, and *zhè bèi mǔ* (Bulbus Fritillariae Thunbergii) 15g, to drain dampness and resolve phlegm.

(2) Liver Constraint

【Syndrome Characteristics】

Longstanding depression or irascibility, irregular menses, profuse or scanty bleeding, swelling pain of the lower abdomen following menstruation, hypochondriac pain or breast distention, a pale red tongue with a thin white or yellow coating, and a wiry and rapid pulse.

【Treatment Principle】

Course the Liver, resolve constraint, and regulate the penetrating vessel.

【Commonly Used Medicinals】

Select *chái hú* (Radix Bupleuri), *zhī zǐ* (Fructus Gardeniae), *yù jīn* (Radix Curcumae), *dāng guī* (Radix Angelicae Sinensis), *xiāng fù* (Rhizoma Cyperi), *chuān liàn zǐ* (Fructus Toosendan), *zhǐ qiào* (Fructus Aurantii), *bái sháo* (Radix Paeoniae Alba) and *huáng qín* (Radix Scutellariae).

【Representative Formula】

Zī Shuǐ Qīng Gān Yǐn (滋水清肝饮).

【Ingredients】

柴胡	chái hú	10g	Radix Bupleuri
当归	dāng guī	12g	Radix Angelicae Sinensis
白芍	bái sháo	12g	Radix Paeoniae Alba
栀子	zhī zǐ	10g	Fructus Gardeniae
生地黄	shēng dì huáng	12g	Radix Rehmanniae
牡丹皮	mǔ dān pí	10g	Cortex Moutan
山茱萸	shān zhū yú	12g	Fructus Corni
茯苓	fú líng	12g	Poria
泽泻	zé xiè	10g	Rhizoma Alismatis
山药	shān yào	20g	Rhizoma Dioscoreae
大枣	dà zǎo	5pieces	Fructus Jujubae

Decoct in 500ml of water until 100ml of liquid remains. Take half warm, twice daily.

【Formula Analysis】

Chái hú (Radix Bupleuri) and *bái sháo* (Radix Paeoniae Alba) course the Liver and regulate qi; *zhī zǐ* (Fructus Gardeniae) and *mǔ dān pí* (Cortex Moutan) clear heat and nourish yin; *shēng dì huáng* (Radix Rehmanniae), *shān zhū yú* (Fructus Corni), *shān yào* (Rhizoma Dioscoreae) and *dà zǎo* (Fructus Jujubae) tonify the Kidney and nourish blood; *fú líng* (Poria) and *zé xiè* (Rhizoma Alismatis) disinhibit water and percolate dampness. The main function of this formula is to course the Liver, resolve constraint, and regulate the penetrating vessel.

【Modifications】

➢ For Liver constraint affecting the Spleen, with symptoms such as shortness of breath and poor appetite, add *huáng qí* (Radix Astragali) 20g, and *bái zhú* (Rhizoma Atractylodis Macrocephalae) 12g, to strengthen the Spleen and tonify qi.

➢ For heat constraint damaging yin, with symptoms such as dry mouth, vexation and constipation, add *zhì shǒu wū* (Radix Polygoni Multiflori Praeparata cum Succo Glycines Sotae) 12g, *xuán shēn* (Radix Scrophulariae) 12g, and *sāng jì shēng* (Herba Taxilli) 12g, to nourish yin and blood.

(3) Spleen Deficiency

【Syndrome Characteristics】

Profuse and prolonged bleeding, shortness of breath, lassitude, a pale complexion, edema of the face and limbs, cold extremities, poor appetite, loose stools, a pale tongue with a thin white coating, and a weak or deep pulse.

【Treatment Principle】

Invigorate the Spleen and tonify qi, nourish blood and regulate menses.

【Commonly Used Medicinals】

Select *huáng qí* (Radix Astragali), *dǎng shēn* (Radix Codonopsis), *gān cǎo* (Radix et Rhizoma Glycyrrhizae), *bái zhú* (Rhizoma Atractylodis Macrocephalae), *fú líng* (Poria), *shān yào* (Rhizoma Dioscoreae), *shēng má* (Rhizoma Cimicifugae), *shā rén* (Fructus Amomi), *shén qū* (Massa

Medicata Fermentata), *gǔ yá* (Fructus Setariae Germinatus), *mài yá* (Fructus Hordei Germinatus), *zhǐ qiào* (Fructus Aurantii), *lái fú zǐ* (Semen Raphani), *shān zhā* (Fructus Crataegi) and *yuǎn zhì* (Radix Polygalae).

【Representative Formula】

Gù Běn Zhǐ Bēng Tāng (固本止崩汤) plus added *shēng má* (Rhizoma Cimicifugae), *shān yào* (Rhizoma Dioscoreae), *dà zǎo* (Fructus Jujubae) and *wū zéi gǔ* (Endoconcha Sepiae).

【Ingredients】

人参	rén shēn	12g	Radix et Rhizoma Ginseng
黄芪	huáng qí	15g	Radix Astragali
白术	bái zhú	12g	Rhizoma Atractylodis Macrocephalae
熟地黄	shú dì huáng	12g	Radix Rehmanniae Praeparata
当归	dāng guī	12g	Radix Angelicae Sinensis
黑姜	hēi jiāng	6g	Rhizoma Zingiberis
升麻	shēng má	10g	Rhizoma Cimicifugae
山药	shān yào	20g	Rhizoma Dioscoreae
大枣	dà zǎo	5pieces	Fructus Jujubae

Decoct in 500ml of water until 100ml of liquid remains. Take half warm, twice daily.

【Formula Analysis】

In this formula, *rén shēn* (Radix et Rhizoma Ginseng), *huáng qí* (Radix Astragali) and *bái zhú* (Rhizoma Atractylodis Macrocephalae) tonify qi to bank the source and secure the center to contain blood; *dāng guī* (Radix Angelicae Sinensis) and *shú dì huáng* (Radix Rehmanniae Praeparata) nourish yin and blood; *hēi jiāng* (Carbonized Rhizoma Zingiberis) warms the middle jiao to arrest bleeding; *shēng má* (Rhizoma Cimicifugae) upbears qi; *shān yào* (Rhizoma Dioscoreae) and *dà zǎo* (Fructus Jujubae) warms the middle jiao and tonifies blood. *Wū zéi gǔ* (Endoconcha Sepiae) astringes blood and secures the penetrating vessel.

【Modifications】

➤ For blood deficiency, add *zhì shǒu wū* (Radix Polygoni Multiflori Praeparata cum Succo Glycines Sotae) 15g, *bái sháo* (Radix Paeoniae Alba) 12g and *sāng jì shēng* (Herba Taxilli) 12g, to both nourish blood and tonify the Kidney and Liver.

➤ For palpitation and insomnia, add *suān zǎo rén* (Semen Ziziphi Spinosae) 12g, *yè jiāo téng* (Caulis Polygoni Multiflori) 30g and *wǔ wèi zǐ* (Fructus Schisandrae) 10g to nourish blood and calm the spirit.

Additional Treatment Modalities

1. Chinese Patent Medicine

(1) Medicinals for the Bleeding Stage:

1) *Shēn Mài Zhù Shè Yè* (参麦注射液)

Intramuscular injection, 2-4ml, twice daily. Or 5-10ml added into 250ml 5% glucose solution. Treats both shock and irregular heartbeat, regulates immunity, and relieves inflammation. Indicated for DUB reversal and deficiency patterns.

2) *Yì Gōng Zhǐ Xuè Kǒu Fú Yè* (益宫止血口服液)

Three times daily, 20ml. Indicated for DUB with qi and yin deficiency patterns.

3) *Qīng Jīng Kē Lè* (清经颗粒)

5g per dose, twice daily, only take in the absence of bleeding during the post-menstrual period, 15 days constitutes one course of treatment. Indicated for DUB with blood-heat patterns.

4) *Shēng Sān Qī Jiāo Náng* (生三七胶囊)

Three pills, 1-2 times daily. Indicated for DUB with blood stasis patterns.

5) *Xuè Jié Jiāo Náng* (血竭胶囊)

Three times daily, 4-6 tablets. 15 days constitutes one course of treatment. The main functions are to treat inflammation and pain, invigorate blood and dispel stasis, astringe to stanch bleeding, generate flesh, and close sores. The consumption of acidic foods is prohibited. This formula is also contraindicated in pregnancy.

6) *Gōng Xuè Níng* (宫血宁)

Prescribe during the bleeding stage or menstruation cycle. 1-2 pills three times daily. The main functions are to stimulate the uterus, arrest bleeding, and relieve inflammation. Indicated for flooding and spotting, profuse menses, and continuous postpartum bleeding. This formula is contraindicated in pregnancy.

7) *Yún Nán Bái Yào* (云南白药)

Powdered, 0.2-0.3g per dose, not to exceed 0.5g. Take every 4 hours, or more often for acute conditions. Capsules, 0.25-0.5g per dose, four times daily with warm water. This formulas arrests bleeding, stimulates the uterus, and relieves inflammation. Indicated for DUB due to qi and blood stagnation or blood-heat patterns. This medicinal is contraindicated in pregnant woman. Intake of fish, beans, or sour and cold foods is also prohibited. Use with caution in patients presenting either cardiac arrhythmias or allergies. Discontinue immediately with the appearance of any allergic reaction. With the appearance of epigastric discomfort, heartburn, or nausea, reduce dosage or discontinue completely. If prescribed long-term and recurrent bleeding appears, perform CBC. With decreased platelet counts, discontinue use.

8) *Hé Yè Wán* (荷叶丸)

1 pill, 2-3 times daily. Take with warm water on an empty stomach. Indicated for patterns of flooding and spotting with blood-heat. Consumption of spicy or greasy foods is prohibited.

9) *Shēn Qiàn Gù Jīng Chōng Jì* (参茜固经冲剂)

1 bag per dose, twice daily. Begin one week before the onset of menstruation through the the end of the cycle. Indicated for DUB associated with qi and yin deficiency patterns with blood stasis.

10) *Níng Xuè Sǎn* (宁血散)

8g, 3-4 times daily. Indicated for blood-heat patterns.

11) *Duàn Xuè Liú Piàn* (断血流片)

3-6 pills, 3-4 times daily. Granules 6.5g, 3 times daily. Indicated for blood-heat patterns.

12) *Shí Huī Sǎn* (十灰散)

9g, twice daily. Indicated for blood-heat patterns.

13) *Gōng Tài Chōng Jì* (宫泰冲剂)

1-2 bags, 2-3 times daily. Indicated for qi and yin deficiency with blood stasis.

(2) Medicinals for the Non-bleeding Stage:

1) *Zǐ Hé Chē Jiāo Náng* (紫河车胶囊)

Take 1-5 tablets, 1-3 times daily after meals. Indicated for insufficiency of both Kidney essence and blood. This formula acts to promote follicular development by replenishing Kidney essence.

2) *Yù Cōng Róng Kǒu Fú Yè* (御苁蓉口服液)

10ml, twice daily. Take on an empty stomach. Indicated for Kidney deficiency patterns.

3) *Fù Fāng Ē Jiāo Jiāng* (复方阿胶浆)

20ml, three times daily. Indicated for qi and blood deficient DUB with symptoms such as dizziness, palpitation, insomnia, poor appetite, leucopenia, or anemia.

4) *Dìng Kūn Dān* (定坤丹)

One or one-half big honeyed pill per dose. Indicated for DUB with qi and blood deficiency and stagnation.

5) *Chūn Xuè Ān Jiāo Náng* (春血安胶囊)

4 tablets, three times daily, or take under the doctor's supervision. Indicated for DUB in adolescents.

6) *Qǐ Jú Dì Huáng Wán* (杞菊地黄丸)

9g, twice daily. Indicated for deficiency of Liver and Kidney yin with hyperactive yang. Consumption of raw, cold or acidic foods is prohibited.

7) *Yǎng Xuè Dāng Guī Jīng* (养血当归精)

10ml, 2-3 times daily. Indicated for qi and blood deficiency due to uterine bleeding. Raw, cold or spicy foods are prohibited. Contraindicated when feverish sensations or wind cold conditions are present.

8) *Shēng Mài Yǐn* (生脉饮)

10ml, three times daily. Indicated for DUB with qi and yin deficiency. Contraindicated when exterior or excess syndromes are present.

9) *Guī Pí Wán* (归脾丸)

Water-honeyed pill, 6g, three times daily. Large honeyed pill, 1 pill three times daily. Indicated for Heart and Spleen qi deficiency during the bleeding stage, and also for the regulation of menstruation after the abnormal bleeding has resolved.

10) *Tóng Rén Wū Jī Bái Fèng Kǒu Fú Yè* (同仁乌鸡白凤口服液)

10ml, 3 times daily, or take under the supervision of a doctor. Indicated for DUB with qi and blood deficiency. Contraindicated when feverish sensations or wind cold symptoms are present.

2. ACUPUNCTURE AND MOXIBUSTION

(1) Deficiency

【Treatment Principle】
Tonify deficiency and support the upright.

【Point Selection】

RN 4	guān yuán	关元
SP 6	sān yīn jiāo	三阴交
BL 23	shèn shù	肾俞
KI 8	jiāo xìn	交信

【Point Modification】
- For qi deficiency, select RN 6 (*qì hǎi*), BL 20 (*pí shù*), BL 43 (*gāo huāng shù*) and ST 36 (*zú sān lǐ*).
- For yang deficiency, select RN 6, DU 4 (*mìng mén*), and KI 7 (*fù liū*).

➢ For yin deficiency, select KI 2 (*rán gǔ*) and KI 10 (*yīn gǔ*).

【Manipulation】

Needle all points with reinforcement. Moxibustion is applicable.

(2) Excess

【Treatment Principle】

Drain excess evils.

【Point Selection】

RN 6	qì hǎi	气海
SP 6	sān yīn jiāo	三阴交
SP 1	yǐn bái	隐白

【Point Modification】

➢ For blood-heat, select SP 10 (*xuè hǎi*) and KI 5 (*shuǐ quán*).

➢ For damp-heat, add RN 3 (*zhōng jí*) and SP 9 (*yīn líng quán*).

➢ For qi constraint, select LV 3 (*tài chōng*), SJ 6 (*zhī gōu*), and LV 1 (*dà dūn*).

➢ For blood stasis, select SP 8 (*dì jī*), SP 8 (*qì chōng*), and SP 12 (*chōng mén*).

【Manipulation】

Needle all points with drainage.

(3) Auricular Therapy

【Point Selection】

uterus		耳穴子宫
cavitas pelvis	TF5	盆腔
subcortex	AT4	皮质下
endocrine	CO18	内分泌
adrenal gland	TG2p	肾上腺
shenmen	TF4	神门

brain stem	AT3, 4i	脑干
Liver	CO12	肝
Spleen	CO13	脾
Stomach	CO4	胃
Kidney	CO10	肾

【Manipulation】

Apply ear seeds to the points and secure with adhesive tape. Press 3-4 times daily 3-5 minutes each time. During the bleeding stage, change seeds every 2 days, alternating ears. After 3-5 treatments, once per week is sufficient. Effects may be expected after 1-4 weeks.

(4) Auricular Acupuncture

【Point Selection】

uterus		子宫
endocrine	CO18	内分泌
Liver	CO12	肝
Kidney	CO10	肾
shenmen	TF4	神门

【Manipulation】

Choose 3-4 points, treat with moderate stimulation once daily or every other day. Retain the needles for 30-60 minutes. Embedding needles are applicable.

3. SIMPLE PRESCRIPTIONS AND EMPIRICAL FORMULAS

(1) Simple Prescriptions

1) *Chǎo jīng jiè suì* (Dry-fried Spica Schizonepetae) 25g, decocted. Indicated for flooding with blood-heat patterns.

2) *Xiān zhù má gēn* (Fresh Radix Boehmeriae) 30g, 1 dose daily for 2

days. Indicated for flooding and spotting with blood-heat patterns.

3) *Wǔ bèi zǐ* (Galla Chinensis), one-half raw and half prepared. Grind into a powder, and take 6g with cool water on an empty stomach. Its main function is to arrest bleeding.

4) *Xiān yì mǔ cǎo* (Herba Leonuri Recens) 50g, consume as a juice. Indicated for flooding with associated blood stasis patterns.

5) *Xiāng fù* (Rhizoma Cyperi) 250g, dry-fry until charred, and grind into a powder. Take 10g with warm wine, twice daily for 10 days. Indicated for spotting due to qi stagnation with abdominal distention and pain.

6) *Ài yè* (Folium Artemisiae Argyi) 5g, dry-fry with vinegar. Mix with 2 egg yolks and remove the dregs. To be taken warm before meals. Indicated for spotting associated with yang deficiency patterns.

7) Vinegar 300g, add 100g calcinated iron to vinegar and steep for 30 minutes, remove the dregs before consuming. Indicated for flooding and spotting.

(2) Empirical Formulas

1) *Lián Qí Yì Xuè Tāng* (莲芪益血汤)

黄芪	huáng qí	30g	Radix Astragali
党参	dǎng shēn	30g	Radix Codonopsis
地榆	dì yú	30g	Radix Sanguisorbae
仙鹤草	xiān hè cǎo	30g	Herba Agrimoniae
旱莲草	hàn lián cǎo	30g	Herba Ecliptae
白术	bái zhú	15g	Rhizoma Atractylodis Macrocephalae
生地黄	shēng dì huáng	15g	Radix Rehmanniae
当归	dāng guī	6g	Radix Angelicae Sinensis
升麻	shēng má	6g	Rhizoma Cimicifugae
三七	sān qī	6g	Radix Notoginseng
坤草	kūn cǎo	6g	Herba Leonuri

| 蒲黄 | pú huáng | 10g | Pollen Typhae |

Indicated during menopause for qi deficiency and blood stasis with blood-heat.

2) *Kǔ Jiǔ Jiān* (苦酒煎)

生地榆	shēng dì yú	250g	Radix Sanguisorbae Cruda
水	shuǐ	250ml	Water
醋	cù	250ml	Vinegar

Indicated for menopausal DUB with blood-heat patterns.

3) *Zhǐ Bēng Tāng* (止崩汤)

炙黄芪	zhì huáng qí	30g	Radix Astragali Praeparata cum Melle
党参	dǎng shēn	15g	Radix Codonopsis
白术	bái zhú	10g	Rhizoma Atractylodis Macrocephalae
怀山药	huái shān yào	15g	Rhizoma Dioscoreae
炙升麻	zhì shēng má	10g	Rhizoma Cimicifugae (fried with liquid)
白芍	bái sháo	15g	Radix Paeoniae Alba
熟地黄	shú dì huáng	20g	Radix Rehmanniae Praeparata
阿胶	ē jiāo	20g	Colla Corii Asini
海螵蛸	hǎi piāo xiāo	12g	Endoconcha Sepiae
赤石脂	chì shí zhī	12g	Halloysitum Rubrum
芡实	qiàn shí	15g	Semen Eutyales
续断	xù duàn	15g	Radix Dipsaci
益母草	yì mǔ cǎo	15g	Herba Leonuri
甘草	gān cǎo	5g	Radix et Rhizoma Glycyrrhizae

Indicated for DUB due to qi and yin deficiency with blood stasis.

4) *Zhǐ Bēng Tāng* (止崩汤)

| 太子参 | tài zǐ shēn | 30g | Radix Pseudostellariae |
| 黄芪 | huáng qí | 30g | Radix Astragali |

生地黄	shēng dì huáng	20g	Radix Rehmanniae
白术	bái zhú	12g	Rhizoma Atractylodis Macrocephalae
白芍	bái sháo	12g	Radix Paeoniae Alba
海螵蛸	hǎi piāo xiāo	12g	Endoconcha Sepiae
茜草炭	qiàn cǎo tàn	12g	Radix Rubiae Carbonisata
女贞子	nǚ zhēn zǐ	15g	Fructus Ligustri Lucidi
旱莲草	hàn lián cǎo	15g	Herba Ecliptae
地榆炭	dì yú tàn	15g	Radix Sanguisorbae Carbonisata
棕榈炭	zōng lǚ tàn	10g	Trachycarpus (carbonized)
阿胶（烊化）	ē jiāo	10g	Colla Corii Asini (dissolved)
甘草	gān cǎo	10g	Radix et Rhizoma Glycyrrhizae

Indicated for qi deficiency and blood-heat with blood stasis.

5) *Zhǐ Bēng Tāng* (止崩汤)

生地榆	shēng dì yú	100g	Radix Sanguisorbae Cruda
牡蛎	mǔ lì	40g	Concha Ostreae
陈醋	chén cù	100ml	Aged Vinegar

Indicated for flooding and spotting associated with blood-heat patterns.

6) Modified *Wēn Jīng Tāng* (温经汤)

当归	dāng guī	10g	Radix Angelicae Sinensis
白芍	bái sháo	10g	Radix Paeoniae Alba
牡丹皮	mǔ dān pí	10g	Cortex Moutan
熟地黄	shú dì huáng	15g	Radix Rehmanniae Praeparata
麦冬	mài dōng	15g	Radix Ophiopogonis
桂枝	guì zhī	6g	Ramulus Cinnamomi
吴茱萸	wú zhū yú	6g	Fructus Evodiae
三七粉（冲服）	sān qī fěn	6g	Radix Notoginseng Powder (infused)
甘草	gān cǎo	6g	Radix et Rhizoma Glycyrrhizae
川芎	chuān xiōng	8g	Rhizoma Chuanxiong

阿胶（烊化）	ē jiāo	12g	Colla Corii Asini (dissolved)
鹿角胶（烊化）	lù jiǎo jiāo	12g	Colla Cornus Cervi (dissolved)
乌贼骨	wū zéi gǔ	30g	Endoconcha Sepiae

Indicated for Kidney deficiency with blood stasis patterns.

7) *Gù* Chōng *Tāng* (固冲汤)

乌贼骨	wū zéi gǔ	30g	Endoconcha Sepiae
煅龙骨	duàn lóng gǔ	30g	Fossilia Ossis Mastodi (calcined)
煅牡蛎	duàn mǔ lì	30g	Concha Ostreae (calcined)
茜草根	qiàn cǎo gēn	15g	Radix et Rhizoma Rubiae
熟地黄	shú dì huáng	15g	Radix Rehmanniae Praeparata
五倍子	wǔ bèi zǐ	15g	Galla Chinensis
黑芥穗	hēi jiè suì	10g	Spica Schizonepetae Carbonisata
炒白术	chǎo bái zhú	12g	Rhizoma Atractylodis Macrocephalae (dry-fried)

Indicated for yin deficiency patterns.

8) *Jǔ* Xiàn *Tāng* (举陷汤)

党参	dǎng shēn	25g	Radix Codonopsis
白术	bái zhú	15g	Rhizoma Atractylodis Macrocephalae
黄芪	huáng qí	30g	Radix Astragali
升麻	shēng má	10g	Rhizoma Cimicifugae
柴胡	chái hú	10g	Bupleurum Chinens
藁本	gǎo běn	10g	Rhizoma Ligustici
防风	fáng fēng	10g	Radix Saposhnikoviae
芥穗炭	jiè suì tàn	10g	Spica Schizonepetae Carbonisata
当归	dāng guī	15g	Radix Angelicae Sinensis
白芍	bái sháo	25g	Radix Paeoniae Alba
山药	shān yào	25g	Rhizoma Dioscoreae
熟地黄	shú dì huáng	25g	Radix Rehmanniae Praeparata

Indicated for qi deficiency patterns.

9) *Yì Qì Shè Xuè Tāng* (益气摄血汤)

黄芪	huáng qí	50g	Radix Astragali
白术	bái zhú	40g	Rhizoma Atractylodis Macrocephalae
阿胶（烊化）	ē jiāo	40g	Colla Corii Asini (dissolved)
益母草	yì mǔ cǎo	40g	Herba Leonuri
茜草炭	qiàn cǎo tàn	40g	Radix Rubiae Carbonisata
乌贼骨	wū zéi gǔ	30g	Endoconcha Sepiae
生地黄	shēng dì huáng	15g	Radix Rehmanniae
佛手	fó shǒu	15g	Fructus Citri Sarcodactylis
升麻	shēng má	15g	Rhizoma Cimicifugae
炙甘草	zhì gān cǎo	6g	Radix et Rhizoma Glycyrrhizae Praeparata cum Melle

Indicated for DUB with qi deficiency patterns.

10) *Tiáo Jīng Tāng* (调经汤)

女贞子	nǚ zhēn zǐ	50g	Fructus Ligustri Lucidi
旱莲草	hàn lián cǎo	25g	Herba Ecliptae
生地黄	shēng dì huáng	25g	Radix Rehmanniae
山药	shān yào	25g	Rhizoma Dioscoreae
侧柏叶	cè bǎi yè	15g	Cacumen Platycladi
白芍	bái sháo	25g	Radix Paeoniae Alba
乌梅	wū méi	15g	Fructus Mume
地榆炭	dì yú tàn	50g	Radix Sanguisorbae Carbonisata
黄芩	huáng qín	15g	Radix Scutellariae
黑芥穗	hēi jiè suì	15g	Spica Schizonepetae Carbonisata

Indicated for Kidney deficiency and Liver constraint patterns.

11) *Tiáo Jīng Tāng* (调经汤)

地榆	dì yú	30g	Radix Sanguisorbae
乌贼骨	wū zéi gǔ	30g	Endoconcha Sepiae

生地黄	shēng dì huáng	24g	Radix Rehmanniae
地骨皮	dì gǔ pí	20g	Cortex Lycii
山萸肉	shān yú ròu	10g	Fructus Corni
麦冬	mài dōng	10g	Radix Ophiopogonis
杭白芍	háng bái sháo	25g	Radix Paeoniae Alba
女贞子	nǚ zhēn zǐ	10g	Fructus Ligustri Lucidi
旱莲草	hàn lián cǎo	10g	Herba Ecliptae
栀子炭	zhī zǐ tàn	10g	Fructus Gardeniae Carbonisata
牡丹皮	mǔ dān pí	10g	Cortex Moutan
阿胶（烊化）	ē jiāo	10g	Colla Corii Asini
元参	yuán shēn	10g	Radix Scrophulariae
龟板	guī bǎn	10g	Testudinis Plastrum

Indicated for patterns of yin deficiency with blood-heat.

12) *Ān Chōng Tāng* (安冲汤)

白术	bái zhú	Rhizoma Atractylodis Macrocephalae
生黄芪	shēng huáng qí	Radix Astragali Cruda
生龙骨	shēng lóng gǔ	Fossilia Ossis Mastodi Cruda
生牡蛎	shēng mǔ lì	Concha Ostreae Cruda
大生地	dà shēng dì	Radix Rehmanniae
生白芍	shēng bái sháo	Radix Paeoniae Alba (raw)
海螵蛸	hǎi piāo xiāo	Endoconcha Sepiae
山茱萸	shān zhū yú	Fructus Corni
茜草	qiàn cǎo	Radix Rubiae
川断	chuān xù duàn	Radix Dipsaci

Indicated for DUB with qi deficiency.

13) *Fù Fāng Xuè Jiàn Chóu Fāng* (复方血见愁方)

| 血见愁 | xuè jiàn chóu | 50g | Acalyphae Astralis |
| 仙鹤草 | xiān hè cǎo | 50g | Herba Agrimoniae |

| 益母草 | yì mǔ cǎo | 50g | Herba Leonuri |

Indicated for DUB due to blood stasis.

14) *Xī Hóng Jiān* (惜红煎)

乌梅	wū méi	30g	Fructus Mume
怀山药	huái shān yào	30g	Rhizoma Dioscoreae
炒白术	chǎo bái zhú	30g	Rhizoma Atractylodis Macrocephalae (dry-fried)
白芍	bái sháo	15g	Radix Paeoniae Alba
炒荆芥穗	chǎo jīng jiè suì	15g	Spica Schizonepetae (dry-fried)
五味子	wǔ wèi zǐ	6g	Fructus Schisandrae
地榆炭	dì yú tàn	30g	Radix Sanguisorbae Carbonisata
甘草	gān cǎo	5g	Radix et Rhizoma Glycyrrhizae
贯众炭	guàn zhòng tàn	15g	Cyrtomii Rhizoma (carbonized)

Indicated for DUB with qi and yin deficiency patterns.

15) *Yì Qì Jiàn Pǐ Huà Yū Tāng* (益气健脾化瘀汤)

党参	dǎng shēn	25g	Radix Codonopsis
黄芪	huáng qí	25g	Radix Astragali
炒白术	chǎo bái zhú	25g	Rhizoma Atractylodis Macrocephalae (dry-fried)
炒地榆	chǎo dì yú	15g	Radix Sanguisorbae (dry-fried)
生山药	shēng shān yào	25g	Rhizoma Dioscoreae (raw)
生龙骨 (先煎)	shēng lóng gǔ	30g	Fossilia Ossis Mastodi Cruda (decocted first)
生牡蛎 (先煎)	shēng mǔ lì	30g	Concha Ostreae Cruda (decocted first)
黑芥穗	hēi jiè suì	10g	Spica Schizonepetae Carbonisata
茜草	qiàn cǎo	10g	Radix Rubiae
鸡内金	jī nèi jīn	10g	Gigeriae Galli
三七末 (冲)	sān qī mò	3g	Radix Notoginseng Powder (infused)

Indicated for DUB due to qi deficiency with blood stasis.

16) *Shèng Yù Sān Cǎo Tāng* (圣愈三草汤)

朝鲜参	cháo xiǎn shēn	15g	Radix Ginseng Coreensis
炙黄芪	zhì huáng qí	30g	Radix Astragali Praeparata cum Melle
熟地	shú dì huáng	30g	Radix Rehmanniae Praeparata
仙鹤草	xiān hè cǎo	30g	Herba Agrimoniae
茜草	qiàn cǎo	30g	Radix Rubiae
旱莲草	hàn lián cǎo	30g	Herba Ecliptae
炒白芍	chǎo bái sháo	12g	Radix Paeoniae Alba (dry-fried)
当归	dāng guī	6g	Radix Angelicae Sinensis
川芎	chuān xiōng	6g	Rhizoma Chuanxiong

Indicated for DUB with qi deficiency and blood stasis.

17) *Jì Duàn Wū Zéi Qiàn Cǎo Tāng* (寄断乌贼茜草汤)

桑寄生	sāng jì shēng	12g	Herba Taxilli
川续断	chuān xù duàn	12g	Radix Dipsaci
乌贼骨	wū zéi gǔ	12g	Endoconcha Sepiae
茜草炭	qiàn cǎo tàn	12g	Radix Rubiae Carbonisata

Indicated for Kidney deficiency patterns.

18) *Tiáo Gān Bǔ Shèn Jīng Yàn Fāng* (调肝补肾经验方)

川续断	chuān xù duàn	15g	Radix Dipsaci
怀山药	huái shān yào	15g	Rhizoma Dioscoreae
全当归	quán dāng guī	15g	Radix Angelicae Sinensis
杭白芍	háng bái sháo	15g	Radix Paeoniae Alba
炒白术	chǎo bái zhú	15g	Rhizoma Atractylodis Macrocephalae (dry-fried)
阿胶珠	ē jiāo zhū	10g	Colla Corii Asini Pilula
女贞子	nǚ zhēn zǐ	10g	Fructus Ligustri Lucidi
生地炭	shēng dì tàn	10g	Radix Rehmanniae Carbonisata
杜仲炭	dù zhòng tàn	10g	Cortex Eucommiae Carbonisata
旱莲草	hàn lián cǎo	10g	Herba Ecliptae

| 黄芩炭 | huáng qín tàn | 10g | Radix Scutellariae Carbonisata |
| 香附末 | xiāng fù mò | 6g | Rhizoma Cyperi Powder |

Indicated for Kidney deficiency and Liver constraint with blood-heat.

19) *Jiā Wèi Guì Zhī Lóng Gŭ Mŭ Lì Tāng* (加味桂枝龙骨牡蛎汤)

桂枝	guì zhī	10g	Ramulus Cinnamomi
丝瓜络	sī guā luò	10g	Retinervus Luffae Fructus
芍药	sháo yào	12g	Paeonia
生姜	shēng jiāng	3pieces	Rhizoma Zingiberis Recens
大枣	dà zǎo	7pieces	Fructus Jujubae
煅龙骨	duàn lóng gǔ	30g	Fossilia Ossis Mastodi (calcined)
煅牡蛎	duàn mǔ lì	30g	Concha Ostreae (calcined)
川续断	chuān xù duàn	15g	Radix Dipsaci
金樱子	jīn yīng zǐ	15g	Fructus Rosae Laevigatae
杜仲	dù zhòng	15g	Cortex Eucommiae

Indicated for DUB due to Kidney deficiency with congealing cold.

20) *Jiàn Pí Yì Shèn Tāng* (健脾益肾汤)

生黄芪	shēng huáng qí	30g	Radix Astragali Cruda
紫石英	zǐ shí yīng	30g	Fluoritum
党参	dǎng shēn	15g	Radix Codonopsis
菟丝子	tù sī zǐ	15g	Semen Cuscutae
白术	bái zhú	12g	Rhizoma Atractylodis Macrocephalae
茯苓	fú líng	10g	Poria
山萸肉	shān yú ròu	10g	Fructus Corni
香附	xiāng fù	10g	Rhizoma Cyperi
阿胶	ē jiāo	10g	Colla Corii Asini
陈皮	chén pí	10g	Pericarpium Citri Reticulatae

Indicated for DUB due to Spleen and Kidney deficiency patterns.

21) *Shuāng Tiáo Hé Jì* (双调合剂)

炙黄芪	zhì huáng qí	Radix Astragali Praeparata cum Melle
炒白术	chǎo bái zhú	Rhizoma Atractylodis Macrocephalae (dry-fried)
紫石英	zǐ shí yīng	Fluoritum
鹿角霜	lù jiǎo shuāng	Cornu Cervi Degelatinatum
旱莲草	hàn lián cǎo	Herba Ecliptae
炒杜仲	chǎo dù zhòng	Cortex Eucommiae (dry-fried)
阿胶	ē jiāo	Colla Corii Asini
当归	dāng guī	Radix Angelicae Sinensis
柴胡	chái hú	Bupleurum Chinens
升麻	shēng má	Rhizoma Cimicifugae
白茅根	bái máo gēn	Rhizoma Imperatae
炒五灵脂	chǎo wǔ líng zhī	Faeces Trogopterori (dry-fried)
炒蒲黄	chǎo pú huáng	Pollen Typhae (dry-fried)

Indicated for DUB due to Spleen and Kidney deficiency patterns, Kidney deficiency with Liver constraint, and deficiency patterns with blood stasis.

22) *Shān Yú Tù Sī Tāng* (山萸菟丝汤)

山萸肉	shān yú ròu	60g	Fructus Corni
菟丝子	tù sī zǐ	30g	Semen Cuscutae
女贞子	nǚ zhēn zǐ	15g	Fructus Ligustri Lucidi
旱莲草	hàn lián cǎo	15g	Herba Ecliptae
五味子	wǔ wèi zǐ	15g	Fructus Schisandrae
益母草	yì mǔ cǎo	10g	Herba Leonuri
茜草	qiàn cǎo	10g	Radix Rubiae

Indicated for DUB due to Kidney deficiency and blood stasis.

PROGNOSIS

When DUB occurs during adolescence, it is often of the non-ovulatory type. However, the development and functions of the hypothalamic-pituitary-ovarian axis naturally mature over time. Although proper treatment may re-establish normal ovulatory menstruation cycles, some cases may require a longer course of treatment. There is a possibility of recurrence due to many causes, including reactions to other medications.

In patients of childbearing age, the condition may be self-limiting in the absence of other organic diseases. The treatment goal is to primarily arrest bleeding and then to establish normal ovulatory cycles.

Menopausal DUB patients may recover in a relatively short period of time. In these cases, we may then focus on treating the deficiency patterns in order to support the patient through the transition.

PREVENTIVE HEALTHCARE

Lifestyle Modification

During the bleeding period the patient should refrain from sexual activities and also be careful to avoid vaginal infections. It is also important to avoid exposure to rain and cold weather, to balance both work and rest, and to maintain regular sleeping habits. Contraceptive drugs and surgery may both adversely affect this condition.

Dietary Recommendation

Cold, raw or spicy foods are prohibited during the bleeding period. Generally limit the intake of all spicy foods in the diet.

(1) *Hé Bàng Ròu Bái Guŏ Rén Tāng* (河蚌肉白果仁汤)

鲜河蚌肉	xiān hé bàng ròu	60g	Fresh Swan-mussel
白果仁	bái guǒ rén	15g	Semen Ginkgo Kernel
北芪	běi qí	15g	Radix Astragali
党参	dǎng shēn	12g	Radix Codonopsis

血余炭（布包）	xuè yú tàn	10g	Crinis Carbonisatus (wrap-boiled)

Decoct with brown sugar. Indicated for DUB with patterns of deficient qi unable to contain blood. Once daily, 7-8 doses per course.

(2) *Wū Jī Guì Yuán Ròu Tāng* (乌鸡桂园肉汤)

Prepare and clean one black-boned chicken. Stuff with *dāng guī* (Radix Angelicae Sinensis) 5g, *shú dì huáng* (Radix Rehmanniae Praeparata) 5g, *guì yuán ròu* (Arillus Longan) 5g, *bái sháo* (Radix Paeoniae Alba) 5g and *zhì gān cǎo* (Radix et Rhizoma Glycyrrhizae Praeparata cum Melle) 10g. Cook in a large pot with high heat for 90 minutes. Indicated for shortened cycles with profuse bleeding of thin menses, lassitude, fright palpitations and a downbearing sensation in the lower abdomen.

(3) *Lǎo Sī Guā Chá* (老丝瓜茶)

白茅根	bái máo gēn	15g	Rhizoma Imperatae
老丝瓜	lǎo sī guā	9g	Luffae Fructus
旱莲草	hàn lián cǎo	9g	Herba Ecliptae

Decocted 1 dose daily for 4-5 days. Indicated for DUB with frenetic movement of blood-heat patterns.

(4) *Chǎo Xiān Qín Cài Lián Gēn* (炒鲜芹菜莲根)

Prepare sliced celery and fresh lotus root, 120g each. Heat cooking oil, add celery and lotus root with salt, and cook for 5 minutes. Indicated for shortened cycles with profuse menses that is thick, viscous, and purplish in color.

(5) *Hēi Mù Ěr Táng Shuǐ* (黑木耳糖水)

Cook 30g *hēi mù ěr* (Auricularia) on low heat until sweet-smelling. Then add 500ml boiled water and 15g brown sugar. Indicated for prolonged or profuse menstruation, dark purple and viscous menses with clotting, distending abdominal or lumbar pain, vexation, thirst, and dark yellow urine.

(6) Yì Mǔ Cǎo Jī Dàn Tāng (益母草鸡蛋汤)

益母草	yì mǔ cǎo	50-60g	Herba Leonuri
香附	xiāng fù	15g	Rhizoma Cyperi
鸡蛋	jī dàn	2	Eggs

Cook thoroughly in water, remove eggshells and simmer. Remove the dregs and eat once daily for 4-5 days. Indicated for DUB with qi stagnation and blood stasis.

(7) Mù Ěr Ǒu Jié Zhū Ròu Dùn Bīng Táng (木耳藕节猪肉炖冰糖)

木耳	mù ěr	15g	Auricularia
藕节	ǒu jié	30g	Nodus Nelumbinis Rhizomatis
冰糖	bīng táng	15g	Crystal Sugar
猪肉	zhū ròu	100g	Pork

Mix with water in a cooking pot and stew. Take twice daily for 5-7 days. Indicated for Liver and Kidney yin deficiency patterns.

(8) Cù Dòu Fǔ (醋豆腐)

Cook 150g tofu with 100ml vinegar. Take before meals, once daily for 7-10 days. Avoid spicy foods.

Regulation of Emotional and Mental Health

A balanced emotional state is very beneficial to reproductive health. Consciously cultivating a pleasant mood and a positive attitude as well as maintaining an active lifestyle during treatment may prove beneficial to recovery.

CLINICAL EXPERIENCE OF RENOWNED PHYSICIANS

Empirical Formulas

1. JIĀO ÀI SÌ WÙ TĀNG (胶艾四物汤) MODIFIED WITH CHÁI HÚ FOR THE TREATMENT OF FLOODING AND SPOTTING DUE TO SUDDEN RAGE (SHI JIN-MO)

【Ingredients】

鹿角胶（另烊化兑服）	lù jiǎo jiāo	10g	Colla Cornus Cervi (dissolved)
砂仁	shā rén	3g	Fructus Amomi
醋柴胡	cù chái hú	5g	Radix Bupleui (fried with vinegar)
阿胶珠	ē jiāo zhū	10g	Colla Corii Asini Pilula
生地黄	shēng dì huáng	6g	Radix Rehmanniae
熟地黄	shú dì huáng	6g	Radix Rehmanniae Praeparata
杭白芍	háng bái sháo	10g	Radix Paeoniae Alba
酒川芎	jiǔ chuān xiōng	5g	Rhizoma Chuanxiong (prepared with wine)
当归身	dāng guī shēn	6g	Radix Angelicae Sinensis
醋祈艾	cù qí ài	6g	Folium Artemisiae Argyi (fried with vinegar)
白蒺藜	bái jí lí	12g	Fructus Tribuli
炒远志	chǎo yuǎn zhì	10g	Radix Polygalae (dry-fried)
炙甘草	zhì gān cǎo	3g	Radix et Rhizoma Glycyrrhizae Praeparata cum Melle

【Indications】

Flooding due to sudden rage impairing the Liver.

【Formula Analysis】

Sudden rage impairs the Liver and often leads to flooding. *Jiāo Ài Sì Wù Tāng* (胶艾四物汤) with *chái hú* (Radix Bupleuri) both course the Liver and regulate blood. *Lù jiǎo jiāo* (Colla Cornus Cervi) tonifies blood and arrests bleeding. *Bái jí lí* (Fructus Tribuli) and *chǎo yuǎn zhì* (Dry-fried

Radix Polygalae) both promote contraction of the uterus.

(Zhu Shen-yu, et al. *Collection of Shi Jin-mo's Clinical Experience* 施今墨临床经验集 . Beijing: People's Medical Publishing House, 1982. 183-184)

2. Empirical Formulas Treating Menopausal DUB (Xia Gui-cheng)

【Ingredients】

鹿衔草	lù xián cǎo	30g	Herba Pyrolae
钩藤	gōu téng	15g	Ramulus Uncariae Cum Uncis
黄芪	huáng qí	15g	Radix Astragali
党参	dǎng shēn	15g	Radix Codonopsis
牡丹皮	mǔ dān pí	10g	Cortex Moutan
黑山栀	hēi shān zhī	10g	Fructus Gardeniae
炒白术	chǎo bái zhú	10g	Rhizoma Atractylodis Macrocephalae (dry-fried)
茯苓	fú líng	10g	Poria
炙远志	zhì yuǎn zhì	10g	Radix Polygalae (fried with liquid)
炒五灵脂	chǎo wǔ líng zhī	10g	Faeces Trogopterori (dry-fried)
炒蒲黄(包)	chǎo pú huáng	10g	Pollen Typhae (dry-fried, wrapped)
炒川断	chǎo chuān xù duàn	10g	Radix Dipsaci (dry-fried)
广木香	guǎng mù xiāng	6g	Radix Aucklandiae

【Indications】

Clear the Liver, invigorate the Spleen and dispel blood stasis. Indicated for menopausal DUB.

【Formula Analysis】

Gōu téng (Ramulus Uncariae Cum Uncis), *mǔ dān pí* (Cortex Moutan), *shān zhī* (Fructus Gardeniae), *lù xián cǎo* (Pyrolae Herba) and *zhì yuǎn zhì* (Fried with liquid Radix Polygalae) drain the Liver and pacify the Heart. *Huáng qí* (Radix Astragali), *dǎng shēn* (Radix Codonopsis), *bái zhú* (Rhizoma Atractylodis Macrocephalae), *fú líng* (Poria) and *mù xiāng* (Radix Aucklandiae) invigorate the Spleen and regulate qi. *Wǔ líng zhī* (Faeces Trogopterori), *pú huáng* (Pollen Typhae) and *chuān xù duàn* (Radix

Dipsaci) dispel stasis and stanch bleeding.

【Modifications】

➢ For excessive heat signs, add *xià kū cǎo* (Spica Prunellae) 10g and *kǔ dīng chá* (Ilex Latifolia) 10g.

➢ For yin deficiency signs, add *nǚ zhēn zǐ* (Fructus Ligustri Lucidi) 15g, *zhì guī bǎn* (Fried with liquid Testudinis Plastrum, decoct first) 15g and *hàn lián cǎo* (Herba Ecliptae) 15g.

➢ For profuse bleeding, add *dà jì* (Herba Cirsii Japonici) 15g, *xiǎo jì* (Herba Cirsii) 15g, *qiàn cǎo tàn* (Carbonized Radix Rubiae) 15g, and *dì yú tàn* (Carbonized Radix Sanguisorbae) 10g.

➢ For yang deficiency, add *bā jǐ tiān* (Radix Morindae Officinalis) 10g, *zǐ shí yīng* (Fluoritum, decocted first) 10g and *bǔ gǔ zhī* (Fructus Psoraleae) 10g.

➢ For excessive damp-heat, add *mǎ biān cǎo* (Herba Verbanae) 30g and *bài jiàng cǎo* (Herba Patriniae) 30g.

➢ For vexation and insomnia, add *yè jiāo téng* (Caulis Polygoni Multiflori) 10g, *hé huān pí* (Cortex Albiziae) 10g, and *chǎo zǎo rén* (Dry-fried Semen Ziziphi Spinosae) 10g.

➢ For lumbar pain, add *chǎo dù zhòng* (Dry-fried Cortex Eucommiae) 10g, and *sāng jì shēng* (Herba Taxilli) 10g.

(Li Yong-sheng. Draining the Liver, Invigorating the Spleen and Dispelling Stasis Methods in the Treatment of 68 Cases of Menopausal DUB 清肝健脾化瘀法治疗更年期功能性子宫出血 68 例. *Zhejiang Journal of Traditional Chinese Medicine* 浙江中医杂志. 1999, 34(1)：8)

3. Gōng Xuè Yǐn (功血饮) in the Treatment of DUB (Wu Xi)

【Ingredients】

金樱子	jīn yīng zǐ	15g	Fructus Rosae Laevigatae
制首乌	zhì shǒu wū	15g	Radix Polygoni Multiflori Praeparata cum Succo Glycines Sotae

赤地利	chì dì lì	15g	Polygonum Chinensis
荔枝壳	lì zhī ké	15g	Litchi Chinensis Sonn
仙鹤草	xiān hè cǎo	15g	Herba Agrimoniae

【Indications】

Clear heat and dispel blood stasis, secure the penetrating vessel and contain blood. Indicated for DUB.

【Formula Analysis】

Chì dì lì (Polygonum Chinensis) both invigorates and detoxifies blood, and *zhì shǒu wū* (Radix Polygoni Multiflori Praeparata cum Succo Glycines Sotae) tonifies the Kidney and secures the penetrating vessel. *lì zhī ké* (Litchi Chinensis Sonn) rectifies qi and dispels blood stasis. *Jīn yīng zǐ* (Fructus Rosae Laevigatae) and *xiān hè cǎo* (Herba Agrimoniae) secure the penetrating vessel and astringe to stanch bleeding.

【Modifications】

➤ For blood-heat patterns, add *shēng dì huáng* (Radix Rehmanniae), *mài dōng* (Radix Ophiopogonis), *dì gǔ pí* (Cortex Lycii), *shā shēn* (Radix Adenophorae seu Glehniae) and *hēi shān zhī* (Carbonized Fructus Gardeniae).

➤ For blood stasis, add *dān shēn* (Radix Salviae Miltiorrhizae) and *tǔ niú xī* (Radix et Rhizome Achyranthes).

➤ For Spleen deficiency, add *dǎng shēn* (Radix Codonopsis), *huáng qí* (Radix Astragali) and *bái zhú* (Rhizoma Atractylodis Macrocephalae).

➤ For Kidney yang deficiency, add *xiān máo* (Rhizoma Curculiginis), *yín yáng huò* (Herba Epimedii) and *pào jiāng* (Rhizoma Zingiberis Praeparata).

➤ For Kidney yin deficiency, add *nǚ zhēn zǐ* (Fructus Ligustri Lucidi), *hàn lián cǎo* (Herba Ecliptae) and *zhì huáng jīng* (Rhizoma Polygonati Praeparata).

(Wu Xi. *A Review of Wu Xi's Gynecology · Volume One* 吴熙妇科溯洄第

一集 . Xiamen: Xiamen University Publishing House, 1994. 312-313)

Selected Case Studies

1. MEDICAL RECORDS OF QIAN BO-XUAN: FLOODING AND SPOTTING DUE TO DEFICIENCY OF THE SPLEEN AND KIDNEY

【Initial Visit】

Ms. Ren, age 19. First visit June 28th 1962.

Chief complaint: irregular menstruation cycles with profuse bleeding for more than 5 years.

Menstruation had been irregular since the onset of menarche at age 14. Patient suffered profuse menses for 7-10 days accompanied by severe distention and pain of the lower abdomen. After exercising heavily during a menstrual period at age 16, an episode of profuse bleeding occurred that lasted for over 50 days. Bleeding ceased after dilatation and curettage, and normal cycles were artificially induced. 3 episodes of severe bleeding had occurred in the previous 3 years, with over 50 days of continuous bleeding. Chinese herbal decoctions, *Yún Nán Bái Yào* (云南白药), *sān qī fěn* (Radix Notoginseng Powder), and injected medications to stanch bleeding had no effect.

She presented symptoms and signs of dizziness, palpitation, a white complexion, vexation, spontaneous sweating, poor appetite, thirst, lumbar pain and lassitude. The tongue appeared pale with a light yellow greasy coating with small prickles in the center. Her pulse was both thready and rapid.

【Pattern Differentiation】

Qi and blood deficiency of the Spleen and Kidney, insecurity of the penetrating and conception vessels.

【Treatment Principle】

Nourish qi and yin, secure the penetrating and conception vessels.

【Prescription】

Modified *Bǔ Zhōng Yì Qì Tāng* (补中益气汤加减)

炙黄芪	zhì huāng qí	15g	Radix Astragali Praeparata cum Melle
人参	rén shēn	6g	Radix et Rhizoma Ginseng
白术	bái zhú	9g	Rhizoma Atractylodis Macrocephalae
甘草	gān cǎo	6g	Radix et Rhizoma Glycyrrhizae
升麻	shēng má	3g	Rhizoma Cimicifugae
生地黄	shēng dì huáng	12g	Radix Rehmanniae
白芍	bái sháo	9g	Radix Paeoniae Alba
阿胶	ē jiāo	2g	Colla Corii Asini
赤石脂	chì shí zhī	15g	Halloysitum Rubrum
禹余粮	yǔ yú liáng	15g	Limonitum
生牡蛎	shēng mǔ lì	15g	Concha Ostreae Cruda
河车粉（冲服）	hé chē fěn	3g	Placenta Hominis Powder (infused)

【Second Visit】

On July 7th, bleeding ceased after 3 doses. Following 5 more doses, the patient complained of dizziness, palpitation, thirst and a dry mouth. Her shortness of breath had improved. Her tongue was pale, with a greasy coating and red prickles. Her pulse was thin, slippery and rapid. The *chi* pulse was weak.

The modified prescription contained the following.

黄芪	huáng qí	15g	Radix Astragali
炙甘草	zhì gān cǎo	9g	Radix et Rhizoma Glycyrrhizae Praeparata cum Melle
升麻	shēng má	3g	Rhizoma Cimicifugae
大生地	dà shēng dì	12g	Radix Rehmanniae
白芍	bái sháo	9g	Radix Paeoniae Alba
阿胶	ē jiāo	12g	Colla Corii Asini
生牡蛎	shēng mǔ lì	15g	Concha Ostreae Cruda
赤石脂	chì shí zhī	15g	Halloysitum Rubrum

禹余粮	yǔ yú liáng	15g	Limonitum
川石斛	chuān shí hú	12g	Herba Dendrobii
紫河车粉 （冲服）	zǐ hé chē fěn	3g	Placenta Hominis Powder (infused)

【Third Visit】

On July 28th, dizziness and blurry vision had improved, with headaches less frequent. Tongue appeared pale with a central crack and a thin white coating on the root. The left pulse was thready and slightly slippery, the *chi* position deep and thready. The right pulse was wiry, thready, and slightly rapid. These symptoms were caused by qi and yin deficiency, and severe impairment of the Spleen and Kidney.

The modified prescription was to tonify qi and yin, consolidate the Spleen and Kidney, and secure the penetrating and conception vessels.

党参	dǎng shēn	9g	Radix Codonopsis
白术	bái zhú	9g	Rhizoma Atractylodis Macrocephalae
炙甘草	zhì gān cǎo	3g	Radix et Rhizoma Glycyrrhizae Praeparata cum Melle
山药	shān yào	9g	Rhizoma Dioscoreae
熟地黄	shú dì huáng	9g	Radix Rehmanniae Praeparata
萸肉	yú ròu	6g	Fructus Corni
阿胶	ē jiāo	9g	Colla Corii Asini
艾叶	ài yè	4.5g	Folium Artemisiae Argyi
生杜仲	shēng dù zhòng	9g	Cortex Eucommiae (raw)
川断	chuān xù duàn	12g	Radix Dipsaci
女贞子	nǚ zhēn zǐ	9g	Fructus Ligustri Lucidi
禹余粮	yǔ yú liáng	15g	Limonitum
河车粉	hé chē fěn	90g (take 3g twice daily)	Placenta Hominis Powder

【Fourth Visit】

On September 14th, menses were profuse, thin, and bright red with small clots. She also complained of coldness and pain in the lower abdomen and lumbus, with a dry mouth. The tongue appeared pale with center crack, and with a thin white greasy coating. The pulse was both thready and rapid. These symptoms were caused by severe impairment of qi and yin, and dysfuction of the penetrating and conception vessels.

The modified prescription was to tonify qi and yin, and secure the penetrating and conception vessels.

人参	rén shēn	6g	Radix et Rhizoma Ginseng
白术	bái zhú	6g	Rhizoma Atractylodis Macrocephalae
炙甘草	zhì gān cǎo	3g	Radix et Rhizoma Glycyrrhizae Praeparata cum Melle
熟地	shú dì huáng	12g	Radix Rehmanniae Praeparata
白芍	bái sháo	9g	Radix Paeoniae Alba
阿胶	ē jiāo	9g	Colla Crii Asini
艾叶	ài yè	4.5g	Folium Artemisiae Argyi
龟板胶	guī bǎn jiāo	12g	Testudinis Plastri Colla
赤石脂	chì shí zhī	15g	Halloysitum Rubrum
禹余粮	yǔ yú liáng	15g	Limonitum
生龙骨	shēng lóng gǔ	15g	Fossilia Ossis Mastodi Cruda
生牡蛎	shēng mǔ lì	15g	Concha Ostreae Cruda
乌贼骨	wū zéi gǔ	15g	Endoconcha Sepiae
河车粉 （冲服）	hé chē fěn	3g	Placenta Hominis Powder (infused)
仙鹤草	xiān hè cǎo	9g	Agrimoniae Herba

【Fifth Visit】

On September 20th, bleeding ceased with this decoction. This cycle lasted 9 days in total. The patient was in good spirits, and complained only of slight dizziness and a dry mouth. Her tongue appeared with a thin, greasy yellow coating. The pulse was thready and rapid. Longstanding bleeding had further depleted qi and blood. Treatment was to tonify qi and blood, and secure the secure the penetrating and conception vessels.

Prescribed *Rén Shēn Guī Pí Wán* (人参归脾丸) 10 pills, one pill nightly. *Hé chē fěn* (Placenta Hominis Powder) 30g, 1.5g twice daily.

【**Sixth Visit**】

On September 29th, patient reported an improved mood with no other complaints. The tongue appeared with a central crack and a yellow greasy coating on the root. The pulse was thready and slightly rapid.

The modified prescription was to tonify the Liver and Kidney, and consolidate the penetrating and conception vessels.

地黄	dì huáng	12g	Radix Rehmanniae
白芍	bái sháo	9g	Radix Paeoniae Alba
女贞子	nǚ zhēn zǐ	9g	Fructus Ligustri Lucidi
沙苑子	shā yuàn zǐ	9g	Semen Astragali Complanati
桑寄生	sāng jì shēng	12g	Herba Taxilli
龟板胶	guī bǎn jiāo	6g	Colla Plastri Testudinis
生龙骨	shēng lóng gǔ	15g	Fossilia Ossis Mastodi Cruda
生牡蛎	shēng mǔ lì	15g	Concha Ostreae Cruda
砂仁	shā rén	1.8g	Fructus Amomi
橘皮	jú pí	3g	Pericarpium Citri Reticulatae
夜交藤	yè jiāo téng	12g	Caulis Polygoni Multiflori

Hé chē fěn (Placenta Hominis Powder) 30g, 1.5g once daily and once nightly.

【**Seventh Visit**】

On October 13th, profuse watery leucorrhea for 3 days, with frequent urination and lumbar pain. The tongue appeared with a central crack and a thin yellow coating, and the pulse was both wiry and thready. These symptoms were caused by qi and yin deficiency and dysfunction of the penetrating and conception vessels.

The modified prescription contained the following.

地黄	dì huáng	12g	Radix Rehmanniae

白芍	bái sháo	9g	Radix Paeoniae Alba
女贞子	nǚ zhēn zǐ	9g	Fructus Ligustri Lucidi
金樱子	jīn yīng zǐ	9g	Fructus Rosae Laevigatae
桑螵蛸	sāng piāo xiāo	12g	Oötheca Mantidis
川断	chuān xù duàn	12g	Radix Dipsaci
生牡蛎	shēng mǔ lì	15g	Concha Ostreae Cruda
制香附	zhì xiāng fù	6g	Rhizoma Cyperi Praeparata
阿胶珠	ē jiāo zhū	6g	Colla Corii Asini Pilula
橘皮	jú pí	3g	Pericarpium Citri Reticulatae

Hé chē fěn (Placenta Hominis Powder) 30g, 1.5g daily and nightly.

【Eighth Visit】

A moderate flow of bright red menses was reported on October 20th. On October 23rd, she complained of frequent urination, but with no lumbar pain present. The tongue appeared with a thin yellow coating and a central crack. The pulse was both thready and wiry.

The modified prescription contained the following.

地黄	dì huáng	12g	Radix Rehmanniae
白芍	bái sháo	9g	Radix Paeoniae Alba
女贞子	nǚ zhēn zǐ	9g	Fructus Ligustri Lucidi
金樱子	jīn yīng zǐ	9g	Fructus Rosae Laevigatae
桑螵蛸	sāng piāo xiāo	12g	Oötheca Mantidis
川断	chuān xù duàn	12g	Radix Dipsaci
生牡蛎	shēng mǔ lì	15g	Concha Ostreae Cruda
阿胶珠	ē jiāo zhū	9g	Colla Corii Asini Pilula
橘皮	jú pí	30g	Pericarpium Citri Reticulatae
赤石脂	chì shí zhī	15g	Halloysitum Rubrum
禹余粮	yǔ yú liáng	15g	Limonitum

【Ninth Visit】

On October 26th, patient reported a normal 5 days menstrual cycle. However she suffered influenza with headache and a sore, dry throat. The tongue appeared with a central crack and a thin yellow coating. The pulse was both thready and rapid.

This relatively acute condition indicated treating the branch by prescribing *Yín Qiào Jiě Dú Wán* (银翘解毒丸), to dispel wind-heat. One pill each morning and afternoon.

Comments:

This case manifested as flooding and spotting that persisted for over 5 years. Because of a congenital deficiency of Kidney qi, the penetrating and conception vessels were unable to function with regularity. So abnormal bleeding appeared that alternated between flooding and spotting. As a result, a severe qi and yin deficiency had developed. The treatment principle in this case is to first strongly tonify the original qi in order to contain blood. Then follow by strengthening the Spleen and Kidney while securing the penetrating and conception vessels. Finally, tonify the Liver and Kidney while continuing to secure the penetrating and conception vessels. This patient gradually recovered after 4 months of treatment.

(Chinese Medicine Research Institute Xi Yuan Hospital. *Qian Bo-xuan's Medical Record of Gynecology* 钱伯煊妇科医案 . Beijing: People's Medical Publishing House, 1980. 14-16)

2. Medical Records of Zhu Xiao-nan: Flooding and Spotting Associated with Yin Deficiency and Hyperactive Fire in Patients of Childbearing Age

【Initial Visit】

Ms. Hu, age 34, married.

Chief complaint: Painful and irregular menstruation with spotting for more than 20 days.

Reported menarche with menstrual pain at age 17. After marriage, her cycles became both prolonged and slightly advanced, presenting patterns of both flooding and spotting. Spotting and abnormal bleeding would typically begin 2 weeks before the normal menstruation date, and were often accompanied by a yellow discharge.

At first visit, the patient reported spotting for over 20 days with associated complaints of dizziness and palpitation, pain and soreness of the lumbus and limbs, and a dry mouth. Also suffered a long history of aversion to cold, with tidal fever in the late afternoon. Cheeks appeared red, eyes swollen, with a yellow and greasy tongue coating. The pulse was hollow and rapid. No improvement was seen after previous dilatation and curettage, so a hysterectomy was recommended. The patient had refused surgery and sought Chinese medicinal treatment instead.

【Pattern Differentiation】

Hyperactive fire due to yin deficiency.

【Treatment Principle】

Invigorate water to restrain fire.

【Prescription】

潞党参	lù dǎng shēn	9g	Radix Codonopsis
归身	guī shēn	6g	Radix Angelicae Sinensis
生地	shēng dì huáng	9g	Radix Rehmanniae
白芍	bái sháo	9g	Radix Paeoniae Alba
山萸肉	shān yú ròu	9g	Fructus Corni
女贞子	nǚ zhēn zǐ	9g	Fructus Ligustri Lucidi
焦白术	jiāo bái zhú	6g	Rhizoma Atractylodis Macrocephalae (scorch-fried)
青蒿	qīng hāo	6g	Herba Artemisiae Annuae
盐水炒黄柏	yán shuǐ chǎo huáng bǎi	9g	Cortex Phellodendri Chinensis (fried with saline)
蒲黄炭	pú huáng tàn	9g	Pollen Typhae (carbonized)
熟军炭	shú jūn tàn	3g	Radix et Rhizoma Rhei (carbonized)
陈皮	chén pí	6g	Pericarpium Citri Reticulatae

Spotting ceased after 4 doses, however the yellow leucorrhea persisted. This complaint was eventually improved by invigorating the

Spleen to constrain discharge. Menstrual cycles were stabilized after one year of treatment. At a 3 year follow-up, no recurring symptoms were reported.

Comments:

This patient complained of flooding and spotting that lasted for more than 10 years. Due to yin and blood deficiency, abnormal bleeding occurred along with associated symptoms such as dizziness and palpitation. In cases such as this, significant heat signs may appear such as a dry mouth, a red complexion, tidal fever, a hollow and rapid pulse, and a yellow greasy tongue coating.

Dǎng shēn (Radix Codonopsis), *bái zhú* (Rhizoma Atractylodis Macrocephalae) and *chén pí* (Pericarpium Citri Reticulatae) were prescribed to tonify qi and invigorate the Spleen. *Dāng guī* (Radix Angelicae Sinensis) and *shēng dì huáng* (Radix Rehmanniae) tonify blood. *Bái sháo* (Radix Paeoniae Alba), *shān yú ròu* (Fructus Corni) and *nǚ zhēn zǐ* (Fructus Ligustri Lucidi) nourish Kidney yin. *Qīng hāo* (Herba Artemisiae Annuae) and *huáng bǎi* (Cortex Phellodendri Chinensis) are indicated to clear excessive heat. *Pú huáng* (Pollen Typhae) and *shú jūn tàn* (Carbonized Radix et Rhizoma Rhei) were perscribed to clear heat and dispel blood stasis. The symptoms of flooding were resolved mainly through applying both purging and tonification methods. After the successful treatment of the internal evils, tonifying foods and herbs were recommended to regulate blood and secure the Kidney.

(Zhu Nan-sun, Zhu Rong-da. *Selected Experiences in Gynecology of Zhu Nan-sun* 朱南孙妇科经验选 . Beijing: People's Medical Publishing House, 1981. 19-21)

3. MEDICAL RECORDS OF LIU FENG-WU: ANOVULAR DUB ASSOCIATED WITH QI DEFICIENCY AND BLOOD STASIS IN PATIENTS OF CHILDBEARING AGE

【Initial Visit】

Ms. Yang, age 28. First visit: August 23rd 1975.

Chief complaint: Abnormal uterine bleeding for over 50 days.

Her last menstrual cycle began June 2^{nd,} when decreased menses appeared for 7 days. Menstrual spotting appeared July 1st.

A previous diagnosis of proliferative endometrium was determined by diagnostic curettage. Spotting had persisted since the surgery for more than 50 days, and pregnancy had been ruled out. Menstrual blood appeared purple with some clotting present. The tongue appeared with a thin white coating, and the pulse was both thready and slow in quality.

【Pattern Differetiation】

Blood deficiency with stasis, disorder of penetrating and conception vessels.

【Treatment Principle】

Nourish and invigorate blood, dispel blood stasis and regulate menstruation.

【Prescription】

Modified *Shēng Huà Tāng* (生化汤加减)

当归	dāng guī	9g	Radix Angelicae Sinensis
川芎	chuān xiōng	4.5g	Rhizoma Chuanxiong
桃仁	táo rén	3g	Semen Persicae
红花	hóng huā	3g	Flos Carthami
益母草	yì mǔ cǎo	6g	Herba Leonuri
泽兰	zé lán	6g	Herba Lycopi
丹参	dān shēn	6g	Radix Salviae Miltiorrhizae
赤芍	chì sháo	6g	Radix Paeoniae Rubra
没药	mò yào	4.5g	Myrrha
柴胡	chái hú	3g	Radix Bupleuri
炒荆芥穗	chǎo jīng jiè suì	6g	Spica Schizonepetae (dry-fried)
蒲黄炭	pú huáng tàn	6g	Pollen Typhae (carbonized)

Spotting ceased after 5 doses, and 3 more doses were taken to consolidate the effect. Follow up showed normal cycles for 3 months with no abnormal bleeding.

Comments:

Due to the presence of stasis, blood may not be contained in the vessels. In this formula, *dāng guī* (Radix Angelicae Sinensis), *chuān xiōng* (Rhizoma Chuanxiong), *yì mǔ cǎo* (Herba Leonuri), *mò yào* (Myrrha), *zé lán* (Herba Lycopi) and *táo rén* (Semen Persicae) nourish and invigorate blood. *Hóng huā* (Flos Carthami) dispels blood stasis, yet nourishes in small doses. *Chì sháo* (Radix Paeoniae Rubra) and *dān pí* (Cortex Moutan) cool and invigorate blood while dispelling blood stasis. *Pú huáng tàn* (Carbonized Pollen Typhae) invigorates blood, dispels stasis and arrests bleeding. *Chái hú* (Radix Bupleuri) and *jīng jiè suì* (Spica Schizonepetae) upbears yang, eliminates dampness, and resolves blood-heat. The main function of this formula is nourish and invigorate blood, resolve blood-heat, dispel stasis, and engender blood.

(Beijing Chinese Medical Hospital. *Gynecological Experiences of Liu Feng-wu* 刘奉五妇科经验 . Beijing: People's Medical Publishing House, 1982. 106)

4. MEDICAL RECORDS OF PU FU-ZHOU: FLOODING AND SPOTTING ASSOCIATED WITH QI DEFICIENCY AND BLOOD-HEAT IN PATIENTS OF CHILDBEARING AGE

【Initial Visit】

Ms. Dai, age 28. First visit: March 2nd, 1957.

Chief complaint: Profuse menstrual bleeding.

Menstruation was 7-9 days late, with profuse purplish-black menses and small clots. She also complained of a downbearing abdominal pain, dizziness, and cold sweats. Her tongue coating appeared yellow and greasy. The pulse was large and wiry in both *chi* positions, the *guan* and *cun* positions were deep and weak.

【Pattern Differentiation】

Qi deficiency with blood-heat.

【Treatment Principle】

Tonify Qi to stanch bleeding.

【Prescription】

Modified *Bā Zhēn Tāng* (八珍汤加减)

当归	dāng guī	4.5g	Radix Angelicae Sinensis
川芎	chuān xiōng	4.5g	Rhizoma Chuanxiong
白芍	bái sháo	9g	Radix Paeoniae Alba
熟地	shú dì huáng	9g	Radix Rehmanniae Praeparata
黄芪	huáng qí	15g	Radix Astragali
党参	dǎng shēn	9g	Radix Codonopsis
炒艾叶	chǎo ài yè	3g	Folium Artemisiae Argyi (dry-fried)
阿胶（烊化）	ē jiāo	9g	Colla Corii Asini (dissolved)
川断	chuān xù duàn	6g	Radix Dipsaci
白术	bái zhú	6g	Rhizoma Atractylodis Macrocephalae
地骨皮	dì gǔ pí	9g	Cortex Lycii

【Second Visit】

The excessive bleeding improved after 3 doses, with less red menses and no abdominal discomfort. She complained of poor appetite, distending headache, and profuse yellow leucorrhea with a foul smell. Both *cun* and *chi* pulse positions were deep. Right *guan* position was deep and slow, with the left *guan* deep and wiry.

Treatment was given to harmonize the Liver and Spleen.

党参	dǎng shēn	6g	Radix Codonopsis
白术	bái zhú	6g	Rhizoma Atractylodis Macrocephalae
茯苓	fú líng	9g	Poria
炙甘草	zhì gān cǎo	3g	Radix et Rhizoma Glycyrrhizae Praeparata cum Melle
当归	dāng guī	6g	Radix Angelicae Sinensis

白芍	bái sháo	9g	Radix Paeoniae Alba
制香附	zhì xiāng fù	6g	Rhizoma Cyperi Praeparata
砂仁（打）	dǎ shā rén	4.5g	Fructus Amomi (thrashed)
柴胡	chái hú	4.5g	Radix Bupleuri
吴萸	wú zhū yú	2.4g	Fructus Evodiae
生姜	shēng jiāng	3pieces	Rhizoma Zingiberis Recens
大枣	dà zǎo	3pieces	Fructus Jujubae

【Third Visit】

After 3 doses, thick foul-smelling discharge appeared. The patient complained of a frontal headache, lassitude, and profuse leucorrhea. However, her lumbar and abdominal discomfort had been relieved, with no bleeding present. The tongue coating appeared thinner, and the pulse was both slow and wiry. These signs indicated a Spleen and Stomach disharmony.

Treatment was given to invigorate the Spleen and harmonize the middle jiao.

党参	dǎng shēn	6g	Radix Codonopsis
白术	bái zhú	6g	Rhizoma Atractylodis Macrocephalae
茯苓	fú líng	9g	Poria
炙甘草	zhì gān cǎo	3g	Radix et Rhizoma Glycyrrhizae Praeparata cum Melle
陈皮	chén pí	6g	Pericarpium Citri Reticulatae
砂仁	shā rén	4.5g	Fructus Amomi
制香附	zhì xiāng fù	6g	Rhizoma Cyperi Praeparata
官桂（去粗皮）	guān guì	2.4g	Cortex Cinnamomi (peeled)
乌贼骨	wū zéi gǔ	15g	Endoconcha Sepiae
黄柏（酒炒）	huáng bǎi	2.4g	Cortex Phellodendri Chinensis (fried with wine)
怀山药	huái shān yào	9g	Rhiizoma Dioscoreae
炮生姜	pào shēng jiāng	3pieces	Rhizoma Zingiberis Praeparata

【**Fourth Visit**】

Profuse menses appeared for two days on the 29th of the previous month. Afterward, normal menstruation continued with some slight clotting. Her abdominal pain had been relieved. Patient complained of headache, poor appetite, and an uncomfortable downbearing sensation in the sacral area. Her tongue coating appeared yellow and greasy, and the pulse was wiry, slippery and forceful. This indicated patterns of blood-heat and dampness obstruction.

Treatment was given to harmonize blood and clear damp-heat.

当归	dāng guī	4.5g	Radix Angelicae Sinensis
白芍	bái sháo	6g	Radix Paeoniae Alba
川芎	chuān xiōng	4.5g	Rhizoma Chuanxiong
茯苓皮	fú líng pí	9g	Poria Cocos
黄芩	huáng qín	4.5g	Radix Scutellariae
苏梗	sū gěng	6g	Caulis Perillae
木香	mù xiāng	6g	Radix Aucklandiae
艾叶	ài yè	3g	Folium Artemisiae Argyi
川断	chuān xù duàn	6g	Radix Dipsaci
乌贼骨	wū zéi gǔ	12g	Endoconcha Sepiae

3 doses decocted.

Comments:

Due to the presence of both qi deficiency and deficient heat, blood may not be contained in the vessels. In this case, the appearance of profuse menses is directly associated with flooding disorder. When the presenting symptoms are acute, it is important that we treat them first. After they have been resolved, we may then approach the root causes of the condition.

Shèng Yù Tāng (圣愈汤) combined with *Jiāo Ài Sì Wù Tāng* (胶艾四物汤) may be prescribed to invigorate the Spleen and tonify qi, nourish blood and stanch bleeding. *Dì gǔ pí* (Cortex Lycii) clears deficient heat from the blood aspect, and *chuān xù duàn* (Radix Dipsaci) regulates and tonifies the penetrating and conception vessels. *Xiāo Yáo Sǎn* (逍 遥 散) with modified *Sì Jūn Zǐ Tāng* (四君子汤) may be used to address the root cause by both invigorating the Spleen and harmonizing the Liver.

5. MEDICAL RECORDS OF PU FU-ZHOU: SPOTTING ASSOCIATED WITH SPLEEN AND STOMACH PATTERNS IN PATIENTS OF CHILDBEARING AGE

【Initial Visit】

Ms. Guo, age 36. First visit July 5th, 1956.

Chief complaint: intermenstrual bleeding.

Patient complained of spotting accompanied by lumbar pain, mental depression, a dry mouth, frequent diarrhea, headache, and poor digestion. Her complexion appeared yellowish, with a yellow and greasy tongue coating in the center. Both *chi* pulse positions were deep and weak, and both *guan* pulse positions were surging and wiry.

【Pattern Differentiation】

Disorder of qi and blood, Spleen and Stomach disharmony.

【Treatment Principle】

Regulate the Spleen and Stomach, harmonize qi and blood.

【Prescription】

Modified *Bā Zhēn Tāng* (八珍汤加味)

红参	hóng shēn	9g	Radix Ginseng Rubra
炒白术	chǎo bái zhú	9g	Rhizoma Atractylodis Macrocephalae (dry-fried)
茯苓	fú líng	9g	Poria
炙甘草	zhì gān cǎo	6g	Radix et Rhizoma Glycyrrhizae Praeparata cum Melle
当归	dāng guī	6g	Radix Angelicae Sinensis
川芎	chuān xiōng	9g	Rhizoma Chuanxiong
白芍	bái sháo	6g	Radix Paeoniae Alba
生地	shēng dì huáng	9g	Radix Rehmanniae
川断	chuān xù duàn	6g	Radix Dipsaci

茜草	qiàn cǎo	6g	Radix Rubiae
香附	xiāng fú	6g	Rhizoma Cyperi
乌贼骨	wū zéi gǔ	15g	Endoconcha Sepiae
益母草	yì mǔ cǎo	9g	Herba Leonuri

3 doses. Decoct until 200ml of liquid remains. Repeat. Take twice daily.

【Second Visit】

She reported improved sleep after one dose, with good spirits the next day. Although the spotting had ceased and her appetite has improved, she still experienced depression and vexation. Her tongue and pulse were unchanged.

Treatment was given to harmonize the Stomach and nourish the Heart.

【Prescription】

红参	hóng shēn	9g	Radix Ginseng Rubra
炒枣仁	chǎo zǎo rén	15g	Semen Ziziphi Spinosae (dry-fried)
茯神	fú shén	9g	Poriae Sclerotium Pararadicis
远志（炙）	yuǎn zhì	6g	Radix Polygalae (fried with liquid)
柏子仁	bǎi zǐ rén	12g	Semen Platycladi
小麦（炒）	xiǎo mài	15g	Triticum Aestivum (dry-fried)
法半夏	fǎ bàn xià	6g	Rhizoma Pinelliae Praeparatum
知母（炒）	zhī mǔ	9g	Rhizoma Anemarrhenae (dry-fried)
宣木瓜	xuān mù guā	6g	Fructus Chaenomelis
建曲	jiàn qū	9g	Massa Medicata Fermentata
荷叶	hé yè	9g	Folium Nelumbinis
炙甘草	zhì gān cǎo	6g	Radix et Rhizoma Glycyrrhizae Praeparata cum Melle
桂园肉	guì yuán ròu	15g	Arillus Longan

3 doses. Decoct until 200ml of liquid remains. Repeat. Take twice daily.

【Third Visit】

No appearance of spotting. Sleeping had improved but with occasional nightmares. Her nighttime urination had been reduced, her appetite improved, and stools appeared well-formed. The tongue coating was now thinner, and the pulse was wiry and slightly rapid.

Treatment was given to nourish the Heart and calm the spirit.

Bǎi Zǐ Yǎng Xīn Wán (柏子养心丸) 200g was prescribed, taken on an empty stomach twice daily.

Comments:

This patient presented symptoms of poor digestive function such as loose stools and a yellowish complexion. Long-term bleeding often leads to both Spleen qi and nutrient-blood deficiencies. Modified *Bā Zhēn Tāng* (八珍汤加味) was then perscribed. *Yì mǔ cǎo* (Herba Leonuri) and *wū zéi gǔ* (Endoconcha Sepiae) arrest bleeding, dispel stasis, and tonify by freeing the vessels. Cooling blood is not indicated in this case, since this particular flooding and spotting pattern is not associated with blood-heat.

6. Medical Records of Pu Fu-zhou: Menopausal Flooding and Spotting Due to Insecurity of the Penetrating and Conception Vessels

【Initial Visit】

Patient: Ms.Du, age 47, first visit on May 25th, 1967.

Chief complaint: Abnormal vaginal bleeding for 43 days.

Profuse red-colored menses with some clotting present. Patient had a history of chronic nephritis and angiocardiopathy, with no tumors present. Urination and stools were normal, and slight edema of the limbs was observed. The tongue appeared pale, with a thin white and greasy coating. The pulse was deep, weak, thready, and rough.

【Pattern Differentiation】

Kidney deficiency with insecurity of the penetrating and conception vessels.

【Treatment Principle】

Regulate the penetrating and conception vessels, tonify qi and stanch bleeding.

【Prescription】

党参	dǎng shēn	30g	Radix Codonopsis
熟地	shú dì huáng	30g	Radix Rehmanniae Praeparata
生杜仲	shēng dù zhòng	9g	Cortex Eucommiae (raw)
川断	chuān xù duàn	9g	Radix Dipsaci
炮姜炭	pào jiāng tàn	3g	Rhizoma Zingiberis Praeparata (carbonized)
鹿角霜	lù jiǎo shuāng	21g	Cornu Cervi Degelatinatum

3 doses, decocted twice. Take half with *Shí Huī Sǎn* (十 灰 散) 1.5g. Add a few drops of vinegar, and take twice daily.

【Second Visit】

Spotting was infrequent and menses were light in color. Urination, stools, and appetite were normal, but sleep quality was poor. The tongue appeared pale with a slightly greasy coating, and the pulse was both deep and slow. Her condition was relatively stable, so treatments were continued to secure the penetrating and conception vessels.

Removed *pào jiāng* (Rhizoma Zingiberis Praeparata), and prescribed 3 doses.

Comments:

At the age of 47, this patient naturally showed some deficiency of the penetrating and conception vessels. She also exhibited a congenitally weak constitution with a history of chronic nephritis. Therefore, *Dǎng shēn* (Radix Codonopsis) and *shú dì huáng* (Radix Rehmanniae Praeparata) were given in relatively large dosages to both tonify qi and secure the Kidney.

(Chinese Medicine Research Institution. *Pu Fu-zhou's Medical Experience* 蒲辅周医疗经验 . Beijing: People's Medical Publishing House, 1976, 199-202)

7. Medical Records of Shi Jin-mo: Adolescent Flooding and Spotting Associated with Spleen Deficiency and Liver Constraint

【Initial Visit】

Patient: Ms. Zang, female, age 20.

Chief complaint: Spotting for 2 months.

Menarche was at age 16, with a history of regular menstrual cycles. Over the past 6 months her cycles had become gradually prolonged, with spotting for the previous 2 months. Patient complained of dizziness, palpitation, shortness of breath, poor appetite, lassitude, lumbar pain, and oppression and distention of the chest. Urination, stool, and sleep were normal. Her tongue appeared normal with a thin white coating. The pulse was deep, thready and forceful.

【Pattern Differentiation】

Spleen deficiency with Liver constraint.

【Treatment Principle】

Tonify qi to contain blood, strengthen the Spleen to reinforce the middle jiao, regulate Liver qi.

【Prescription】

黑升麻	hēi shēng má	3g	Rhizoma Cimicifugae (carbonized)
生牡蛎（布包）	shēng mǔ lì	10g	Concha Ostreae Cruda (wrapped)
生龙齿（布包）	shēng lóng chǐ	10g	Dens Draconis (raw) (wrapped)
五倍子（捣碎）	wǔ bèi zǐ	3g	Galla Chinensis (pounded)
五味子（捣碎）	wǔ wèi zǐ	3g	Fructus Schisandrae (pounded)
黑芥穗	hēi jiè suì	6g	Spica Schizonepetae Carbonisata
白蒺藜	bái jí lí	10g	Fructus Tribuli

沙蒺藜	shā jí lí	10g	Semen Astragali Complanati
生地 （砂仁 3g 同捣）	shēng dì huáng	6g	Radix Rehmanniae (pounded with Fructus Amomi 3g and Radix Rehmanniae Praeparata 6g)
杭白芍 （柴胡 5g 同炒）	háng bái sháo	10g	Radix Paeoniae Alba (dry-fried with Radix Bupleuri 5g)
鹿角胶 （另溶兑服）	lù jiǎo jiāo	6g	Colla Cornus Cervi (dissolved, infused)
阿胶珠	ē jiāo zhū	10g	Colla Corii Asini Pilula
山萸炭	shān yú tàn	15g	Fructus Corni (carbonized)
茅根炭	máo gēn tàn	15g	Imperatae Rhizoma (carbonized)
米党参	mǐ dǎng shēn	6g	Radix Codonopsis (fried with rice)
厚朴花	hòu pò huā	6g	Flos Magnoliae Officinalis
玫瑰花	méi guī huā	6g	Flos Rosae Rugosae
柏叶炭	bǎi yè tàn	10g	Cacumen Platycladi (carbonized)
莲房炭	lián fáng tàn	10g	Receptaculum Nelumbinis (carbonized)
炒建曲	chǎo jiàn qū	10g	Massa Medicata Fermentata (dry-fried)

【Second Visit】

Her bleeding markedly decreased after 2 doses, with some persistent spotting. Palpitation, shortness of breath, dizziness, poor appetite, oppression and distention of the chest remained. Her pulses were unchanged. Modifications to the formula were as follows.

黑升麻	hēi shēng má	3g	Rhizoma Cimicifugae (carbonized)
川杜仲	chuān dù zhòng	10g	Cortex Eucommiae
黑芥穗	hēi jiè suì	6g	Spica Schizonepetae Carbonisata
川续断	chuān xù duàn	10g	Radix Dipsaci
生牡蛎（生 龙齿 10g 同打 同布包）	shēng mǔ lì	10g	Concha Ostreae Cruda (thrashed and wrapped with Dens Dragonis 10g)

阿胶珠	ē jiāo zhū	10g	Colla Corii Asini Pilula
生地（砂仁 5g 同炒）	shēng dì huáng	6g	Radix Rehmanniae (dry-fried with Fructus Amomi 5g and Radix Rehmanniae Praeparata 6g)
杭白芍（醋 柴胡 5g 同炒）	háng bái sháo	10g	Radix Paeoniae Alba (dry-fried with Radix Bupleui, prepared with vinegar 5g)
山萸炭	shān yú tàn	15g	Fructus Corni (carbonized)
厚朴花	hòu pò huā	6g	Flos Magnoliae Officinalis
莱菔子	lái fú zǐ	6g	Semen Raphani
仙鹤草（炒）	xiān hè cǎo	12g	Herba Agrimoniae (dry-fried)
玫瑰花（炒）	méi guī huā	6g	Flos Rosae Rugosae (dry-fried)
莱菔英	lái fú yīng	6g	Raphanus Sativus
麦芽	mài yá	10g	Fructus Hordei Germinatus
茅根炭	máo gēn tàn	15g	Imperatae Rhizoma (carbonized)
谷芽	gǔ yá	10g	Fructus Setariae Germinatus
酒黄连	jiǔ huáng lián	3g	Rhizoma Coptidis (fried with wine)
沙蒺藜	shā jí lí	10g	Semen Astragali Complanati
炒远志	chǎo yuǎn zhì	6g	Radix Polygalae (dry-fried)
酒黄芩	jiǔ huáng qín	6g	Radix Scutellariae (fried with wine)
白蒺藜	bái jí lí	10g	Fructus Tribuli

3 doses.

The abnormal bleeding had ceased completely. Her appetite had improved, and abdominal distention had been relieved. Patient continued to complain of dizziness, palpitation, shortness of breath, and vexing heat in the afternoon. The pulse had also become stronger. Continued tonification of qi and blood was indicated.

Rén Shēn Guī Pí Wán (人参归脾丸) was prescribed, 1 pill each morning and at noon. Also *Yù Yè Jīn Dān* (玉液金丹), 1 pill in the evening for 30 days.

Comments:

For patients with prolonged menstruation and spotting, the general treatment principles are to tonify qi, strengthen the Spleen and Kidney, and secure the penetrating and conception vessels. In this case, Liver blood deficiency led to constraint of Liver qi. Medicinals such as *chái hú* (Radix Bupleuri), *hòu pò huā* (Flos Magnoliae Officinalis), *méi guī huā* (Flos Rosae Rugosae), *lái fú zǐ* (Semen Raphani) and *lái fú yīng* (Raphanus Sativus) were selected to promote the free flow of Liver qi. The proper formula can disperse while securing, and tonify without causing stagnation.

On the second visit, *huáng qín* (Radix Scutellariae) and *huáng lián* (Rhizoma Coptidis) were added in order to prevent stagnation from transforming into Liver fire, and to avoid further menstrual irregularities. *Huáng qín* (Radix Scutellariae) and *huáng lián* (Rhizoma Coptidis) were mixed with wine to reduce their cold and bitter natures. *Chái hú* (Radix Bupleuri) courses the Liver while lifting and upbearing. *Shēng má* (Rhizoma Cimicifugae) and *jiè suì* (Spica Schizonepetae) were carbonized to more strongly stanch bleeding.

(Zhu Shen-yu. *Collected Clinical Experiences of Shi Jin-mo* 施今墨临床经验集 . Beijing: People's Medical Publishing House, 1982. 180-184)

8. MEDICAL RECORDS OF WU XI: ADOLESCENT FLOODING AND SPOTTING WITH SPLEEN AND KIDNEY DEFICIENCY PATTERNS

【Initial Visit】

Patient: Ms. Li, age 15. First visit on December 31st, 1994.

Chief complaint: Profuse menses for more than 1 year, abnormal bleeding for 28 days.

Patient reported incessant bleeding for 28 days, with profuse menses for more than 1 year. Menarche occurred at age 13, with typical 7-8 day periods on a 30-35 day cycle. Her last period had begun on December 3rd. Ultrasound exam revealed median uterus, slightly small. She complained of dizziness, lassitude, and poor appetite. Her tongue appeared pale, with a thin white coating. The pulse was both thready and weak.

【Pattern Differentiation】

Spleen and Kidney insufficiency.

【Treatment Principle】

Tonify the Spleen and Kidney, secure the penetrating vessel.

【Prescription】

鹿衔草	lù xián cǎo	30g	Herba Pyrolae
生地黄	shēng dì huáng	15g	Radix Rehmanniae
阿胶	ē jiāo	15g	Colla Crii Asini
棕榈炭	zōng lǚ tàn	15g	Petiolus Trachycarpus (carbonized)
炮姜炭	pào jiāng tàn	10g	Rhizoma Zingiberis Praeparata (carbonized)
黄芩炭	huáng qín tàn	8g	Radix Scutellariae (carbonized)
煅乌贼骨	duàn wū zéi gǔ	20g	Endoconcha Sepiae (calcined)
黄芪	huáng qí	15g	Radix Astragali
白术	bái zhú	10g	Rhizoma Atractylodis Macrocephalae

【Second Visit】

On January 2nd, 1995, abnormal bleeding patterns had ceased completely. Her appetite, energy levels and the pulse had also improved. *Huáng qí* (Radix Astragal) and *bái zhú* (Rhizoma Atractylodis Macrocephalae) were removed, and two more doses were prescribed. At a three month follow up exam, no recurrence was reported.

Comments:

In the treatment of adolescent DUB, the main priority is to stanch bleeding effectively. According to the principles of "Se Liu, Cheng Yuan, and Fu Jiu", the correct prescription focuses on both dispelling stasis and arresting bleeding, with an emphasis on the treatment of the blood stasis pattern. In this formula, *lù xián cǎo* (Pyrolae Herba) is used in great dosage to calm the spirit, secure the penetrating vessel, and conduct blood back to the vessels. *Shēng dì huáng* (Radix Rehmanniae) and *ē jiāo* (Colla Crii Asini) tonify the Kidney, nourish yin-blood and arrest bleeding. In this case, these three medicinals were used to apply the

"Cheng Yuan" (Treat the root) method.

The combination of *zōng lǚ tàn* (Carbonized Petiolus Trachycarpi), *pào jiāng tàn* (Carbonized Rhizoma Zingiberis Praeparata), *huáng qín tàn* (Carbonized Radix Scutellariae) and *duàn wū zéi gǔ* (Calcined Endoconcha Sepiae) were used to apply the "Se Liu" (stanch bleeding) method.

(Wu Xi. *A Review of Wu Xi's Gynecology · Volume Three* 吴熙妇科溯洄第三集 . Xiamen: Xiamen University Publishing House, 1997. 117-118)

Discussions

1. Luo Yuan-kai's Perspectives on the Treatment of Flooding and Spotting

Kidney yin deficiency and Spleen qi deficiency are the root causes of flooding and spotting disorder. In addition, blood-heat and blood stasis may also be involved in many cases. The main symptoms of flooding and spotting involve profuse or chronic bleeding occurring outside of the normal menstrual cycle. However, longstanding blood loss leads to blood deficiency, qi deficiency, and in severe cases, even shock or collapse. In treatment, patterns of blood-heat or blood stasis must be also addressed concurrently. However, for severe flooding and spotting, the priority is to stanch bleeding. This symptomatic approach is referred to as Se Liu (stanch bleeding). In all cases, we should eventually combine this with the Cheng Yuan method (treat the root).

Most cases of flooding and spotting are associated with deficiency patterns, so tonification may be the primary principle of treatment. However, in some cases it is appropriate to first address the excess symptoms, and then follow with tonification. Draining and tonifying methods may also be used simultaneously.

With the presence of internal heat, we may select a formula that includes medicinals that clear heat and nourish yin. In general, cold and bitter medicinals that clear heat are not commonly indicated.

With blood stasis patterns, medicinals that dispel stasis and generate new blood may be combined with medicinals that nourish and invigorate blood.

The main pathomechanism of flooding patterns is an insecurity of the penetrating and conception vessels with qi being unable to contain blood in the vessels, whether or not heat or blood stasis is present. So tonifying qi to contain blood is emphasized in most flooding patterns, where the heat and stasis patterns are addressed later in treatment.

In the empirical formula *Zī Yīn Gù Qì Tāng* (滋阴固气汤), *tù sī zǐ* (Semen Cuscutae) and *shān yú ròu* (Fructus Corni) are selected to nourish the Liver and Kidney. *Dǎng shēn* (Radix Codonopsis), *huáng qí* (Radix Astragali), *bái zhú* (Rhizoma Atractylodis Macrocephalae) and *zhì gān cǎo* (Radix et Rhizoma Glycyrrhizae Praeparata cum Melle) strengthen the Spleen and tonify qi. *Ē jiāo* (Colla Corii Asini) and *lù jiǎo shuāng* (Cornu Cervi Degelatinatum) astringe to stop bleeding. *Hé shǒu wū* (Radix Polygoni Multiflori) with *bái sháo* (Radix Paeoniae Alba) are prescribed to nourish blood and emolliate the Liver. *Xù duàn* (Radix Dipsaci) is selected to secure the Kidney. This formula treats the Kidney, Liver, and Spleen. It can effectively stanch bleeding while nourishing both yin and blood.

If chronic flooding and spotting has led to a deficiency of both yin and yang, *zōng lǘ tàn* (Carbonized Petiolus Trachycarpi), *chì shí zhī* (Halloysitum Rubrum) and *pào jiāng tàn* (Carbonized Rhizoma Zingiberis Praeparata) may be added, and the dosage of *rén shēn* (Radix et Rhizoma Ginseng), *huáng qí* (Radix Astragali) and *bái zhú* (Rhizoma Atractylodis Macrocephalae) should be greatly increased in order to tonify qi to stanch bleeding.

At the same time, SP 1 (*yǐn bái*), LV 1 (*dà dūn*), and SP 6 (*sān yīn jiāo*) may be treated with moxibustion. Moxa SP 1 and LV 1 alternately, three times daily.

If there is blood stasis, add *yì mǔ cǎo* (Herba Leonuri) and *pú huáng tàn* (Carbonized Pollen Typhae), to dispel stasis and stanch bleeding.

Our primary approach should be to secure the Kidney while treating the root. *Xiān líng pí* (Herba Epimedii), *bā jǐ tiān* (Radix Morindae Officinalis), *dù zhòng* (Cortex Eucommiae), *bǔ gǔ zhī* (Fructus Psoraleae) and *gǒu qǐ zǐ* (Fructus Lycii) are often selected to tonify the Kidney and nourish blood. Tonification of the Kidney aims to regulate the menses while also promoting ovulation.

Spotting is most often associated with patterns of Liver and Kidney yin deficiency leading to internal stirring of the ministerial fire. We may encounter complex presentations involving blood stasis or damp-heat as well. The treatment of spotting is more challenging than flooding patterns because it is necessary to generate sufficient yin and blood within a short period of time. Recurrence is also more prevalent than in flooding cases.

The primary treatment principle for spotting is to nourish the Liver and Kidney. Clearing deficient heat or dispelling blood stasis may also be indicated. *Zuǒ Guī Yǐn* (左归饮) with modified *Èr Zhì Wán* (二至丸) may be selected.

With blood stasis, add *yì mǔ cǎo* (Herba Leonuri) and *qiàn cǎo tàn* (Carbonized Radix Rubiae).

With damp-heat, add *cán shā* (Faeces Bombycis) and *chǎo huáng qín* (Dry-fried Radix Scutellariae).

With excessive Heart fire and symptoms of vexation or insomnia, add *wǔ wèi zǐ* (Fructus Schisandrae), *bǎi zǐ rén* (Semen Platycladi) and *hé shǒu wū* (Radix Polygoni Multiflori).

With predominate yin deficiency symptoms without signs of heat or stasis, add *tù sī zǐ* (Semen Cuscutae) and *lù jiǎo jiāo* (Colla Cornus Cervi).

After abnormal bleeding patterns have ceased, our primary approach is to both emolliate the Liver and secure the Kidney in order to regulate menstruation.

Medicinals to treat the blood aspect: During the bleeding period, medicinals that are moving in nature such as *dāng guī* (Radix Angelicae Sinensis) and *chuān xiōng* (Rhizoma Chuanxiong) should not be prescribed. Their pungent and warm nature increases the risk of exacerbating the condition.

If menstruation is irregular or delayed, *dāng guī* (Radix Angelicae Sinensis) or *chuān xiōng* (Rhizoma Chuanxiong) may then be chosen to invigorate blood and promote menses. Again, these medicinals are contraindicated during menstruation.

To both to stanch bleeding and cool blood, *mǔ dān pí* (Cortex Moutan), *dì yú* (Radix Sanguisorbae), *jiāo zhī zǐ* (Scorch-fried Fructus Gardeniae) and *ǒu jié* (Nodus Nelumbinis Rhizomatis) may be selected.

To warm the channels and stanch bleeding, select *pào jiāng tàn* (Carbonized Rhizoma Zingiberis Praeparata), *ài yè* (Folium Artemisiae Argyi), *lù jiǎo shuāng* (Cornu Cervi Degelatinatum) and *pò gù zhǐ* (Fructus Psoraleae).

To nourish blood and stanch bleeding, select *gāng niǎn gēn* (Radix Rhodomyrti), *dì niǎn gēn* (Melastoma dodecandrum Lour) and *ē jiāo* (Colla Corii Asini).

To nourish yin and stanch bleeding, select *nǚ zhēn zǐ* (Fructus Ligustri Lucidi), *guī bǎn jiāo* (Colla Plastri Testudinis) and *hàn lián cǎo* (Herba Ecliptae).

To dispel blood stasis and stanch bleeding, select *yì mǔ cǎo* (Herba Leonuri), *pú huáng* (Pollen Typhae), *tián qī* (Radix Notoginseng) and *dà huáng tàn* (Carbonized Radix et Rhizoma Rhei).

To astringe to stanch bleeding select *chì shí zhī* (Halloysitum Rubrum), *wū méi* (Fructus Mume) and *wǔ bèi zǐ* (Galla Chinensis).

Use caution with carbonized herbs to arrest bleeding because overuse may cause stasis.

(Luo Yuan-kai. The Essentials of Gynecology 女科述要 . *New Journal of Traditional Chinese Medicine* 新中医 . 1992, (5)：16-17)

2. ZHU XIAO-NAN'S EXPERIENCE IN THE TREATMENT OF FLOODING AND SPOTTING

Empirically effective medicinals:

(1) *Guàn zhòng* (Rhizoma Cyrtomii) and *yuǎn zhì* (Radix Polygalae Tenuifoliae) are very effective in the treatment of abnormal uterine bleeding.

(2) For chronic flooding and spotting where prescriptions that tonify qi to contain blood are ineffective, blood stasis dispelling and heat clearing medicinals should be combined with those that tonify qi.

Select *shú jūn tàn* (Carbonized Radix et Rhizoma Rhei), *pú huáng tàn* (Carbonized Pollen Typhae), *yì mǔ cǎo* (Herba Leonuri), and *shēn sān qī* (Radix Notoginseng). *Shú jūn tàn* (Carbonized Radix et Rhizoma Rhei) is the most effective. The formula *Zhèn Líng Dān* (震灵丹) contains *yǔ yú liáng* (Limonitum), *zǐ shí yīng* (Fluoritum), *dài zhě shí* (Haematitum), *chì shí zhī* (Halloysitum Rubrum), *rǔ xiāng* (Olibanum), *mò yào* (Myrrha), *wǔ líng zhī* (Faeces Trogopterori) and *zhū shā* (Cinnabaris). Prescribe up to 3g each per dose.

(3) *Xiān hè cǎo* (Herba Agrimoniae) and *xiān táo cǎo* (Herba Euphorbiae Humifusae) are both effective for acute and sudden flooding. 12g per dose.

To rectify chronic flooding and spotting, select viscous medicinals like *ē jiāo* (Colla Corii Asini), *guī bǎn jiāo* (Colla Plastri Testudinis), *huáng míng jiāo* (Oxhide Gelatin) and *niú jiǎo sāi* (Bovis Cornus Os) which may be prepared as a paste by combining them with medicinals that strengthen the Spleen, harmonize the Stomach, and tonify to stanch bleeding. This preparation functions to arrest bleeding directly when taken daily. Since the digestive function of chronic patients is often impaired, and due to the sweet and greasy nature of this preparation, medicinals that strengthen the Spleen and Stomach should be added.

(Zhu Nan-sun, Zhu Rong-du and Dong Ping. *Gynecology Experience of Zhu Xiao-nan* 朱小南妇科经验选 . Beijing: People's Medical Publishing House, 1981. 18-23)

3. WANG WEI-CHUAN'S EXPERIENCE IN THE TREATMENT OF FLOODING AND SPOTTING

Although there are a variey of patterns associated with flooding and spotting, they all share the common symptom of profuse bleeding. Care should be taken to avoid qi and blood depletion. Follow the general principle of treating the symptoms in acute cases, and treating the origin in chronic cases.

Regarding sudden flooding, we must take care to avoid qi and blood desertion by securing qi and rescuing yang. *Dú Shēn Tāng* (独参汤) with added *tóng biàn* (Urina Hominis) may be prescribed. Relatively large doses of *dǎng shēn* (Radix Codonopsis), *huáng qí* (Radix Astragali), *xiān hè cǎo* (Herba Agrimoniae), *zōng lǘ tàn* (Carbonized Petiolus Trachycarpi), guàn zhòng tàn (Carbonized Rhizoma Osmundae) and *guǎng sān qī* (Radix Notoginseng) are often used to secure the qi, prevent desertion and stanch bleeding.

For chronic cases, treatment should be based on accurate pattern differentiation with an greater emphasis on Cheng Yuan (treating the root) with Se Liu (stanch bleeding). We must first assess the condition of the Liver, Spleen and Kidney, and then treat accordingly. Nourish in cases of insufficient Liver yang, and course when Liver qi is in excess. Warm in cases of insufficient Kidney yang, while nourish and emolliate in deficient Spleen yin patterns.

Four principles for the treatment of flooding:

(1) Flooding patterns in young patients are usually due to Liver qi stagnation associated with disturbances of the seven effects. The

treatment principle is to emolliate the Liver and relieve qi stagnation, calm the spirit and cool blood. Ectopic pregnancy should first be ruled out.

(2) Flooding patterns in mature patients typically show a decline of Kidney qi with an insecurity of the penetrating and conception vessels. Deficiency of the middle qi impairs the Spleens ability of containment, as well as the Liver's function of storage. This leads to impairment of the Kidney and the penetrating and conception vessels. The best approach is to secure and regulate qi, nourish the Kidney, and harmonize the penetrating vessel. Structural diseases such as cervical cancer and hysteromyoma should be ruled out.

(3) Flooding and spotting preceding delivery is often associated with Liver and Kidney heat constraint leading to the frenetic movement of blood. The treatment principles of Cheng Yuan (treat the root) with Se Liu (stanch bleeding) should be applied here. Cheng Yuan method may prevent miscarriage by treating the underlying causes, where Se Liu treats the abnormal bleeding pattern directly.

(4) Flooding and spotting following delivery is often associated with malnourishment, overwork, or intemperate sexuality. In these cases we should regulate qi and secure blood. We must of course stanch bleeding immediately to prevent qi and blood desertion.

Pattern differentiation and formulas:

(1) Qi Deficiency

Select modified *Rén Shēn Yǎng Róng Tāng* (人参养荣汤).

1) To nourish blood and stanch bleeding, add *xiān hè cǎo* (Herba Agrimoniae) 60g, *xià kū cǎo* (Spica Prunellae) 60g, *dà jì* (Herba Cirsii Japonici) 12g, *xiǎo jì* (Herba Cirsii) 12g and *ē jiāo* (Colla Corii Asini) 9-30g.

2) To warm the Kidney to benefit qi absorbtion, add *shā rén* (Fructus Amomi) 6g, *kòu rén* (FructusAmomi Rotundus) 6g and *bái sháo* (Radix Paeoniae Alba) 9g.

3) To relieve headache and dizziness, add *tiān má* (Rhizoma Gastrodiae) 24g and *yuǎn zhì* (Radix Polygalae) 9g.

4) For Stomach cold, add *wú zhū yú* (Fructus Evodiae) 9g.

5) For yang deficiency, add *shú fù piàn* (Radix Aconitila Teralis Preparata) 24-60g (decocted first, for two hours).

6) For severe qi deficiency, add *jí lín shēn* (Radix et Rhizoma Ginseng) 9-60g.

7) For qi and blood deficiency due to chronic spotting, add *lù róng* (Cornu Cervi Pantotrichum) 3g (infused), *xuè yú tàn* (Crinis Carbonisatus) 9g, *wū zéi gǔ* (Endoconcha Sepiae) 12g and *zōng lǘ tàn* (Carbonized Petiolus Trachycarpi) 9g.

(2) Blood Deficiency

Select *Guī Pí Tāng* (归脾汤).

1) To nourish blood and tonify qi, select *dǎng shēn* (Radix Codonopsis) 24-60g, *shēng huáng qí* (Radix Astragali Cruda) 24-60g, *bái zhú* (Rhizoma Atractylodis Macrocephalae) 9g, *lù jiǎo jiāo* (Colla Cornus Cervi) 9-30g (infused) and *mù xiāng* (Radix Aucklandiae) 6g.

2) To tonify the Heart, select *běi wǔ wèi zǐ* (Fructus Schisandrae Chinensis) 12g, *shān yú ròu* (Fructus Corni) 12g, *shú zǎo rén* (Semen Ziziphi Spinosae) 9g (dry-fried), *lóng yǎn ròu* (Arillus Longan) 24g and *fú shén* (Poriae Sclerotium Pararadicis) 9g.

(3) Yang Deficiency

Select *Hé Jiān Dì Huáng Yǐn Zī* (河间地黄饮子).

1) To warm the Kidney and free the yang, select *shú fù piàn* (Radix Aconitila Teralis Preparata) 24-60g (decocted first, for two hours), *gǒu qǐ* (Fructus Lycii) 12g, *dǎng shēn* (Radix Codonopsis) 24-60g, *shēng huáng qí* (Radix Astragali Cruda) 24-60g and *háng bā jǐ* (Radix Morindae Officinalis) 12g.

2) With spontaneous sweating, add *jīn yīng zǐ* (Fructus Rosae Laevigatae) 60g, *lóng gǔ* (Fossilia Ossis Mastodi) 9g, *mǔ lì* (Concha Ostreae) 12g, and *fú xiǎo mài* (Fructus Tritici Levis) 24g.

(4) Yin Deficiency

Select *Yī Guàn Jiān* (一贯煎).

1) To nourish the Kidney and emolliate the Liver, select *běi shā shēn* (Radix Glehniae) 9g, *mài dōng* (Radix Ophiopogonis) 9g, *chuān liàn zǐ* (Fructus Toosendan) 9g, *shēng dì huáng* (Radix Rehmanniae) 12g, *gǒu qǐ* (Fructus Lycii) 12g, *bái jí lí* (Fructus Tribuli) 9g, *nǚ zhēn zǐ* (Fructus Ligustri Lucidi) 24g, *hàn lián cǎo* (Herba Ecliptae) 24g, *sāng jì shēng* (Herba Taxilli) 15g and *tù sī zǐ* (Semen Cuscutae) 15g.

2) With hypochondriac pain, add *xià kū huā* (Spica Prunellae) 12g, *xiè bái* (Bulbus Allii Macrostemonis) 12g, *chái hú* (Bupleuri Radix) 9g and *dān shēn* (Radix Salviae Miltiorrhizae) 9g. *Chái hú* (Bupleuri Radix) should be discontinued after 1 or 2 doses due to its yang-upbearing nature.

3) With tidal fever, add *yù zhú* (Rhizoma Polygonati Odorati) 9g, *biē jiǎ* (Carapax Trionycis) 24g, *shēng guī bǎn* (Raw Testudinis Plastrum) 30g (decocted first for two hours), *féi zhī mǔ* (Raw Rhizoma Anemarrhenae) 9g, and *dì gǔ pí* (Cortex Lycii) 9g

4) With severe insufficiency of body fluids, add *dǎng shēn* (Radix Codonopsis) 9g and *tiān mén dōng* (Radix Asparagi) 9g.

5) With dry mouth and a bitter taste, add *huáng lián* (Rhizoma Coptidis) 9g.

6) For flooding and spotting with clotting, add *sān qī fěn* (Radix Notoginseng Powder) 9g (infused), *pú huáng tàn* (Carbonized Pollen Typhae) 9g and *xuè jié* (Sanguis Draconis) 9g.

(5) Blood Stasis

Select Modified *Xuè Fǔ Zhú Yū Tāng* (加减血府逐瘀汤).

桃仁	táo rén	9g	Semen Persicae
土红花	tǔ hóng huā	9g	Herba Cirsii Japonici
三棱	sān léng	9g	Rhizoma Sparganii
莪术	é zhú	9g	Rhizoma Curcumae
水蛭	shuǐ zhì	9g	Hirudo
当归	dāng guī	9g	Radix Angelicae Sinensis
生蒲黄	shēng pú huáng	9g	Pollen Typhae Crudum
血竭	xuè jié	6g	Sanguis Draconis
炒五灵脂	chǎo wǔ líng zhī	12g	Faeces Trogopterori (dry-fried)
三七粉（冲服）	sān qī fěn	3g	Radix Notoginseng Powder (infused)

(6) Liver Qi Stagnation

Select *Zī Shuǐ Qīng Gān Yǐn* (滋水清肝饮).

1) To regulate qi, relieve constraint and nourish yin, select *dāng guī* (Radix Angelicae Sinensis) 9g, *shēng dì huáng* (Radix Rehmanniae) 12g, *zé xiè* (Rhizoma Alismatis) 9g, *fú líng* (Poria) 9g, *bái sháo* (Radix Paeoniae Alba) 9g, *chái hú* (Bupleuri Radix) 9g, *shān zhī* (Fructus Gardeniae) 9g, and *dān pí* (Cortex Moutan) 9g.

2) With epigastric pain, add *chuān liàn zǐ* (Fructus Toosendan) 9g, *tái wū* (Radix Linderae) 9g and *jiǔ xiāng chóng* (Aspongopus) 9g.

3) With lumbar pain, add *dù zhòng* (Cortex Eucommiae) 9g, *xù duàn* (Radix Dipsaci) 24-60g and *qiāng huó* (Rhizoma et Radix Notopterygii) 9g.

(7) Phlegm-damp

Select *Liù Jūn Zǐ Tāng* (六君子汤) or *Juān Yǐn Liù Shén Tāng* (蠲饮六神汤)

1) To percolate dampness and resolve phlegm, select *jú hóng* (Exocarpium Citri Rubrum) 9g, *shí chāng pǔ* (Rhizoma Acori Talarinowii) 9g, *zhì dǎn nán xīng* (Prepared Arisaema Cum Bile) 9g, *bàn xià* (Rhizoma Pinelliae) 9g, *máo zhú* (Dry-fried Rhizoma Atractylodis) 9g, *chén pí*

(Pericarpium Citri Reticulatae) 9g, *bái zhǐ* (Radix Angelicae Dahuricae) 9g and *huò xiāng* (Herba Agastachis) 6g.

2) With yellow foul-smelling leucorrhea, add *chūn gēn pí* (Cortex Ailanthi) 9g, *hóng téng* (Caulis Sargentodoxae) 24g and *pú gōng yīng* (Herba Taraxaci) 24g.

3) With leucorrhea, add *fú róng huā* (Hibisci Mutabilis) 9g, *hóng téng* (Caulis Sargentodoxae) 24g, and *pú gōng yīng* (Herba Taraxaci) 24g.

4) With excessive phlegm-heat, body fluid failing to transport, shortness of breath and vexation, add *zhú lì* (Succus Bambusae) 15g (infused 3 times).

5) With asthma due to phlegm, add *shān yú ròu* (Fructus Corni) 12g, *jī xuè téng gāo* (Spatholobi paste) 12g, *hǎi fú shí* (Pumice) 9g and *má róng* (Shredded Herba Ephedrae) 3g.

6) With a dry throat and a dark red tongue, add *chuān bèi mǔ* (Bulbus Fritillariae Cirrhosae) 9g (infused).

(8) Accumulation of Damp-heat

Select *Yín Jiǎ Hé Jì* (银甲合剂).

1) To clear heat and eliminate dampness, select *yín huā* (Flos Lonicerae) 9g, *lián qiào* (Fructus Forsythiae) 9g, *hóng téng* (Caulis Sargentodoxae) 24g, *pú gōng yīng* (Herba Taraxaci) 24g, *dà qīng yè* (Folium Isatidis) 9g, *zǐ huā dì dīng* (Herba Violae) 12g, *shēng biē jiǎ* (Raw Carapax Trionycis) 24g, and *chūn gēn pí* (Cortex Ailanthi) 9g.

2) In patterns of flooding and spotting with profuse leucorrhea, indicating predominate dampness. Add *cāng zhú* (Rhizoma Atracylodis) 9g, *chǎo huáng bǎi* (Dry-fried Cortex Phellodendri Chinensis) 9g and *zōng lǘ tàn* (Carbonized Petiolus Trachycarpi) 9g.

3) In patterns with bright red menses, sudden flooding, dry throat with a bitter taste, and feverish sensations when bleeding, indicating predominate heat. Add *bái máo gēn* (Rhizoma Imperatae) 9g, *shēng dì tàn*

(Carbonized Radix Rehmanniae) 12g and *shí hú* (Herba Dendrobii) 9g.

4) With frequent, scant urination with a downbearing or prickling sensation, add *hǔ pò mò* (Succinum Powder) 6g (infused or wrapped).

(Wang Wei-chuan. *Wang Wei-chuan's Selected Experience of Stubborn Diseases* 王渭川疑难病症治验选. Chengdu: Sichuan Science and Technology Publishing House, 1984. 226-231)

4. Liu Min-ru's Perspective on Flooding and Spotting

According to Dr. Liu, the etiology of flooding and spotting is associated with disorders of both qi and blood occurring together. The entire viscera may be involved, yet the root cause is primarily associated with the Kidney. Kidney insecurity often leads to general deficiencies of both qi and yin. The emphasis in clinic is to nourish qi and yin while tonifying the Kidney to secure the origin.

(Chengdu Chinese Medical College. Department of Gynecology. *Gynecology of Chinese Medicine* 中医妇科学. Beijing: People's Medical Publishing House, 1986. 127-143）

5. Yang Jia-lin's Discussion on the Etiology and Progression of Flooding and Spotting Disorder

(1) Rather than etiology, deficient qi and yin-blood is seen usually as a result of flooding and spotting.

In the early stages of the disease, the patient's constitution is usually healthy and the zheng qi (right qi) is far from prostration. As chronic disease consumes yin and blood, qi may eventually become exhausted. Serious qi and blood deficiency patterns may appear in longstanding cases.

DUB patients with a congenital deficiency of yin often show signs of both yin deficiency and blood-heat. This heat results from yin-depletion due to blood loss. In many cases, the primary cause of the disease is not directly related to the presenting symptoms.

In some cases, overwork and taxation may impair Spleen qi, which in turn leads to an insecurity of the penetrating and conception vessels as well as a dual deficiency of qi and blood.

Flooding and spotting may be also due to yin deficiency with internal heat. This can result in qi-depletion, which leads to further deficient conditions of qi and yin. However, most qi and yin-blood deficiencies are a direct result of the excessive blood loss in the course of flooding and spotting.

(2) Qi and yin deficiency that results from flooding and spotting tends to further exacerbate the abnormal bleeding condition. Since the main symptom of flooding and spotting is vaginal bleeding, the ebb and flow of both qi and blood must be clearly observed.

The primary causes of this disorder are more obvious in the early stages, when the supply of qi and blood is relatively sufficient. As the disease progresses, however, the consumption of yin and blood leads to a more serious deficiency of qi and yin. This is the most commonly seen cause and effect progression, where the resulting qi and blood deficiency becomes an aggravating factor in the vaginal bleeding disorder. Furthermore, patterns of blood stasis and stagnation also may prevent new blood from entering the vessels. In these cases, blood stasis is not only a direct cause of flooding and spotting, but also a likely result of other causes. This is another typical cause and effect cycle in the transformation and progression of flooding and spotting.

(3) Each case presents a clinical decision as to whether focus on the underlying cause of the pattern, or to treat based on the symptomatic effects that can be observed. When it is impossible to find the primary cause, or if the present symptoms have no direct relationship to the primary cause, the treatment should focus on the effects of the disease progression.

The treatment of acute bleeding should focus primarily on the symptoms. The general treatment principle is to first stanch bleeding, while tonifying qi. This especially applies in cases of and flooding and spotting associated with qi and yin deficiency.

Commonly used formulas:

1) Qi and Yin Deficiency

Select *Shēng Mài Sǎn* (生脉散) with *Shàng Hǎi Jiǎ Fāng* (上海甲方)

白芍	bái sháo	Radix Paeoniae Alba
生地	shēng dì huáng	Radix Rehmanniae
女贞子	nǚ zhēn zǐ	Fructus Ligustri Lucidi
旱莲草	hàn lián cǎo	Herba Ecliptae
大蓟	dà jì	Herba Cirsii Japonici
小蓟	xiǎo jì	Herba Cirsii
炒蒲黄	chǎo pú huáng	Pollen Typhae (dry-fried)
炒槐花	chǎo huái huā	Flos Sophorae (dry-fried)
茜草	qiàn cǎo	Radix Rubiae

2) Qi and Blood Deficiency

Select *Jǔ Yuán Jiān* (举元煎) and *Dì Sháo Gǒu Qǐ Èr Zhì Wán* (地芍枸杞二至丸) with added medicinals to stanch bleeding.

3) Longstanding Qi Deficiency Impairing Yang

Select *Gù Běn Zhǐ Bēng Tāng* (固本止崩汤) with added *bǔ gǔ zhī* (Fructus Psoraleae), *jiāo ài* (Scorch-fried Folium Artemisiae Argyi) and *xuè yú tàn* (Crinis Carbonisatus).

4) Profuse Bleeding

Prescribe *Dú Shēn Tāng* (独参汤), 2 doses daily.

In cases of spotting, we may treat both the cause and effect together.

This approach is also appropriate when bleeding is mild, or at the stage where it has ceased completely.

(Yang Jia-lin. Discussion on the Etiology and Progression of Flooding and Spotting disorder 试论崩漏病程中的因果转化. *Sichuan Journal of Traditional Chinese Medicine* 四川中医. 1988, (4)：6-7)

6. Wu Xi's Experience in Flooding and Spotting Treatment

(1) Etiologies

Flooding and spotting disorders can be clearly differentiated in most cases. Most patterns of flooding are excess conditions, while spotting is usually associated with deficiency. However, chronic flooding eventually results in deficiency, where chronic spotting may lead to blood stasis. In some patients, these two symptoms may appear alternately. Proper pattern differentiation is primarily based on changes in the quantity, quality, and color of the bleeding. Along with the tongue and pulse, we must consider the course and progression of the condition as well.

(2) Pathomechanisms

1) Damage due to the seven affects and five emotions may transform into fire which leads to a disorder of the penetrating and conception vessels, with blood failing to stay in the vessels. Pensiveness or over-thinking impair the Spleen, where sorrow damages the Lung, and anger causes stagnation of Liver qi. Resultant blood stasis in the uterine collaterals may also lead to blood failing to stay in the vessels.

2) Overwork and taxation also may lead to deficient Spleen qi that is unable to contain blood, and the Liver's function of blood storage may also be affected. Both of these conditions may lead to flooding and spotting disorder.

3) Congenital deficiencies and intemperate sexuality often lead to

Kidney qi deficiency with an insecurity of the penetrating and conception vessels. Insufficient Kidney yin leads to frenetic ministerial fire that may distress blood.

4) Overeating generally damages the Spleen and Stomach, where an excess of spicy foods may create an accumulation of internal heat, causing deficient Spleen unable to contain, or damp-heat pouring downwards. When this heat converges with Kidney fire, flooding and spotting disorders may occur.

5) Blood stasis collecting internally: Cold or heat evils may invade the uterus, both of which can lead to blood stasis. Deficiency and stagnation of qi also affect the free movement of blood. In childbearing patients, a persistent flow of lochia may also result in obstruction which may lead to blood failing to stay in the vessels.

(3) Treatment

Clinical treatment may be divided into three steps.

1) Determine the Severity of Bleeding.

Since abnormal bleeding is the primary symptom of flooding and spotting, we must consider using the Se Liu (stanch bleeding) method. Acute symptoms should be addressed first. In cases of severe flooding, the bleeding condition must be given priority in treatment. In cases of spotting, this may not be necessary. However, we should not only secure and astringe, but also consider selecting medicinals to address the cause. The patterns and medications for Se Liu are as follows.

For qi deficiency, select *Bŭ Zhōng Yì Qì Tāng* (补中益气汤) added with *ē jiāo* (Colla Corii Asini), *chǎo bái sháo* (Dry-fried Radix Paeoniae Alba), *wū zéi gŭ* (Endoconcha Sepiae), *wū méi tàn* (Carbonized Fructus Mume), *yì mŭ căo* (Herba Leonuri) and *zhǐ qiào* (Fructus Aurantii).

For blood deficiency, select *Jiāo Ài Sì Wù Tāng* (胶艾四物汤) plus *xuè yú tàn* (Crinis Carbonisatus), *zōng lǘ tàn* (Carbonized Petiolus Trachycarpi), *hàn lián cǎo* (Herba Ecliptae) and *xiān hè cǎo* (Herba Agrimoniae).

For yang deficiency, select *Yòu Guī Wán* (右归丸) plus *fù pén zǐ* (Fructus Rubi), *chì shí zhī* (Halloysitum Rubrum), *lù jiǎo jiāo* (Colla Cornus Cervi), *jiāng tàn* (Carbonized Rhizoma Zingiberis Recens) and *bǔ gǔ zhī* (Fructus Psoraleae).

For yin deficiency, select *Zuǒ Guī Wán* (左归丸) with *Èr Zhì Wán* (二至丸) plus *guī bǎn* (Testudinis Plastrum) and *lián fáng tàn* (Carbonized Receptaculum Nelumbinis).

For blood-heat, select *Qīng Rè Gù Jīng Tāng* (清热固经汤) plus *cè bǎi tàn* (Carbonized Cacumen Platycladi), *qiàn cǎo tàn* (Carbonized Radix Rubiae) and *huái huā tàn* (Carbonized Flos Sophorae).

For blood stasis, select *Táo Hóng Sì Wù Tāng* (桃红四物汤) fried with *Shī Xiào Sǎn* (失笑散) plus *huā ruǐ shí* (Ophicalcitum), *sān qī fěn* (Radix Notoginseng Powder), *jiāo shān zhā* (Scorch-fried Fructus Crataegi) and *xuè jié* (Sanguis Draconis).

For profuse flooding with a faint pulse, treatment should tonify the original qi. *Shēn Fù Lóng Mǔ Tāng* (参附龙牡汤) may be selected to both tonify and prevent desertion. Medicinals known to contract the uterus may be selected to reinforce the effect of those that arrest bleeding. Select *yì mǔ cǎo* (Herba Leonuri), *zhǐ qiào* (Fructus Aurantii), *zhǐ shí* (Fructus Aurantii Immaturus), *mǎ chǐ xiàn* (Herba Portulacae), *jī xuè téng* (Caulis Spatholobi), *pú huáng* (Pollen Typhae), *wú zhū yú* (Fructus Evodiae), *chōng wèi zǐ* (Fructus Leonuri), *shān zhā* (Fructus Crataegi), *ài yè* (Folium Artemisiae Argyi) and *zǎo rén* (Semen Ziziphi Spinosae). According to modern research, these medicinals contract the uterus and promote both vascular constriction and defluxion of the endometrium. This approach has been shown to effectively shorten the menstrual cycle and reduce abnormal bleeding.

2) Emphasize Pattern Differentiation When Treating the Root.

The Cheng Yuan (treat the root) method requires accurate pattern differentiation. Blood-heat, blood stasis, qi deficiency, Liver qi stagnation and Kidney deficiency should all be carefully considered. Se Liu and Cheng Yuan methods should not be seen as entirely separate methods, as they are usually applied together. In fact, Se Liu may depend on the application of Cheng Yuan, and in some cases, treating the root should be given priority. For instance, a patient that presents chronic scant bleeding with clotting may best be treated by first dispelling blood stasis. After the stasis condition has been addressed, the Se Liu (stanch bleeding) and Fu Jiu (establish and regulate menses) methods may be applied.

3) Establish and Regulate Menses (Fu Jiu)

Treatment should emphasize on the Liver, Kidney, Spleen, and Stomach. The Spleen and Kidney should be specifically addressed.

(4) Three Inadvisable Points in Flooding and Spotting Treatment

1) Treatment should be given in accordance with normal human physiological functions. With spotting that persists for more than 28 days, the correct treatment method is to invigorate blood rather than to stanch bleeding. After menstruation has been re-established, treatment may then focus on the underlying cause.

2) Astringing medicinals should not be prescribed too early in treatment due to the possibility of causing blood stasis.

3) Medicinals of a cold nature should be used with caution in adolescent patients. Cold may create stagnation and thus impair the free flow of blood. This may result in amenorrhea, which is even more difficult to treat.

(5) Flooding and Spotting Treatments in Patients of Different Age Groups.

1) Adolescence

Adolescent women are full of vital force, and their Kidney qi is in a state of growth and development. Therefore, treatments aiming to regulate menstruation are generally not necessary. Treatment should support this natural development and allow the condition to resolve itself over time. When the viscera are in harmony, the individual is in balance. Since the Kidney is in a state of growth, its ability to transform yin and yang is not yet fully developed. When the acquired constitution is affected, the Kidney's function of storage may also be impaired. A resultant insecurity of the penetrating and conception vessels may lead to blood failing to stay in the vessels.

Treatment should tonify the Kidney and secure the penetrating vessel, stanch bleeding, and regulate menses. Select *Yòu Guī Wán* (右归丸) and remove both *ròu guì* (Cortex Cinnamomi) and *dāng guī* (Radix Angelicae Sinensis). Add *zhì huáng qí* (Radix Astragali Praeparata cum Melle), *fù pén zǐ* (Fructus Rubi), *zǐ hé chē* (Placenta Hominis) and *chì shí zhī* (Halloysitum Rubrum).

Kidney deficiency with stagnation of cold may cause obstruction that prevents the blood from returning to the vessels. Such a condition may present purplish menses with clotting and intermittent abdominal pain. Select *zhì rǔ xiāng* (Fried with liquid Olibanum), *zhì mò yào* (Fried with liquid Myrrha) and *wǔ líng zhī* (Faeces Trogopterori).

In patterns of Kidney and Spleen deficiency, the Spleen's warming function as well as its ability to transport and transform may be affected. Associated signs are edema, lassitude, poor appetite and loose stools.

Select *chǎo lù dǎng* (Dry-fried Radix Codonopsis), *chǎo bái zhú* (Dry-fried Rhizoma Atractylodis Macrocephalae), *chūn shā rén* (Fructus

Amomi), *fú líng* (Poria), *huái shān yào* (Rhizoma Dioscoreae) and *pào jiāng tàn* (Carbonized Rhizoma Zingiberis Praeparata).

In adolescent flooding and spotting, it is important to both tonify the Kidney and regulate menses after the cessation of the abnormal bleeding pattern. Normal menstrual function is based on the theory of the mutual transformation of Kidney yin and Kidney yang. After the cessation of bleeding, treatments should be selected in accordance with the timing of the menstrual cycle. During the postmenstrual period, treatment should focus on nourishing blood, tonifying Kidney and replenishing yin-essence. Between periods, treatment should tonify yin to support yang, invigorate blood, and regulate qi while promoting the free flow of qi and blood in the uterine, penetrating and conception vessels. This method promotes the mutual transformation of yin and yang. In the late intermenstrual period, we should tonify Kidney to assist yang and warm the uterus. During the premenstrual period, the primary principle is to regulate qi and blood in order to promote the smooth flow of menses. After proper treatment according to these four phases, Kidney yin should be sufficient, yang qi invigorated, and qi and blood in harmony. Normal menstruation can occur only when yin and yang are able to transform into one another.

2) Childbearing Period

Abnormal bleeding during the childbearing period is often related to pregnancy and delivery. This is usually associated with disorders of the management and storage functions of the Spleen and Liver, respectively. Treatment must regulate the Liver and invigorate the Spleen, stanch bleeding and secure the menses. After abnormal bleeding has ceased, treatment must emphasize nourishing the Kidney, Liver and Spleen in order to address the root cause.

3) Menopausal Period

In women approaching menopause, the root cause is most often associated with deficiency of the Kidney. The most commonly seen patterns are Kidney yin deficiency, with exuberant Heart and Liver fire disturbing the Sea of Blood. Kidney deficiency may also combine with damp-heat and blood stasis conditions. This can lead to obstruction of the penetrating and conception vessels with frenetic blood failing to stay in the vessels. Treatment should nourish the Kidney and clear the Liver, dispel stasis and stanch bleeding.

Select modified *Sì Cǎo Tāng* (四草汤) with *Zuǒ Guī Wán* (左归丸). Medicinals include *mǎ biān cǎo* (Herba Verbanae), *lù xián cǎo* (Herba Pyrolae), *yì mǔ cǎo* (Herba Leonuri), *qiàn cǎo* (Radix Rubiae), *mò hàn lián* (Herba Ecliptae), *dà shēng dì* (Radix Rehmanniae), *shān yú ròu* (Fructus Corni), *huái shān yào* (Rhizoma Dioscoreae), *mǔ dān pí* (Cortex Moutan), *hēi shān zhī* (Carbonized Fructus Gardeniae), *Shī Xiào Sǎn* (失笑散, wrapped), *guī bǎn jiāo* (Colla Plastri Testudinis) (infused), and *sān qī mò* (Radix Notoginseng Powder).

With heat symptoms, add *huáng qín* (Radix Scutellariae) and *huáng bǎi* (Cortex Phellodendri Chinensis).

With Heart fire flaming upward, select *lián zǐ xīn* (Plumula Nelumbinis), *hé huān pí* (Cortex Albiziae) and *qīng lóng chǐ* (Dens Draconis).

For damp-heat and blood stasis patterns that present chronic bleeding of hot, foul-smelling menses, remove *mò hàn lián* (Herba Ecliptae), *guī bǎn jiāo* (Colla Plastri Testudinis). Added *yì yǐ rén* (Semen Coicis), *fú líng* (Poria), *bái zhú* (Rhizoma Atractylodis Macrocephalae), *chuān huáng bǎi* (Cortex Phellodendri Chinensis), *hóng téng* (Caulis Sargentodoxae), *bài jiàng cǎo* (Herba Patriniae), *shēng dà huáng* (Raw Radix et Rhizoma Rhei), *hóng huā* (Flos Carthami) and *Bì Yù Sǎn* (碧玉散) all act to drain excess heat while dispelling blood stasis and stagnation.

(6) Discussion on Treatments and Selection of Medicinals

Generally, treatments include tonifying qi to contain blood, nourishing yin, cooling blood, warming menstruation and dispelling stasis. But tonifying qi to secure menstruation is most essential. The engendering, management and movement of blood all depend on the engendering, transformation and regulation of qi. Nourishing yin, invigorating qi and harmonizing blood may promote blood coagulation and uterine contraction. This may arrest bleeding by inhibiting regional circulation, resulting in defluxion of the endometrium.

Select medicinals such as *shēng dì huáng* (Radix Rehmanniae), *guī bǎn* (Testudinis Plastrum), *ē jiāo* (Colla Corii Asini), *nǚ zhēn zǐ* (Fructus Ligustri Lucidi), *hàn lián cǎo* (Herba Ecliptae), *cè bǎi* (Cacumen Platycladi), and *ǒu piàn* (Sliced Nodus Nelumbinis Rhizomatis).

Tonifying and cooling blood may be seen in terms of modern biomedicine as the regulation of fluid metabolism and the function of blood coagulation. *Huáng qí* (Radix Astragali) and *dǎng shēn* (Radix Codonopsis) tonify qi and blood, which may promote both smooth muscle contraction and constriction of the blood vessels. *Wū zéi gǔ* (Endoconcha Sepiae) and *mǔ lì* (Concha Ostreae) may assist in coagulation through astringing.

Dāng guī (Radix Angelicae Sinensis) and *xiāng fù* (Rhizoma Cyperi) tonify blood and invigorate qi. *Dāng guī* (Radix Angelicae Sinensis) enters the blood aspect, while *xiāng fù* (Rhizoma Cyperi) also regulates qi. They assist one another while balancing the functions of both qi and blood. They may function together to regulate the timing of uterine contractions. *Dāng guī* (Radix Angelicae Sinensis) also may relieve uterine spasm, promote uterine contraction, and promote the normal discharge of blood. The coordinated effects of such medicinals are known to be effective in controlling bleeding by promoting uterine contraction.

The therapeutic methods of invigorating blood, moving qi, relieving pain, and dispelling blood stasis may be associated with increased uterine blood flow, dilation of blood vessels and regular uterine contraction. *Guì xīn* (Cortex Cinnamomi) and *guì zhī* (Ramulus Cinnamomi) warm yang and free the collaterals. Blood moves with warmth, and congeals and stagnates with cold. Stagnation is resolved with warmth. The function of the following medicinals may induce dilation of blood vessels, resulting in improved blood circulation.

Dān shēn (Radix Salviae Miltiorrhizae), *hóng huā* (Flos Carthami) and *táo rén* (Semen Persicae) may dilate vessels and promote uterine contraction. *Zhǐ qiào* (Fructus Aurantii), *xiāng fù* (Rhizoma Cyperi), *wū yào* (Radix Linderae), *mù xiāng* (Radix Aucklandiae) and *yán hú* (Rhizoma Corydalis) rectify qi and remove stagnation. Blood is the mother of qi and qi is the commander of blood, thus the movement qi promotes the movement of blood. So to invigorate blood, we must also promote the free flow of qi. *Pú huáng* (Pollen Typhae) and *wǔ líng zhī* (Faeces Trogopterori) may promote both uterine contraction and blood circulation. They also function to stanch bleeding by astringing and invigorating blood.

(Wu Xi. *A Review of Wu Xi's Gynecology · Volume Three* 吴熙妇科朔洄第三集 . Xiamen: Xiamen University Publishing House, 1997. 140-143)

7. Ban Xiu-wen's Points in Flooding and Spotting Treatment

There are three main characteristics in Dr. Ban's treatment of flooding and spotting.

(1) Treatment is based on etiology and pattern differentiation.

(2) The use of both cooling and warming methods to regulate blood and qi.

(3) Secure the origin and clear the source, while tonifying the Kidney

and regulating menses.

Generally, the pathomechanisms associated with flooding and spotting include cold, heat, deficiency and stasis. They are most often related to disorders of qi and blood, the viscera, or yin and yang. Various conditions may interact one another, involving multiple organs, as well as the penetrating and conception vessels. Treatment is then based on accurate pattern differentiation. Appropriate treatment may apply various methods such as coursing the Liver, invigorating the Spleen, tonifying the Kidney, warming yang, clearing heat, and purging stasis.

(1) Heat Patterns

Heat patterns in this condition usually manifest as deficient fire. Select *Dì Gǔ Pí Yǐn* (地骨皮饮), *Èr Dì Tāng* (二地汤) with *Èr Zhì Wán* (二至丸), *běi shā shēn* (Radix Glehniae) and *mài dōng* (Radix Ophiopogonis). These medicinals are sweet, cooling and yin-nourishing. Cold and bitter medicinals are generally prohibited in order to to avoid possible impairment of Spleen yang or yin blood. To eliminate fire, select *xiān hé yè* (Folium Nelumbinis Recens), *xiān máo gēn* (Imperatae Rhizoma Recens), *zhù má gēn* (Radix Boehmeriae), and *hàn lián cǎo* (Herba Ecliptae).

(2) Cold Patterns

For cold patterns, select medicinals that are warm and moist in nature such as *ài yè* (Folium Artemisiae Argyi), *ròu guì* (Cortex Cinnamomi), *bā jǐ tiān* (Radix Morindae Officinalis), *suǒ yáng* (Herba Cynomorii) and *tù sī zǐ* (Semen Cuscutae), which both nourish yin and downbear fire.

(3) Deficiency Patterns

With deficiency patterns, select *Rén Shēn Yǎng Róng Tāng* (人参养荣汤), modified *Zuǒ Guī Wán* (左归丸) and modified *Yòu Guī Wán* (右归丸). Treatment emphasizes tonifying qi to contain blood, while invigorating both Spleen and Kidney yang. Once yin and yang have been engendered, the blood will stay in the vessels.

(4) Stasis Patterns

To dispel stasis without damaging the right qi, and to arrest bleeding without causing stagnation, select medicinals that invigorate blood such as *jī xuè téng* (Caulis Spatholobi), *yì mǔ cǎo* (Herba Leonuri), *shān zhā* (Fructus Crataegi), *sān qī* (Radix Notoginseng) and *zé lán* (Herba Lycopi).

Dr. Ban considers abnormal bleeding to be associated primarily with the syndrome of blood failing to stay in the vessels. For stasis patterns, astringing medicinals should be prescribed with caution. The most commonly selected medicinals are those that both resolve stasis and arresting bleeding, such as *qiàn gēn* (Radix Rubiae), *yì mǔ cǎo* (Herba Leonuri), *xiān hè cǎo* (Herba Agrimoniae) and *chǎo shān zhā* (Dry-fried Fructus Crataegi).

When chronic bleeding patterns with deficiency of the right qi has progressed into of efflux desertion, select *duàn lóng gǔ* (Calcined Fossilia Ossis Mastodi), *duàn mǔ lì* (Calcined Concha Ostreae), *wǎ lèng zì* (Concha Arcae), *hǎi piāo xiāo* (Endoconcha Sepiae), *fú lóng gān* (Terra Flava Usta) and *bǎi cǎo shuāng* (Fuligo Plantae). These medicinals effectively astringe without causing stagnation.

Dr. Ban commonly prescribes *Wǔ Zǐ Yǎn Zōng Wán* (五子衍宗丸) to tonify the Kidney.

For Kidney yang deficiency, add *bǔ gǔ zhī* (Fructus Psoraleae), *bā jǐ tiān* (Radix Morindae Officinalis), *chuān xù duàn* (Radix Dipsaci), *dù zhòng* (Cortex Eucommiae) and *sāng piāo xiāo* (Vaginal Ovorum Mantidis), which warm the Kidney and benefit essence.

For Kidney yin deficiency, select *nǚ zhēn zǐ* (Fructus Ligustri Lucidi), *běi shā shēn* (Radix Glehniae), *mài dōng* (Radix Ophiopogonis) and *shǒu wū* (Radix Polygoni Multiflori).

For qi and blood deficiency, remove *wŭ wèi zǐ* (Fructus Schisandrae) and *chē qián zǐ* (Semen Plantaginis), then add *Shèng Yù Tāng* (圣愈汤) or *Rén Shēn Yǎng Róng Tāng* (人参养荣汤) to warm and strenghten the Spleen and Kidney, and tonify qi to engender blood.

With blood stasis, remove *wŭ wèi zǐ* (Fructus Schisandrae) and add *jī xuè téng* (Caulis Spatholobi), *táo rén* (Semen Persicae), *zé lán* (Herba Lycopi), *sū mù* (Lignm Sappan) and *huáng qí* (Radix Astragali) which warm the Kidney, tonify qi, and invigorate blood.

As for the regulation of the menstruation cycle, Dr. Ban emphasizes both warming the Kidney and tonifying the Spleen during the postmenstrual period. This approach benefits the storage function of the uterus, while nourishing the source of menses. During the premenstrual period, primarily invigorate qi and harmonize blood. During the menstrual cycle, tonify blood and strengthten the Kidney in order to disinhibit uterine discharge.

(Lu Hui-ling. Selections from Professor Ban Xiu-wen's Experience with Menstrual Disorders 班秀文教授论治月经病经验拮萃 . *Liaoning Journal of Traditional Chinese Medicine* 辽宁中医杂志 . 1993, 5 : 6-9)

8. LIU FENG-WU'S TREATMENT OF INTERMENSTRUAL BLEEDING

Vaginal bleeding during the ovulation period is often due to latent damp-heat in the penetrating and conception vessels. Following the ovulation period, the functions of those vessels gradually increase. These functions are associated with yang, which may become exuberant and trigger the latent damp-heat. A common manifestation of damp-heat pouring downward is the appearance of profuse leucorrhea. When damp-heat enters the collaterals, blood will be damaged and move frenetically, out of the penetrating and conception vessels. For this bleeding pattern, treatment must clear heat and disinhibit dampness while invigorating qi and blood.

(Beijing Chinese Medical Hospital and Beijing Chinese Medical School. *Gynecological Experience of Liu Feng-wu* 刘奉五妇科经验 . Beijing: People's Medical Publishing House, 1982. 103-137)

9. TIAN XUE-MING'S PERSPECTIVE ON ARRESTING PATTERNS OF FLOODING

Dr. Tian considers the word "zhong" (middle) in the term "beng zhong lou xia" (flooding and spotting) to refer to an underlying deficiency of the middle jiao with a failure to manage and contain blood. "Xia" refers to the fall of the central qi. When deficient qi fails to contain, blood and qi may collapse. "Xia" can also refer to a deficiency or impairment of the lower origin. Therefore, the root treatment to stanch flooding is based primarily on tonification of the Spleen and Kidney.

After the cessation of abnormal bleeding, blood should be stabilized. With Spleen deficiency, we must secure the origin of Spleen qi. With lower origin deficiency and impairment, nourish Kidney water to generally reinforce the treatment effect. To stanch flooding, it is often improper to apply astringing medicinals. In clinic, tenacious and recurrent flooding and spotting patterns are usually caused by the misuse of astringent medicinals such as *wū zéi gǔ* (Endoconcha Sepiae) and *chūn gēn pí* (Cortex Ailanthi). The astringing method should only be applied as a branch treatment during emergency, or as a supplement to treating the root condition.

The most common clinical patterns of flooding and spotting are associated with deficiency, especially deficient heat. While clearing the source, cold medicinals should be prescribed with caution due to the possibility of damage to Stomach qi, which may lead to blood failing to return to the vessels.

(Tian Wei-zhong, Tian Wei-dong. Tian Xue-ming's Treatment on Arresting Patterns of Flooding 田学明老中医谈止崩之法 . *Tianjin Journal of Traditional Chinese Medicine* 天津中医 . 1997, 14 (1)：4-5)

10. Chai Song-yan's Experience in the Treatment of Flooding and Spotting

The pathomechanisms of flooding and spotting include:

(1) Spleen and Kidney insufficiency, with impairment of the penetrating and conception vessels.

(2) Latent heat in the sea of blood, with frenetic movement of blood-heat.

(3) Stagnation obstructing the uterus and blood failing to stay in the vessels.

Prescribe medicinals in accordance with the bleeding and non-bleeding stages, based on pattern differentiation.

(1) Blood-heat

1) Excessive Heat Patterns

Medicinals for the bleeding stage are as follows.

生牡蛎	shēng mǔ lì	30g	Concha Ostreae Cruda
柴胡	chái hú	4g	Radix Bupleuri
坤草	kūn cǎo	4g	Herba Leonuri
白芍	bái sháo	10g	Radix Paeoniae Alba
生地	shēng dì huáng	15g	Radix Rehmanniae
侧柏炭	cè bǎi tàn	15g	Cacumen Platycladi (carbonized)
荷叶	hé yè	10g	Folium Nelumbinis
椿皮	chūn pí	10g	Cortex Ailanthi
仙鹤草	xiān hè cǎo	12g	Herba Agrimoniae
大蓟	dà jì	12g	Herba Cirsii Japonici
小蓟	xiǎo jì	12g	Herba Cirsii
黄芩	huáng qín	8g	Radix Scutellariae

For profuse bleeding with slight abdominal pain, add *sān qī fěn* (Radix Notoginseng Powder) 3g (infused).

For dry bound stools, add *quán guā lóu* (Fructus Trichosanthis) 20g. Medicinals for the non-bleeding stage are as follows.

柴胡	chái hú	4g	Radix Bupleuri
荷叶	hé yè	6g	Folium Nelumbinis
麦冬	mài dōng	10g	Radix Ophiopogonis
椿皮	chūn pí	10g	Cortex Ailanthi
地骨皮	dì gǔ pí	10g	Cortex Lycii
白芍	bái sháo	12g	Radix Paeoniae Alba
女贞子	nǚ zhēn zǐ	15g	Fructus Ligustri Lucidi
茅根	máo gēn	20g	Rhizoma Imperatae

For persistent abnormal bleeding for over 25 days, use the medicinals indicated for the bleeding stage. Begin treatment on the second day of the regular menstrual cycle.

For an intermenstrual period of less than 22 days, add *shēng mǔ lì* (Concha Ostreae) 20g.

For delayed menstruation, add *yì mǔ cǎo* (Herba Leonuri) 10g.

2) Deficient Heat Patterns

Medicinals for the bleeding stage are as follows.

沙参	shā shēn	30g	Radix Adenophorae seu Glehniae
生牡蛎	shēng mǔ lì	30g	Concha Ostreae Cruda
生地	shēng dì huáng	15g	Radix Rehmanniae
仙鹤草	xiān hè cǎo	15g	Herba Agrimoniae
女贞子	nǚ zhēn zǐ	15g	Fructus Ligustri Lucidi
地骨皮	dì gǔ pí	10g	Cortex Lycii
椿皮	chūn pí	10g	Cortex Ailanthi
白芍	bái sháo	10g	Radix Paeoniae Alba
阿胶珠	ē jiāo zhū	10g	Colla Corii Asini Pilula
莲须	lián xū	10g	Stamen Nelumbinis
坤草	kūn cǎo	6g	Herba Leonuri

Medicinals for the non-bleeding stage are as follows.

枸杞子	gǒu qǐ zǐ	12g	Fructus Lycii
白芍	bái sháo	12g	Radix Paeoniae Alba
旱莲草	hàn lián cǎo	12g	Herba Ecliptae
百合	bǎi hé	12g	Bulbus Lilii
女贞子	nǚ zhēn zǐ	12g	Fructus Ligustri Lucidi
地骨皮	dì gǔ pí	10g	Cortex Lycii
沙参	shā shēn	10g	Radix Adenophorae seu Glehniae
覆盆子	fù pén zǐ	10g	Fructus Rubi
香附	xiāng fù	6g	Rhizoma Cyperi
柴胡	chái hú	5g	Radix Bupleuri

(2) Spleen and Kidney Qi Deficiency Pattern

Medicinals for bleeding stage are as follows.

太子参	tài zǐ shēn	20g	Radix Pseudostellariae
生牡蛎	shēng mǔ lì	30g	Concha Ostreae Cruda
仙鹤草	xiān hè cǎo	12g	Herba Agrimoniae
覆盆子	fù pén zǐ	12g	Fructus Rubi
莲须	lián xū	12g	Stamen Nelumbinis
首乌	shǒu wū	10g	Radix Polygoni Multiflori
阿胶珠	ē jiāo zhū	10g	Colla Corii Asini Pilula
枸杞	gǒu qǐ	12g	Fructus Lycii
白术	bái zhú	10g	Rhizoma Atractylodis Macrocephalae
柴胡	chái hú	6g	Radix Bupleuri
坤草	kūn cǎo	4g	Herba Leonuri

Medicinals for non-bleeding stage are as follows.

柴胡	chái hú	3g	Radix Bupleuri
太子参	tài zǐ shēn	12g	Radix Pseudostellariae
怀山药	huái shān yào	12g	Rhizoma Dioscoreae
阿胶珠	ē jiāo zhū	10g	Colla Corii Asini Pilula
覆盆子	fù pén zǐ	10g	Fructus Rubi

内金	jī nèi jīn	10g	Gigeriae Galli
枸杞子	gǒu qǐ zǐ	10g	Fructus Lycii
香附	xiāng fù	10g	Rhizoma Cyperi

For loose stools, add zé xiè (Rhizoma Alismatis).

For insomnia, add *shǒu wū* (Radix Polygoni Multiflori) 10g.

(3) Blood Stasis

柴胡	chái hú	3g	Radix Bupleuri
香附	xiāng fù	10g	Rhizoma Cyperi
坤草	kūn cǎo	10g	Herba Leonuri
茜草炭	qiàn cǎo tàn	10g	Radix Rubiae Carbonisata
杜仲	dù zhòng	10g	Cortex Eucommiae
仙鹤草	xiān hè cǎo	12g	Herba Agrimoniae
阿胶珠	ē jiāo zhū	12g	Colla Corii Asini Pilula
生牡蛎	shēng mǔ lì	15g	Concha Ostreae Cruda

Prognosis according to the pulses: Slippery and large pulses with profuse bleeding imply that the condition may become chronic. This pulse is often associated with heat patterns. Thready, or deep and weak pulses imply a relatively mild condition.

(Geng Jia-wei, Zhang Ming-ju. Introduction to Chai Song-yan's Experience in the Treatment of Flooding and Spotting 柴松岩治疗崩漏临床经验介绍 . *Beijing Journal of Traditional Chinese Medicine* 北京中医 . 1997, (4)：8-9)

11. Xu Shou-tian's Treatment of Adolescent Flooding and Spotting with the Cheng Yuan Method

Dr. Xu points out that proper treatment of DUB in adolescent patients emphasizes Cheng Yuan (treating the root). Medicinals for Se Liu (stanching bleeding) should only be used in acute conditions of severe bleeding. He also holds that freeing the vessels is the most effective approach to the treatment of chronic spotting.

Dr. Xu favors *Shī Xiào Sǎn* (失笑散). In this formula, *wǔ líng zhī* (Faeces Trogopterori) is sweet and warm in nature. It enters the Liver and invigorates blood. *Pú huáng* (Pollen Typhae) is sweet and acrid in nature. It breaks the blood and treats the stagnation of the Jueyin vessels. The combination of these two medicinals both invigorate blood and arrest bleeding while regulating the metabolism.

In clinic, adolescent DUB may present with combined deficient and excess patterns such as Kidney deficiency with blood stasis, or Spleen deficiency with Liver constraint. Thus, correct treatment should emphasize treatment of the the root. After the cessation of abnormal bleeding, it is necessary to regulate menstruation.

(1) Insufficiency of Kidney Qi

Treatment should tonify the Kidney and secure the penetrating vessel. Commonly used medicinals are as follows.

熟地	shú dì huáng	Radix Rehmanniae Praeparata
怀山药	huái shān yào	Rhizoma Dioscoreae
女贞子	nǚzhēn zǐ	Fructus Ligustri Lucidi
旱莲草	hàn lián cǎo	Herba Ecliptae
菟丝子	tù sī zǐ	Semen Cuscutae
枸杞子	gǒu qǐ zǐ	Fructus Lycii
首乌	shǒu wū	Radix Polygoni Multiflori
桑寄生	sāng jì shēng	Herba Taxilli
淫羊藿	yín yáng huò	Herba Epimedii
肉苁蓉	ròu cōng róng	Herba Cistanches

For yin deficiency, add *ē jiāo* (Colla Corii Asini) and *guī bǎn* (Testudinis Plastrum).

For yang deficiency, add *xiān máo* (Rhizoma Curculiginis) and *bā jǐ tiān* (Radix Morindae Officinalis).

(2) Deficient Spleen with Failure of Containment

The treatment principle is to invigorate the Spleen to manage blood. Commonly used medicinals are as follows.

党参	dǎng shēn	Radix Codonopsis
黄芪	huáng qí	Radix Astragali
白术	bái zhú	Rhizoma Atractylodis Macrocephalae
茯苓	fú líng	Poria
怀山药	huái shān yào	Rhizoma Dioscoreae
柏子仁	bǎi zǐ rén	Semen Platycladi
陈皮	chén pí	Pericarpium Citri Reticulatae
半夏	bàn xià	Rhizoma Pinelliae
仙鹤草	xiān hè cǎo	Herba Agrimoniae
炮姜	pào jiāng	Rhizoma Zingiberis Praeparata
大枣	dà zǎo	Fructus Jujubae
炙甘草	zhì gān cǎo	Radix et Rhizoma Glycyrrhizae Praeparata cum Melle

(3) Frenetic Movement of Blood-heat

The treatment principle is to clear heat and cool blood. Commonly used medicinals are as follows.

细生地	xì shēng dì	Radix Rehmanniae
丹皮	dān pí	Cortex Moutan
白芍	bái sháo	Radix Paeoniae Alba
川连	chuān lián	Rhizoma Coptidis
山栀	shān zhī	Fructus Gardeniae
石斛	shí hú	Herba Dendrobii
女贞子	nǚ zhēn zǐ	Fructus Ligustri Lucidi
旱莲草	hàn lián cǎo	Herba Ecliptae
地榆	dì yú	Radix Sanguisorbae
茜草	qiàn cǎo	Radix Rubiae
甘草	gān cǎo	Radix et Rhizoma Glycyrrhizae

(4) Stasis Stagnating in the Uterus

The treatment principle is to invigorate blood and dispel stasis. Commonly used medicinals are as follows.

当归	dāng guī	Radix Angelicae Sinensis
赤芍	chì sháo	Radix Paeoniae Rubra
川芎	chuān xiōng	Rhizoma Chuanxiong
蒲黄	pú huáng	Pollen Typhae
五灵脂	wǔ líng zhī	Faeces Trogopterori
艾叶	ài yè	Folium Artemisiae Argyi
炮姜	pào jiāng	Rhizoma Zingiberis Praeparata
益母草	yì mǔ cǎo	Herba Leonuri
香附	xiāng fù	Rhizoma Cyperi
茜草	qiàn cǎo	Radix Rubiae
红花	hóng huā	Flos Carthami

(Xu Jing-sheng. Xu Shou-tian's Experience in the Treatment of DUB in Adolescence 胥受天老中医诊治青春期功血经验 . *Liaoning Journal of Traditional Chinese Medicine* 辽宁中医杂志 . 1989, (7)：1-2)

12. Xu Run-san's Consideration of Kidney Function in the Treatment of Flood and Spotting

Dr. Xu considers flooding and spotting conditions to be primarily associated with disorders of the Liver and Kidney. In the progression of this disease, uterine blood stagnation appears during particular stages. Qi deficiency and blood-heat are also secondary syndromes that often appear during the bleeding stage. Therefore, effective treatment may be divided into two steps.

(1) Stanch Bleeding

1) Yin Deficiency with Blood-Heat Patterns

Select *Zī Yīn Zhǐ Xuè Fāng* (滋阴止血方).

生地	shēng dì huáng	30g	Radix Rehmanniae
女贞子	nǚzhēn zǐ	30g	Fructus Ligustri Lucidi
旱莲草	hàn lián cǎo	50g	Herba Ecliptae
阿胶	ē jiāo	10g	Colla Corii Asini (dissolved)
生甘草	shēng gān cǎo	6g	Radix et Rhizoma Glycyrrhizae (raw)
当归	dāng guī	10g	Radix Angelicae Sinensis
三七粉	sān qī fěn	3g	Radix Notoginseng Powder (infused)

2) Qi and Yang Deficiency Patterns

Select *Wēn Yáng Zhǐ Xuè Fāng* (温阳止血方).

鹿衔草	lù xián cǎo	60g	Herba Pyrolae
党参	dǎng shēn	50g	Radix Codonopsis
三七粉（分冲）	sān qī fěn	6g	Radix Notoginseng Powder (infused)

For predominate qi deficiency, add *dǎng shēn* (Radix Codonopsis) 100g.

3) Blood Stasis Stagnating in the Uterus

Select *Huà Yū Zhǐ Xuè Fāng* (化瘀止血方)

炒丹参	chǎo dān shēn	20g	Radix Salviae Miltiorrhizae (dry-fried)
党参	dǎng shēn	20g	Radix Codonopsis
益母草	yì mǔ cǎo	15g	Herba Leonuri
当归	dāng guī	10g	Radix Angelicae Sinensis
川芎	chuān xiōng	10g	Rhizoma Chuanxiong
制香附	zhì xiāng fù	10g	Rhizoma Cyperi Praeparata

三七粉（分冲）	sān qī fěn	3g	Radix Notoginseng Powder (infused)

4) Blood Stasis Transforming into Heat

Select *Liáng Xuè Huà Yū Fāng* (凉血化瘀方)

玳瑁	dài mào	10g	Carapax Eretmochelytis
桃仁	táo rén	10g	Semen Persicae
生地	shēng dì huáng	30g	Radix Rehmanniae
生白芍	shēng bái sháo	20g	Radix Paeoniae Alba (raw)
旱莲草	hàn lián cǎo	30g	Herba Ecliptae
丹皮	dān pí	15g	Cortex Moutan
红花	hóng huā	5g	Flos Carthami
三七粉（分冲）	sān qī fěn	3g	Radix Notoginseng Powder (infused)

For profuse bleeding, add blood nourishing medicinals. Select *ē jiāo* (Colla Corii Asini), *dǎng shēn* (Radix Codonopsis) and *tù sī zǐ* (Semen Cuscutae).

(2) Regulate Menses and Establish Ovulation

1) Liver and Kidney Yin Deficiency

Select *Zī Shèn Tiáo Zhōu Fāng* (滋肾调周方).

生地	shēng dì huáng	10g	Radix Rehmanniae
山萸肉	shān yú ròu	10g	Fructus Corni
生白芍	shēng bái sháo	10g	Radix Paeoniae Alba (raw)
当归	dāng guī	10g	Radix Angelicae Sinensis
紫河车	zǐ hé chē	10g	Placenta Hominis
制香附	zhì xiāng fù	10g	Rhizoma Cyperi Praeparata
山药	shān yào	15g	Rhizoma Dioscoreae
枸杞子	gǒu qǐ zǐ	15g	Fructus Lycii
益母草	yì mǔ cǎo	15g	Herba Leonuri
女贞子	nǚ zhēn zǐ	20g	Fructus Ligustri Lucidi

2) Kidney Yang Deficiency

Select *Wēn Shèn Tiáo Zhōu Fāng* (温肾调周方).

仙灵脾	xiān líng pí	12g	Herba Epimedii
仙茅	xiān máo	12g	Rhizoma Curculiginis
紫河车	zǐ hé chē	10g	Placenta Hominis
当归	dāng guī	10g	Radix Angelicae Sinensis
白芍	bái sháo	10g	Radix Paeoniae Alba
制香附	zhì xiāng fù	10g	Rhizoma Cyperi Praeparata
枸杞子	gǒu qǐ zǐ	20g	Fructus Lycii
女贞子	nǚ zhēn zǐ	15g	Fructus Ligustri Lucidi
党参	dǎng shēn	15g	Radix Codonopsis
益母草	yì mǔ cǎo	15g	Herba Leonuri

For qi deficiency, double the dosage of *dǎng shēn* (Radix Codonopsis).

In overweight patients, add *lù jiǎo shuāng* (Cornu Cervi Degelatinatum) 10g.

(Jing Yan, Zhao Hong, Ling Hong-zhi. Pattern Differetiation in Flooding and Spotting 崩漏辨治. *China Journal of Traditional Chinese Medicine and Pharmacy* 中国医药学报 . 1998, 13(6)：75)

PERSPECTIVES OF INTEGRATIVE MEDICINE

Challenges and Solutions

DUB is an acute, severe and stubborn disease in gynecology. Acute conditions refer to the symptoms of profuse vaginal bleeding, or flooding. Severe conditions refer to chronic bleeding patterns that lead to lowered hemoglobin levels, or even hemorrhagic shock. Stubborn refers to the difficulty of both arresting bleeding and restoring menstruation in the long term.

The challenges and solutions are as follows.

CHALLENGE #1: STANCH BLEEDING QUICKLY AND EFFECTIVELY

(1) Examination and Diagnosis of the Pathomechanism Using Pattern Differentiation

The pathomechanisms involved in DUB generally include deficiency, heat and stasis. Effective treatment is rare because these three causes may manifest singly or in combination, as well as interacting with one another. For this reason, DUB is referred to as a tenacious condition. The key to diagnosis and pattern differentiation is to clarify the consequences of treatment at each stage. To be specific, treatment will be fully effective only when determined by the progression of the disease, the course of treatment, the patient's constitution and reactions to medication, and the results of supplementary examination. For patients with no observable symptoms, treatment should be based primarily on the pathomechanisms of deficiency, heat and stasis. For profuse and acute bleeding patterns, treatment should emphasize the securing and lifting of qi. For chronic spotting, treatment should emphasize nourishing blood or dispelling stasis. Misuse of bleeding-arresting medicinals may also cause qi and blood stagnation in the uterus. Although bleeding patterns may cease temporarily, this disease may recur if the underlying cause is not fully addressed.

(2) Selecting Se Liu Treatments According to the Specific Presentation

There are three main methods to stanch bleeding:
1) Arrest bleeding
2) Arrest bleeding and treat the root
3) Treat the root and restore menses.
Effectiveness can be determined in three respective aspects:
1) Reduction or cessation of bleeding
2) Gradual cessation of profuse bleeding

3) Gradual prolongation of the non-bleeding stage, leading to normal menstruation.

(3) Integrate Medical Diagnosis with Both Pattern Differentiation and Therapeutic Method

Ovulatory DUB is known to be often directly associated with hysteromyoma. Therefore, DUB should be clearly differentiated from other diseases so that the underlying cause may be clarified. In the past, profuse vaginal bleeding was always diagnosed as simply flooding and spotting disorder. Modern theory views flooding and spotting disorders as a gynecological disease. In this way, both constitutional and structural conditions may be ruled out. Modern clinical experience shows that profuse vaginal bleeding is in fact often associated with flooding and spotting disorder. However, further examination is indicated to evaluate subsequent courses of treatment.

(4) The Application of Chinese Medicine with Biomedical Approaches

For particularly tenacious DUB where the effect of Chinese medicine is not sufficient, the integration of biomedical treatment is indicated.

(5) Selection of Blood Stanching Medicinals for Specific Blood Patterns

1) Medicinals that Tonify Deficiency and Secure Qi:

Rén shēn (Radix et Rhizoma Ginseng), *tài zǐ shēn* (Radix Pseudostellariae), *huáng qí* (Radix Astragali), *dǎng shēn* (Radix Codonopsis), *shā shēn* (Radix Adenophorae seu Glehniae), *dà zǎo* (Fructus Jujubae) and *shān yào* (Rhizoma Dioscoreae).

2) Medicinals that Clear Heat:

Guàn zhòng (Cyrtomii Rhizoma), *huáng qín* (Radix Scutellariae), *huáng bǎi* (Cortex Phellodendri Chinensis), *dà huáng* (Radix et Rhizoma Rhei), *xià kū cǎo* (Spica Prunellae), *hóng téng* (Caulis Sargentodoxae) and *bái huā shé shé cǎo* (Herba Hedyotis Diffusae).

3) Blood-cooling Medicinals:

Dà jì (Herba Cirsii Japonici), *xiǎo jì* (Herba Cirsii), *huái huā* (Flos Sophorae), *dì yú* (Radix Sanguisorbae), *cè bǎi yè* (Cacumen Platycladi), *bái máo gēn* (Rhizoma Imperatae), *zhù má gēn* (Radix Boehmeriae), *zǐ cǎo* (Radix Arnebiae), *shēng dì huáng* (Radix Rehmanniae) and *mǔ dān pí* (Cortex Moutan).

4) Medicinals that Warm the Vessels:

Chǎo ài yè (Dry-fried Folium Artemisiae Argyi), *chǎo xù duàn* (Dry-fried Radix Dipsaci), *pào jiāng tàn* (Rhizoma Zingiberis Carbonisata), *ròu guì* (Cortex Cinnamomi), *fù piàn* (Radix Aconiti Lateralis Praeparata) and *xiān líng pí* (Herba Epimedii).

5) Medicinals that Dispel Stasis:

Sān qī (Radix Notoginseng), *yì mǔ cǎo* (Herba Leonuri), *qiàn gēn tàn* (Carbonized Radix et Rhizoma Rubiae), *mǔ dān pí* (Cortex Moutan), *pú huáng* (Pollen Typhae), *jiàng xiāng* (Lignum Dalbergiae Odoriferae), *xiāng fù* (Rhizoma Cyperi) and *zhǐ qiào* (Fructus Aurantii).

6) Medicinals that Secure and Astringe:

Mǔ lì (Concha Ostreae), *lóng gǔ* (Fossilia Ossis Mastodi), *zhēn zhū mǔ* (Concha Margaritifera Usta) and *wū zéi gǔ* (Endoconcha Sepiae).

7) Medicinals that Restrain Leakage:

Xiān hè cǎo (Herba Agrimoniae), *jī guān huā* (Flos Celosiae Cristatae), *xuè yú tàn* (Crinis Carbonisatus), *zōng lǘ tàn* (Carbonized Petiolus Trachycarpi), *wū méi* (Fructus Mume), *ǒu jié* (Nodus Nelumbinis Rhizomatis), *huā shēng yī* (Arachis Hypogaea), *jīn yīng zǐ* (Fructus Rosae Laevigatae) and *Shí Huī Sǎn* (十灰散).

8) Medicinals that Tonify Blood:

Ē jiāo (Colla Corii Asini), *lù jiǎo jiāo* (Colla Cornus Cervi), *guī bǎn jiāo* (Colla Plastri Testudinis), *niú jiǎo jiāo* (Colla Cornus Os) and *bái sháo* (Radix Paeoniae Alba).

Challenge #2: Regulate Menses and Promote Ovulation

(1) Patient compliance is needed due to the relatively long term treatment that may be required.

(2) To avoid recurrence, normal ovulatory cycles should be achieved.

(3) When Chinese medicine fails to promote ovulation, integrative biomedical approaches may be indicated.

Treatments to promote ovulation are as follows.

1) Cyclic Treatment in Accordance with Menstruation:

For both adolescent and child bearing age patients, the treatment goal is to re-establish regular ovulation. There are two primary approaches to treatment. First is to regulate the reproductive and endocrine function by stimulating development of the primordial follicle during the non-bleeding stage. Secondly, we aim to control the volume and length of the abnormal bleeding pattern. Formulas that both invigorate the Kidney and dispel blood stasis are indicated. This approach may be used for 2-3 cycles, followed by a semi-cyclic treatment plan. BBT should be monitored throughout treatment.

2) Semi-cyclic Treatment:

Treatment is applied only during the postmenstrual period in anovular patients. Medicinals that both tonify the Kidney and replenish essence are first prescribed to promote follicular development, followed by blood invigorating and qi rectifying medicinals to promote ovulation. Generally, medicinals should be taken for 5 to 10 days beginning on the fifth day of the cycle, or after bleeding has ceased. However, with elevated BBT, medicinals may be discontinued. The semi-cyclic approach may be applied in patients of ovulatory type during the follicular and beta phases. The principle is to primarily tonify Kidney yin in the former, while replenishing essence and tonifying Kidney yang in the latter.

3) Medicinals for Cyclic Treatments:

Formulas that both tonify Kidney yin and replenish essence may function to promote follicular development. Medicinals that rectify qi, invigorate blood, and warm Kidney yang may promote ovulation through their effect on the corpus luteum.

Insight from Empirical Wisdom

1. FACTORS INFLUENCING THE EFFECTIVE TREATMENT OF DUB

There are four aspects to consider during treatment.

(1) The Establishment of a Proper Treatment Plan

DUB is a condition that requires a highly individualized treatment based on a thorough gynecological examination. Appropriate treatment should be determined based on patient history, laboratory examination, and the progression and presenting symptoms of the disease. We may choose to use Chinese medicine, biomedicine, or an integrative approach. All require treatment of the abnormal bleeding patterns as well as the establishment of regular menstrual cycles. The former approach addresses the presenting symptoms, where the latter is the required for a long-term effect. Chronic conditions usually require an extended treatment plan. Therefore it is important to perform a thorough intake to ensure the most effective and efficient treatment.

Ovarian function is generally stable during the childbearing period, where anovulatory conditions are most typical in adolescent and premenopausal patients. Anovulation during adolescence or menopause not only impairs reproductive function, but may also lead to other associated conditions. Ovarian function in adolescent patients is in a state of development, whereas during the menopausal period it is in decline. Although both groups present anovular DUB, each requires its own approach to treatment. In adolescents, the general goal is to arrest bleeding and support ovarian function through tonification of the Kidney. In menopausal patients, we must stanch bleeding while addressing possible anemia. Nourishing blood, strengthening the Spleen, and rectifying qi are the main treatment principles.

(2) The Selection of Biomedicines

An integrative approach to treatment may be required. This includes the application of modern biomedicines in combination with the appropriate Chinese medicinals. Our treatment objectives are to stanch bleeding, relieve symptoms, and also establish regular ovulatory menstrual cycles. Using TCM treatment alone, it is essential to prescribe medicinals in proper combination in order to address multiple patterns. There is a complex relationship between disease diagnosis, pattern differentiation, and medicinal selection. Since the proper approach to treatment is often not completely understood, clinical results may be poor.

For example, it is difficult to quickly and effectively control abnormal bleeding while also attempting to regulate menstruation. Furthermore, clinical reports show a variety of approaches in the choice of medicinals for Se Liu, Cheng Yuan and Fu Jiu. However, during the bleeding stage, the Se Liu and Cheng Yuan methods combined have been shown to be more effective than the application of Se Liu alone.

(3) Consistency of Treatment

1) Treatment in Accordance with the Bleeding Pattern:

It is of course important to determine the proper treatment principle. Typically, we must decide whether to focus on stanching bleeding or removing obstruction. For patients with DUB of recent onset, when bleeding occurs near the normal cycle, treatment should mainly focus on removing obstruction. This is to avoid possible endocrine disturbances of the reproductive axis. This approach provides a good foundation for regulating menstruation in the future. The primary treatment in other cases may emphasize the Se Liu method. For patients with chronic conditions, it is important to be aware of any periodic increase in bleeding. If so, approach the bleeding symptom as a menstrual cycle and treat accordingly. After 3-5 days, the main method is the Se Liu approach. Consistent treatment at that time requires both stanching bleeding and regulating the menses.

2) Treatment in Accordance with the Storage and Release Functions of the Uterus:

The physiological function of uterus involves storing and releasing at regular intervals. The proper manifestation of the release function is seen during menstruation and childbirth. The manifestation of storage is seen during the accumulation of menses and the formation of the embryo. Uterine dysfunction in DUB patients is associated with disorders of storage and release, therefore the stages of uterine function should be considered. These include the storage stage, the release stage, the transition from releasing to storage, and vice versa. The proper approach is to tonify and secure the penetrating and conception vessels during the storage phase, where during the release phase we emphasize the dispelling of stasis. During the transition stages we should combine these approaches accordingly. Only when uterine functions are regulated can the patient fully recover.

Ultrasonic examination may be useful in determining physiological function in anovular DUB patients. Stanching bleeding at the proper time is essential. During the storage stage, the qi and blood of the penetrating and conception vessels tends to be relatively insufficient. Endometrial thickness should also be measured. At 0.2-0.5cm, blood tonification is the primary treatment principle. At 0.6-1.3cm, the qi and blood of the penetrating and conception vessels tends to stagnate. In this case, the correct principle is to invigorate blood.

For patients with a relatively thin endometrium, Se Liu may be applied alone or in combination with Cheng Yuan and Fu jiu methods. For flooding and spotting disorder, the general approach is primarily based on the Se Liu method. However, for sudden flooding, we should stanch bleeding while also considering the root cause. Combining Se Liu and Cheng Yuan methods should be considered in light of the presenting symptoms as well as the severity and progression of the condition. For chronic cases with the absence of clotting or severe symptoms, the primary approach is to dispel blood stasis and arrest bleeding. Ultrasonic examination should be performed to determine endometrial thickness. If the endometrium is relatively thick, this suggests qi and blood stagnation in the uterus and penetrating and conception vessels, despite the absence of clotting or other signs of blood stasis. The treatment principle in this case is to rectify qi, dispel blood stasis, and stanch bleeding while stimulating defluxion of the endometrium. If the endometrium is relatively thin, we should tonify the Kidney and strengthen the Spleen to assist endometrial development. Modifications to the formula should be based on pattern differentiation as well the status of the uterus.

3) DUB due to Asynchronous Ovarian Function:

Generally, only one ovary functions during each menstrual cycle. If both are functioning, 1-2 mature dominant follicles may be produced. Proper functioning of the uterus is shown by the presence of periodic bleeding, or regular monthly cycles. Diphase BBT typically indicates anovulation.

If bilateral ovarian cycles are asynchronous with persistent follicle development, particular clinical manifestations will appear. Follicles from both ovaries may develop at the same time, which may manifest as irregular bleeding patterns. Monophase BBT does not in itself indicate ovulation, as two asynchronous ovulations may appear outside the normal cycle, one often immediately following menstruation. This condition may lead to DUB as well as unintentional pregnancy.

In cases presenting one mature dominant follicle with the concurrent development of several immature follicles, endometrial function may be over stimulated, causing hyperplasia. The dominant ovarian follicle should be supported while the other should be inhibited. Monitor by ultrasonic examination.

2. Regulating Menstruation in Adolescent DUB Patients

At present, there are two approaches to the treatment of adolescents. One method is to first address the abnormal bleeding pattern, followed by treatments to regulate menstruation.

The long-term goal of treatment is to establish regular ovulation. The other is to stanch bleeding while simultaneously attempting to establish normal cycles. This approach more generally supports reproductive functioning and development, which may lead to natural and spontaneous ovulation.

The aim of first approach is to actively treat the symptoms, prevent recurrence, and provide a foundation for reproductive functioning in the future. The second approach lets nature take its course. To avoid the the exhaustion of ovarian follicle, follicle release should be limited to the propose of reproduction during the childbearing period.

Reproductive ovarian functioning peaks during the childbearing period, rather than during adolescence. Since adolescents are not yet mature, it may be more appropriate to allow ovulation to occur naturally, rather than attempting to induce it with medicinals. As a result, reproductive function becomes active at the optimum time. It is more appropriate to allow follicles to remain semi-dormant until the optimum time for reproduction. However, the treatment plan requires a long-term approach with follow-up examinations. If the patient remains anovulatory by the age of 18, ovarian function may be actively stimulated. In Chinese Medicine, ovarian function is directly related to the congenital constitution. If congenital Kidney qi is sufficient, ovulation occurs and reproductive function may remain stable for a long period of time. In treatment, normal ovulatory cycles may be established spontaneously. With congenital deficiency there may be difficulty in establishing normal ovulation, and the childbearing period may be relatively short. Long-term treatment plans should be established in order to regulate the ovarian function. For women younger than 18, especially those with early menarche at ages 11 to 13, only regulation of the menstrual cycles may be needed. Ovaries may remain semi-dormant rather than actively promoted. Treatment for adolescent DUB should be determined based on the congenital constitution, where long-term follow up is indicated for those with deficiencies.

Summary

1. THE ADVANTAGES OF BIOMEDICINE AND CHINESE MEDICINALS

The treatment of DUB may include both biomedical and non-medical methods. Both methods stanch abnormal bleeding patterns and effectively treat the root through the regulation of menstruation.

The advantage of biomedicine is the clarity of the effect and mechanism of action. Menstrual cycles can be restored quickly and effectively with hormone therapy. Supplementary gynecological examinations may be useful for objective evaluation of both the diagnosis and treatment effect. Surgery is very effective for patients with profuse or acute bleeding, and biomedicines that promote ovulation often restore reproductive function more quickly.

The advantage of Chinese medicinal formulas is their ability to promote reproductive function through combining a variety of medicinals. Their effects are stable over time, and there are no side effects when used long term, such as decreased ovarian function. In addition, they may also improve the general function of other physiological systems.

2. CREATING INDIVIDUALIZED TREATMENT PLANS

(1) Individual Treatment Plans

Treatment objectives are based on a variety of factors, particularly the age of the patient. We may divide patients into three specific groups. The first group includes adolescents who have recently begun menstruating, and women approaching menopause. The main treatment goal is to relieve general symptoms, and address possible anemia due to excessive blood loss. The second group includes mature adolescents and menopausal women. Here the aims are to re-establish regular menstruation and relieve menopausal symptoms respectively. The third group includes women in the childbearing period. The goal here is to establish reproductive health. Individualized treatment plans are required for each group.

(2) The Principles of Individualized Treatment Plans

The goals of treatment should first be clear. Both the age of the patient and the congenital constitution should be taken into consideration. Whether or not the patient desires to conceive is also a deciding factor. Other associated disease conditions should be ruled out. Integrative treatment should be considered, as this may be proved to be the most effective approach.

3. SYNERGISTIC EFFECTS OF MEDICINALS THAT REGULATE MENSES AND STIMULATE OVULATION

(1) Estrogen-like Effects of Medicinals and Formulas that Tonify the Kidney

Research shows that herbs and formulas which invigorate the Kidney have estrogen-like effects, which may raise estrogen levels or promote estrogen-like effects. Both show synergistic effects in both the promotion of follicular development and endometrial hyperplasia. Therefore, the application of Kidney tonics may be useful in reducing both the dosages and side effects of estrogen therapy. With appropriate clinical conditions, these medicinals may effectively replace estrogen therapy completely.

(2) Medicinals that Course the Liver and Stanch Bleeding and Their Effects on Ovulation

When combined with Kidney tonics and prescribed in the late follicular phase, these medicinals have been shown to effectively stimulate ovulation.

(3) Stimulation of the Corpus Luteum with Medicinals that Invigorate Blood and Rectify Qi

Research shows that these medicinals may promote the functions of corpus luteum which are also associated with elevated BBT.

(4) Medicinals that Invigorate Blood, Rectify Qi, Dispel Blood Stasis and Free the Channels and Their Effects on Hormone Withdrawal

These medicinals may accelerate defluxion of the endometrium during the progestational stage, particularly during progestin withdrawal. They may also be useful during the proliferative phase at specific estrogen levels.

4. CURETTAGE AND THE USE OF MEDICINALS THAT TONIFY QI, DISPEL BLOOD STASIS, AND CLEAR HEAT

DUB may be associated with single or complex patterns of deficiency, heat, or blood stasis. These pathomechanisms often have relationships of cause and effect. Both deficiency and heat conditions may lead to blood stasis patterns. As a result, new blood is unable to flow in the vessels, which tends to aggravate the abnormal bleeding condition. Chinese medicinals may effectively address the deficiency and heat patterns. However, during the course of treating the blood stasis condition, severe anemia may result from excessive blood loss, and diagnostic curettage may be indicated.

5. Efficacy and Safety in the Integrative Treatment of DUB

Generally speaking, formulas that stanch acute flooding include medicinals that tonify qi, where Kidney tonifying medicinals are also included to regulate menstruation and secure the origin. The main symptom of DUB is the prescence of abnormal bleeding. Since qi and blood share the same source and are rooted in one another, qi moves the blood and blood carries qi. So, excessive blood loss will inevitably be accompanied by qi deficiency or even desertion. Formulas for acute flooding conditions must therefore include medicinals to tonify qi, secure the penetrating and conception vessels, prevent stasis, and also nourish the source of transformation. Being responsible for reproduction, the Kidney is also the foundation of menstrual function. Therefore, medicinals to regulate menstruation are always accompanied by those that strengthen the Kidney.

The safety and efficacy of Chinese medicinals are highly consistent in adolescent DUB treatment. For childbearing age patients who present hormone related conditions such as hysteromyoma and endometriosis, tonifying qi remains a safe and effective treatment method.

However, the long-term effects of both regulating menstruation and nourishing the Kidney are in question. Kidney-tonifying medicinals should therefore be used with caution in patients of childbearing age.

In menopausal patients, the main clinical manifestations involve Kidney deficiency. Although Kidney tonification is indicated, it is inevitable that ovarian function will decline. Androgen and progestin are safer choices for treatment during the menopausal period, as estrogen or estrogen-like treatment may increase the incidence of breast or uterine tumors. They may also be effectively combined with medicinals that both tonify qi and strengthen the Spleen.

SELECTED QUOTES FROM CLASSICAL TEXTS

Spiritual Pivot-Origins of Miscellaneous Diseases ,Chapter 66 (灵枢 • 百
病始生篇第六十六 , *Líng Shū • Bǎi Bìng Shǐ Shēng Piān Liù Shí Liù*):
　"阳络伤则血外溢，阴络伤则血内溢。"

　"Impairment of the yang collaterals leads to blood flooding
outwardly, while impairment of the yin collaterals leads to blood flooding
inwardly."

*Plain Questions-Discussions on the Differences between Yin and Yang,
Chapter 7* (素问 • 阴阳别论篇第七 , *Sù Wèn • Yīn Yáng Bié Lùn Piān Dì Qī*):
　"阴虚阳搏谓之崩。"

　"Exuberant yang due to deficient yin results in flooding."

Fine Formulas for Women-Formulas for Acute Flooding, Chapter 15 (妇人
大全良方 • 崩暴下血不止方论第十五 , *Fù Rén Dà Quán Liáng Fāng • Bēng
Bào Xià Xuè Bù Zhǐ Fāng Lùn Dì Shí Wǔ*):
　"妇人崩中者，由脏腑损伤，冲脉任脉血气俱虚故也。"

　"Flooding in women is associated with impairment of the zang-
fu organs, as well as qi and blood deficiency of the penetrating and
conception vessels."

*Complete Works of Jing-yue-Volume of Gynecology, Flooding and Spotting,
Chapter 12* (景岳全书 • 妇人规 • 崩淋经漏不止十二 , *Jǐng Yuè Quán Shū •
Fù Rén Guī • Bēng Lín Jīng Lòu Bù Zhǐ Shí Èr*):
　"崩漏不止，经乱之甚者也。盖乱则或前或后，漏则不时妄行。"
　"崩淋既久，真阴日亏，多致寒热咳嗽，脉见弦数或豁大等证。此乃元气

亏损，阴虚假热之脉，尤当用参、地、归、术甘温之属，以峻培本源，庶可望生。"

"Flooding and spotting is a severe menstrual disorder. Disorder refers to either a delayed or advanced menstrual cycle, where spotting refers to both irregular and frenetic menstruation."

"Chronic flooding and spotting may lead to a gradual deficiency of true yin. Symptoms include alternating fever and chills, cough, and pulses which may be wiry and rapid, or gaping and large. These pulse qualities indicate a deficiency of the original qi, accompanied by yin deficiency with false heat. Medicinals that are sweet and warm in nature such as *rén shēn* (Radix et Rhizoma Ginseng), *dì huáng* (Radix Rehmanniae), *dāng guī* (Radix Angelicae Sinensis) and *bái zhú* (Rhizoma Atractylodis Macrocephalae) are indicated in order to strongly bank the source, and potentially save the patients' life."

Origin and Indicators of Disease-Miscellaneous Diseases of Gynecology-Indicator for Spotting, Part 2 (诸病源候论 · 妇人杂病诸候二 · 漏下侯 , *Zhū Bìng Yuán Hòu Lùn · Fù Rén Zá Bìng Zhū Hòu Èr · Lòu Xià Hòu*):
"血非时而下淋漓不断，谓之漏下。"

"Longstanding irregular bleeding patterns are referred to as spotting."

Origin and Indicators of Disease-Miscellaneous Diseases of Gynecology-Indicators for flooding and spotting, Part 2 (诸病源候论 · 妇人杂病诸候二 · 崩中漏下侯 , *Zhū Bìng Yuán Hòu Lùn · Fù Rén Zá Bìng Zhū Hòu · Bēng Zhōng Lòu Xià Hòu*):
"崩中之状，是伤损冲任之脉，冲任之脉皆起于胞内，为经脉之海，劳伤过度，冲任气虚，不能制约经血，故忽然崩下，淋沥不断，名曰崩中漏下。"

"Flooding is associated with impairment of the penetrating and conception vessels. Both vessels originate from the uterus, and are considered to be the sea of all vessels. Taxation may lead to deficient qi, failing to contain the menses. Therefore, sudden flooding and persistent spotting develop. This is called flooding and spotting."

Modification of Necessities for Women's Diseases-Flooding, Chapter 8 (女科辑要笺正・第八节血崩, *Nǚ Kē Jí Yào Jiān Zhèng・Dì Bā Jié Xuè Bēng*):

"崩中一证，因火者多，因寒者少，然即使是火，亦是虚火，非实火可比。"

"Most cases of flooding are associated with fire rather than cold. However, this fire results from conditions of deficiency rather than of excess."

Fu Qing-zhu's Studies on Gynecology-Dizziness due to Flooding, Part 6 (傅青主女科・血崩昏暗六, *Fù Qīng Zhǔ Nǚ Kē・Xuè Bēng Hūn Àn Liù*):

"止崩之药不可独用，必须于补阴之中行止崩之法。"

"Medicinals that arrest flooding must be combined with those that nourish yin."

Fu Qingzhu's Studies on Gynecology-Flooding due to Constraint, Part 10 (傅青主女科・郁结血崩十, *Fù Qīng Zhǔ Nǚ kē・Yù Jié Xuè Bēng Shí*):

"妇人有怀抱甚郁，口干舌渴，呕吐吞酸，而血下崩者，人皆以火治之，时而效，时而不效，其故何也？是不识为肝气之郁结也。夫肝主藏血，气结而血亦结，何以反至崩漏？盖肝之性急，气结则其急更甚，更急则血不能藏，故崩不免也。治法宜以开郁为主，……方用平肝开郁止血汤。"

"In women with constrained emotions, symptoms such as dry mouth, thirst, vomiting, and acid regurgitation are commonly seen along with flooding. Treating it as a heat pattern is not always effective, because the actual cause is due to constraint of Liver qi. The Liver governs the storage of blood. Furthermore, constraint of qi often leads to stagnation of blood. But in these cases, the constraint of qi further aggravates the Liver, which may lead to flooding disorder directly. Correct treatment must primarily relieve constraint. *Píng Gān Kāi Yù Zhǐ Xuè Tāng* (平肝开郁止血汤) is indicated."

Golden Mirror of the Medical Tradition-Essential Experience of Gynecology-Flooding and Spotting (医宗金鉴·妇科心法要诀·崩漏门, *Yī Zōng Jīn Jiàn · Fù Kē Xīn Fǎ Yào Jué · Bēng Lòu Mén*):
"妇人经行之后，淋漓不止，名曰经漏。经血忽然大下不止，名为经崩。"

"Persistent inter-menstrual bleeding is called menstrual spotting. Sudden and acute menstrual bleeding is called flooding."

Golden Mirror of the Medical Tradition-Essential Experience of Gynecology-Regulating Menstruation (医宗金鉴·妇科心法要诀·调经证治, *Yī Zōng Jīn Jiàn · Fù Kē Xīn Fǎ Yào Jué · Tiáo Jīng Zhèng Zhì*):
"若血多有块，色紫稠黏，乃内有瘀血，用四物汤加桃仁、红花破之，名桃红四物汤。先期血少浅淡，乃气虚不能摄血也，用当归补血汤补之，其方即当归，黄耆也。若血涩少，其色赤者，乃热盛滞血，用四物汤加姜黄、黄芩、丹皮、香附、延胡通之。"

"Profuse, purplish and thick menses with clotting are associated with blood stasis. Purge with *Táo Hóng Sì Wù Tāng* (桃红四物汤), which consists of *Sì Wù Tāng* (四物汤) with added *táo rén* (Semen Persicae) and *hóng huā* (Flos Carthami)."

"Advanced and scant menses that are light in color indicate deficient qi failing to contain blood. Tonify with *Dāng Guī Bǔ Xuè Tāng* (当归补血

汤) which contains both *dāng guī* (Radix Angelicae Sinensis) and *huáng qí* (Radix Astragali)."

"Inhibited and scant red menses indicates exuberant heat stagnating blood. Free the vessels with *Sì Wù Tāng* (四物汤) plus added *jiāng huáng* (Rhizoma Curcumae Longae), *huáng qín* (Radix Scutellariae), *dān pí* (Cortex Moutan), *xiāng fù* (Rhizoma Cyperi) and *yán hú* (Rhizoma Corydalis)."

Discussion on Blood Patterns, Chapter of Flooding and Discharge (血证论 · 崩带, *Xuè Zhèng Lùn · Bēng Dài*):

"崩漏者，非经期而下血之谓也。"

"古名崩中，谓血乃中州脾土所统摄，脾不摄血，是以崩溃，名曰崩中，示人治崩，必治中州也。"

"Menses that do not appear with regularity are called flooding and spotting."

"The classic name of flooding, "Beng Zhong" (Middle Collapse) refers to the Spleen earth in the central region whose function is to contain blood. Collapse is due to the Spleen failing to contain blood. This illustrates that the treatment of flooding and spotting must always address the middle jiao."

Basic Introduction to Medicine-Gynecology (医学入门 · 妇人门, *Yī Xué Rù Mén · Fù Rén Mén*):

"凡非时血行，淋漓不净，谓之漏下；忽然暴下，若山崩然，谓之崩中。"

"Irregular menstruation that is accompanied by inter-menstrual bleeding is called spotting. Sudden menstruation that occurs like a landslide is called flooding."

Formulas for Common People-Chapter of Flooding and Spotting (济生方 · 崩漏, *Jì Shēng Fāng · Bēng Lòu*):

"崩漏之疾，本乎一证，轻者谓之漏下，甚者谓之崩中。"

"Flooding and spotting are both associated with the same disease. The minor condition is called spotting, and the major condition is called flooding."

Supplement to Zhu Dan-xi's Experience (丹溪心法附余, *Dān Xī Xīn Fǎ Fù Yú*):

"初用止血以塞其流，中用清热凉血以澄其源，末用补血以还其流。若只塞其流不澄其源，则滔天之势不能遏；若只澄其源不复其旧，则孤孑之阳无以立，故本末勿遗，前后不紊，方可言治也。"

"In the earliest stage of the disease course, the treatment principle is to stop bleeding. In the middle stage, the treatment principle is to purge heat and cool blood to treat the source. In the later stage, treatment should nourish blood in order to establish menstruation. By only arresting bleeding without treating the source, flooding may likely not be controlled. Treating only the source also may not establish normal menstruation, therefore the single yang method is not indicated for these conditions. All aspects of the disease process should be considered."

Secrets from the Orchid Chamber-Gynecology (兰室秘藏 · 妇人门, *Lán Shì Mì Cáng · Fù Rén Mén*):

"妇人血崩，是肾水阴虚，不能镇守胞络相火，故血走而崩也。"

"Flooding is associated with yin deficiency of the Kidney which fails to settle the ministerial fire in the uterine collaterals, leading to blood running out of the vessels."

The Jade Ruler of Gynecology-Chapter of Flooding (妇科玉尺 · 崩漏 , *Fù Kē Yù Chǐ · Bēng Lòu*):

"崩漏，究其源，则有六大端：一由火热，二由虚寒，三由劳伤，四由气陷，五由血瘀，六由虚弱。"

"There are six principle causes of flooding and spotting: heat, deficient cold, overwork, qi fall, blood stasis, and general deficiency."

MODERN RESEARCH

Clinical Research

1. PATTERN DIFFERENTIATION AND CORRESPONDING TREATMENT

(1) DUB in Adolescents

In clinical trials, Liu Zheng-jian and his colleagues divided DUB patients into 3 treatment groups. Their respective patterns included qi deficiency, blood-heat with deficiency, and Kidney deficiency. For qi deficiency patterns, the following medicinals were selected.

Dǎng shēn (Radix Codonopsis) 30-60g, *hóng shēn* (Radix et Rhizoma Ginseng Rubra)10g, *huái shān yào* (Rhizoma Dioscoreae) 30g, *huáng jīng* (Rhizoma Polygonati) 30g, *hé shǒu wū* (Radix Polygoni Multiflori) 15g, *shēng huáng qí* (Radix Astragali Cruda) 15g, *hǎi piāo xiāo* (Endoconcha Sepiae) 15g, *huā ruǐ shí* (Ophicalcitum) 20g, *shēng dà huáng* (Raw Radix et Rhizoma Rhei) 10g, *shēng má* (Rhizoma Cimicifugae) 6g and *zhì gān cǎo* (Radix et Rhizoma Glycyrrhizae Praeparata cum Melle) 6g.

For blood-heat patterns, *tài zǐ shēn* (Radix Pseudostellariae) 60g, *xī yáng shēn* (Radix Panacis Quinquefolii) 6g, *shēng huáng qí* (Radix Astragali Cruda) 15g, *hǎi piāo xiāo* (Endoconcha Sepiae) 15g, *hé shǒu wū* (Radix

Polygoni Multiflori) 15g, *bái sháo* (Radix Paeoniae Alba) 15g, *chǎo huáng qín* (Dry-fried Radix Scutellariae) 15g, *dà shēng dì* (Radix Rehmanniae) 30g, *huā ruǐ shí* (Ophicalcitum) 20g, *tù sī zǐ* (Semen Cuscutae) 10g, and *shēng dà huáng* (Raw Radix et Rhizoma Rhei) 10g were selected.

For Kidney deficiency patterns, *tài zǐ shēn* (Radix Pseudostellariae) 30-60g, *dà shēng dì* (Radix Rehmanniae) 30g, *huái shān yào* (Rhizoma Dioscoreae)30g, *huā ruǐ shí* (Ophicalcitum) 20g, *shēng dà huáng* (Raw Radix et Rhizoma Rhei) 10g, *hǎi piāo xiāo* (Endoconcha Sepiae) 15g, *bái sháo* (Radix Paeoniae Alba) 15g, *shān zhū yú* (Fructus Corni) 15g, *chǎo dù zhòng* (Dry-fried Cortex Eucommiae) 15g and *tù sī zǐ* (Semen Cuscutae) 15g were selected. In this formula, *huā ruǐ shí* (Ophicalcitum) was included due to its sour, astringent, and neutral properties. This medicinal may arrest bleeding without causing stasis. *Shēng dà huáng* (Raw Radix et Rhizoma Rhei) has cold and bitter properties which both dispel blood stasis and generate new blood. [1]

According to Dr. Li Jun-you, patterns of deficient yin and excessive fire in adolescents are typically caused by an insufficiency of qi, essence, and Kidney yin. These patterns may cause uterine disturbances which lead to flooding and spotting disorder. Adolescent flooding and spotting is most often associated with blood-heat and yin deficiency patterns. Young people may also tend to consume an excess of cold-natured foods, and also often present with affect damage. These lifestyle conditions almost always lead to patterns involving blood stasis combined with heat.

His formula, modified *Qīng Huà Zhǐ Bēng Tāng* (清化止崩汤) has been shown to be very effective in the treatment of adolescent DUB.

Medicinals include *dāng guī* (Radix Angelicae Sinensis) 12g, *bái sháo* (Radix Paeoniae Alba) 12g, *chuān xù duàn* (Radix Dipsaci) 12g, *shēng dì huáng* (Radix Rehmanniae) 15g, *yì mǔ cǎo* (Herba Leonuri) 15g, *chì sháo* (Radix Paeoniae Rubra) 10g, *mǔ dān pí* (Cortex Moutan)10g, *bái wēi* (Radix et Rhizoma Cynanchi Atrati) 10g, *qiàn căo* (Radix Rubiae) 10g, *zé lán* (Herba Lycopi) 10g, *bái máo gēn* (Rhizoma Imperatae) 30g, and *ŏu jié* (Nodus Nelumbinis Rhizomatis) 30g. Three months constitutes one course of treatment. [2]

Dr. Bi Hua and her colleagues treated 26 cases of DUB with medicinals that invigorate yin and purge yang.

The basic formula contained *zhì guī băn* (Fried with liquid Testudinis Plastrum) 10-24g, *shēng dì huáng* (Radix Rehmanniae) 15g, *dì gŭ pí* (Cortex Lycii) 15g, *zhì nŭ zhēn* (Prepared Fructus Ligustri Lucidi) 15g, *mò hàn lián* (Herba Ecliptae) 15g, *lù xián căo* (Herba Pyrolae) 15g, *huái shān yào* (Rhizoma Dioscoreae) 15g, *shān yú ròu* (Fructus Corni) 10g, *chăo huáng qín* (Dry-fried Radix Scutellariae) 10g, and *chăo huáng băi* (Dry-fried Cortex Phellodendri Chinensis) 10g.

With excessive heat associated with yin deficiency and profuse bleeding, *xiān hè căo* (Herba Agrimoniae), *shēng dì yú* (Raw Radix Sanguisorbae) and *guàn zhòng* (Cyrtomii Rhizoma) were added to further invigorate yin and clear heat.

With yin deficiency and Liver fire, *dān pí* (Cortex Moutan) and *shān zhī* (Fructus Gardeniae) were added.

With profuse bleeding or spotting with epigastric pain, *Shī Xiào Săn* (失笑散), *yì mŭ căo* (Herba Leonuri) 15g and *ŏu jié tàn* (Nodus Nelumbinis Rhizomatis Carbonisata) were added to dispel blood stasis and stanch bleeding.

With qi and yin deficiency due to chronic bleeding, *shēng huáng qí* (Radix Astragali Cruda) and *dăng shēn* (Radix Codonopsis) were added to tonify qi.

With damp summer-heat, and disturbances of the penetrating vessel, *fú líng* (Poria) and *bàn xià* (Rhizoma Pinelliae) were added to calm the spirit and purge heat.

With anxiety, *wŭ wèi zĭ* (Fructus Schisandrae), *hé huān pí* (Cortex

Albiziae) and *yè jiāo téng* (Caulis Polygoni Multiflori) were added to calm the spirit and secure the penetrating vessel.

With constipation, *guā lóu rén* (Semen Trichosanthis) and *xuán shēn* (Radix Scrophulariae) were added to moisten the intestines and unblock the viscera.

Results showed 12 cases fully recovered, 10 cases with excellent response, 2 cases effective, and 2 cases ineffective. The total effective rate reached 83%. [3]

Shi Heng-min used an empirical formula to treat 50 cases of adolescent DUB.

The formula included *hóng shēn* (Radix et Rhizoma Ginseng Rubra) or *dǎng shēn* (Radix Codonopsis) 10g, *mài dōng* (Radix Ophiopogonis) 10g, *yuǎn zhì* (Radix Polygalae) 10g, *ē jiāo* (Colla Corii Asini) 10g, *huáng qí* (Radix Astragali) 15g, *chuān xù duàn* (Radix Dipsaci) 15g, *shēng dì huáng* (Radix Rehmanniae) 15g, *shú dì huáng* (Radix Rehmanniae Praeparata) 15g, *tù sī zǐ* (Semen Cuscutae) 20g, *dì yú tàn* (Radix Sanguisorbae Carbonisata) 30g, *duàn lóng gǔ* (Calcined Fossilia Ossis Mastodi) 30g and *duàn mǔ lì* (Calcined Concha Ostreae) 30g.

Results showed 35 cases fully recovered, 7 cases with excellent response, and 3 cases improved. The total effective rate reached 100%. [4]

Dr. Zhu Pei-yan divided adolescent DUB patients into 2 treatment groups, a qi and blood deficiency group and another presenting internal heat due to yin deficiency. The general treatment principle was to regulate and tonify the penetrating and conception vesssels. With early menstruation, formulas were used to tonify both qi and yin such as *Liù Wèi Dì Huáng Tāng* (六味地黄汤) combined with *Èr Zhì Wán* (二至丸) and *Guī Pí Tāng* (归脾汤).

Commonly selected medicinals included *shān yào* (Rhizoma Dioscoreae), *shú dì huáng* (Radix Rehmanniae Praeparata), *shān zhū yú* (Fructus Corni), *dān pí* (Cortex Moutan), *nǚ zhēn zǐ* (Fructus Ligustri

Lucidi), *hàn lián cǎo* (Herba Ecliptae), *tài zǐ shēn* (Radix Pseudostellariae), *shēng huáng qí* (Radix Astragali Cruda), *dāng guī tàn* (Radix Angelicae Sinensis Carbonisata), *chǎo zǎo rén* (Dry-fried Semen Ziziphi Spinosae). *Huáng qín* (Radix Scutellariae), *hǎi piāo xiāo* (Endoconcha Sepiae), *duàn mǔ lì* (Calcined Concha Ostreae) and *xiān hè cǎo* (Herba Agrimoniae).

After the cessation of bleeding, daily *Guī Pí Tāng* (归脾汤) was prescribed to tonify blood, with *Liù Wèi Dì Huáng Wán* (六味地黄丸) to be taken in the evening. 10-15 days per month constituted one course, after which treatment was discontinued until menstruation resumed. One pill per dose, for 2-3 months. With symptoms of a dry mouth and tongue or sore throat, *Guī Pí Wán* (归脾丸) was reduced to one-half pill per dose. With abdominal distention and poor appetite, *Liù Wèi Dì Huáng Wán* (六味地黄丸) was also reduced by one-half.

Results showed 87 cases with excellent response, 29 cases effective, with 13 cases ineffective. The total effective rate reached 90%. [5]

(2) DUB in Different Age Groups

Gao Li-ping studied a group of 15-56 year old DUB patients that showed abnormal bleeding lasting from 10-62 days. Subjects were divided into five treatment groups.

1) Blood-heat Disturbing the Interior:

Modified *Qín Zhú Sì Wù Tāng* (芩术四物汤) was prescribed.

Medicinals included *dāng guī* (Radix Angelicae Sinensis), *chuān xiōng* (Rhizoma Chuanxiong), *shēng dì huáng* (Radix Rehmanniae), *huáng qín* (Radix Scutellariae), *bái zhú* (Rhizoma Atractylodis Macrocephalae), *chì sháo* (Radix Paeoniae Rubra), *cè bǎi* (Cacumen Platycladi), *shēng dì yú* (Raw Radix Sanguisorbae) and *ǒu jié* (Nodus Nelumbinis Rhizomatis).

With constipation, *quán guā lóu* (Fructus Trichosanthis) was added.

With restlessness and vexation, *xià kū cǎo* (Spica Prunellae) was added.

With yin deficiency signs, *nǔ zhēn zǐ* (Fructus Ligustri Lucidi) and *hàn lián cǎo* (Herba Ecliptae) were added.

2) Deficient Qi Unable to Contain Blood:

Bǔ Zhōng Yì Qì Tāng (补中益气汤) was prescribed.

Medicinals included *dǎng shēn* (Radix Codonopsis), *huáng qí* (Radix Astragali), *chén pí* (Pericarpium Citri Reticulatae), *bái zhú* (Rhizoma Atractylodis Macrocephalae), *shān yào* (Rhizoma Dioscoreae), *hǎi piāo xiāo* (Endoconcha Sepiae), *shēng má* (Rhizoma Cimicifugae), *dāng guī* (Radix Angelicae Sinensis) and *zhì gān cǎo* (Radix et Rhizoma Glycyrrhizae Praeparata cum Melle).

When accompanied by blood stasis, *yì mǔ cǎo* (Herba Leonuri) and *shēng pú huáng* (Pollen Typhae Crudum) were added.

With heat, *huáng qín* (Radix Scutellariae) was added.

3) Kidney Yin Deficiency:

Modified *Zuǒ Guī Yǐn* (左归饮) was prescribed. Medicinals included *huái shān yào* (Rhizoma Dioscoreae), *shān zhū yú* (Fructus Corni), *shú dì huáng* (Radix Rehmanniae Praeparata), *fú líng* (Poria), *gǒu qǐ* (Fructus Lycii), *tù sī zǐ* (Semen Cuscutae), *jīn yīng zǐ* (Fructus Rosae Laevigatae), *nǔ zhēn zǐ* (Fructus Ligustri Lucidi), *ǒu jié* (Nodus Nelumbinis Rhizomatis), *hàn lián cǎo* (Herba Ecliptae) and *zhì gān cǎo* (Radix et Rhizoma Glycyrrhizae Praeparata cum Melle).

With vexation and insomnia, *Jiāo Tài Wán* (交泰丸) was prescribed, or *wǔ wèi zǐ* (Fructus Schisandrae), *yè jiāo téng* (Caulis Polygoni Multiflori) and *lián zǐ xīn* (Plumula Nelumbinis).

4) Kidney Yang Deficiency:

Modified *Yòu Guī Yǐn* (右归饮) was prescribed. Medicinals included *lù jiǎo shuāng* (Cornu Cervi Degelatinatum), *shú dì huáng* (Radix Rehmanniae Praeparata), *shān yào* (Rhizoma Dioscoreae), *shān zhū yú* (Fructus Corni), *gǒu qǐ* (Fructus Lycii), *tù sī zǐ* (Semen Cuscutae), *bǔ gǔ zhī* (Fructus Psoraleae), *chǎo xù duàn* (Dry-fried Radix Dipsaci) and *chì shí zhī* (Halloysitum Rubrum).

With edema, *guì zhī* (Ramulus Cinnamomi) and *fú líng* (Poria) were added.

5) Stasis Stagnating in the Uterus:

Táo Hóng Sì Wù Tāng (桃红四物汤) modified with *Shī Xiào Sǎn* (失笑散). Medicinals included *hóng huā* (Flos Carthami), *chuān xiōng* (Rhizoma Chuanxiong), *dāng guī* (Radix Angelicae Sinensis), *táo rén* (Semen Persicae), *qiàn cǎo* (Radix Rubiae), *shēng dì huáng* (Radix Rehmanniae), *shēng pú huáng* (Pollen Typhae Crudum), *wǔ líng zhī* (Faeces Trogopterori), *yì mǔ cǎo* (Herba Leonuri) and *hǎi piāo xiāo* (Endoconcha Sepiae).

With profuse bleeding, *sān qī fěn* (Radix Notoginseng Powder) and *huā ruǐ shí* (Ophicalcitum) were added.

With a dry mouth, a bitter taste and constipation, *dān pí* (Cortex Moutan) and *shēng dà huáng* (Raw Radix et Rhizoma Rhei) were added.

Results showed 166 cases recovered, 42 cases improved, and 15 cases ineffective. [6]

Dr. Feng Shi-song treated 81 cases of DUB based on pattern differentiation. Ages ranged from 16-50 years, with 30 cases presenting anovulation. There were 38 cases of Kidney qi deficiency, 30 cases of blood-heat, and 31 cases of blood stasis patterns. *Tāi Pán Wū Bèi Sǎn* (胎盘乌贝散) was prescribed at 3-6g per dose, decocted with honey or brown sugar, three times daily. Medicinals included *tāi pán* (Placenta) 2 portions, *wū zéi gǔ* (Endoconcha Sepiae) 1 portion, *zhè bèi mǔ* (Bulbus Fritillariae Thunbergii) 1 portion and *è bái pí* (Cortex Ailanthi) 1 portion.

With symptoms of blood-heat, *kŭ shēn* (Radix Sophorae Flavescentis), *tŭ fú líng* (Rhizoma Smilacis Glabrae) and *dì yú* (Radix Sanguisorbae) were added.

With damp-heat toxin flowing downward with symptoms of pruritus vulvae, the decoction was also applied externally.

In the Spleen and Kidney deficiency group, 26 cases recovered completely, with no recurrence. 9 cases improved, presenting irregular menstruation. 3 cases showed no effect.

In the blood-heat pattern group, 20 cases completely recovered, 9 improved, and 1 case showed no effect.

In the qi deficiency and blood stasis group, 9 cases recovered, 3 cases improved, and 1 showed no effect. [8]

(3) Pattern Differentiation and Treatment in Accordance with Menstruation

In 98 cases of DUB, Dr. Dong Su-qin colleagues applied a cyclic method of treatment based on menstruation. Ages ranged from 11-54 years, with the course of disease lasting from 2 months to 2 years. This group of patients included 31 cases of anovular DUB, with 67 cases ovulatory. 8 cases presented proliferative phases, 2 cases cyst-like hyperplasia, 2 cases adenoma type hyperplasia, and 5 cases of atrophic endometrium. The method first applied was to arrest bleeding, followed by treatment to regulate menses.

1) Kidney Yang Deficiency:

Bleeding stage treatment: The treatment principles during this period were to invigorate Kidney yang and secure the penetrating and conception vessels.

Medicinals included *shú dì huáng* (Radix Rehmanniae Praeparata), *shān yào* (Rhizoma Dioscoreae), *shān zhū yú* (Fructus Corni), *bā jǐ tiān*

(Radix Morindae Officinalis), *dù zhòng* (Cortex Eucommiae) and *lù jiāo jiāo* (Colla Cornus Cervi) 15g each, *nǚ zhēn zǐ* (Fructus Ligustri Lucidi), *hàn lián cǎo* (Herba Ecliptae) and *bǔ gǔ zhī* (Fructus Psoraleae) 12g each, *duàn lóng gǔ* (Calcined Fossilia Ossis Mastodi), *duàn mǔ lì* (Calcined Concha Ostreae), *dì yú tàn* (Radix Sanguisorbae Carbonisata) and *ài tàn* (Folium Artemisiae Argyi Carbonisata) 10g each.

Postmenstrual stage treatment: The treatment principles were to tonify the Kidney, nourish essence, and regulate the penetrating and conception vessels.

Medicinals included *shú dì huáng* (Radix Rehmanniae Praeparata), *shān yào* (Rhizoma Dioscoreae), *bā jǐ tiān* (Radix Morindae Officinalis), *dāng guī* (Radix Angelicae Sinensis) and *dān shēn* (Radix Salviae Miltiorrhizae) 10g each, *nǚ zhēn zǐ* (Fructus Ligustri Lucidi), *hàn lián cǎo* (Herba Ecliptae), *tù sī zǐ* (Semen Cuscutae) and *ròu cōng róng* (Herba Cistanches) 15g each, *zǐ hé chē* (Placenta Hominis) and *jī xuè téng* (Caulis Spatholobi) 20g each.

Intermenstrual treatment: The treatment principles were to tonify Kidney yang, free the collaterals and invigorate blood.

Medicinals included *zǐ hé chē* (Placenta Hominis) 20g, *ròu cōng róng* (Herba Cistanches), *tù sī zǐ* (Semen Cuscutae), *nǚ zhēn zǐ* (Fructus Ligustri Lucidi), *shān yào* (Rhizoma Dioscoreae), *xiāng fù* (Rhizoma Cyperi), *zé lán* (Herba Lycopi), *bā jǐ tiān* (Radix Morindae Officinalis) and *sāng shèn* (Fructus Mori) 15g each, *fù pén zǐ* (Fructus Rubi), *dān shēn* (Radix Salviae Miltiorrhizae) and *huáng qín* (Radix Scutellariae) 10g each.

Premenstrual treatment: The treatment principles were to warm the Kidney and uterus, tonify the Kidney and rectify qi.

Medicinals included *zǐ hé chē* (Placenta Hominis) 20g, *ròu cōng róng* (Herba Cistanches), *tù sī zǐ* (Semen Cuscutae), *nǚ zhēn zǐ* (Fructus Ligustri Lucidi), *gǒu qǐ* (Fructus Lycii), *jī xuè téng* (Caulis Spatholobi), *tiān mén dōng* (Radix Asparagi) and *wǔ wèi zǐ* (Fructus Schisandrae) 15g each, *sāng shèn* (Fructus Mori), *dāng guī* (Radix Angelicae Sinensis), *shǒu wū* (Radix Polygoni Multiflori) and *dān shēn* (Radix Salviae Miltiorrhizae) 10g each.

2) Kidney Yin Deficiency:

Bleeding stage treatment: Medicinals were selected during this period to nourish Kidney yin, clear heat, cool blood, and stanch bleeding.

Medicinals included *nǚ zhēn zǐ* (Fructus Ligustri Lucidi), *hàn lián cǎo* (Herba Ecliptae), *shān zhū yú* (Fructus Corni), and *tiān mén dōng* (Radix Asparagi) 15g each, *jī xuè téng* (Caulis Spatholobi), *zǐ hé chē* (Placenta Hominis), and *wǔ wèi zǐ* (Fructus Schisandrae) 20g each, *cè bǎi tàn* (Carbonized Cacumen Platycladi), *shēng dì tàn* (Radix Rehmanniae Carbonisata), *dì yú* (Radix Sanguisorbae), and *ǒu jié* (Nodus Nelumbinis Rhizomatis) 10g each, plus *wū zéi gǔ* (Endoconcha Sepiae)15g.

Postmenstrual stage treatment: Medicinals were selected during this period to nourish the Liver and Kidney, and to regulate the penetrating and conception vessels.

Medicinals included *dāng guī* (Radix Angelicae Sinensis), *sāng shèn* (Fructus Mori), *shú dì huáng* (Radix Rehmanniae Praeparata), *ē jiāo* (Colla Corii Asini), *shān yào* (Rhizoma Dioscoreae), *dān shēn* (Radix Salviae Miltiorrhizae) 10g each, *nǚ zhēn zǐ* (Fructus Ligustri Lucidi), *zǐ hé chē* (Placenta Hominis), *tù sī zǐ* (Semen Cuscutae), *ròu cōng róng* (Herba Cistanches), *gǒu qǐ zǐ* (Fructus Lycii), and *huáng qín* (Radix Scutellariae) 15g each, plus *jī xuè téng* (Caulis Spatholobi) 30g.

Intermenstrual treatment: Medicinals were selected during this period to nourish the Kidney, tonify qi, and secure the penetrating and conception vessels.

They included *bā jǐ tiān* (Radix Morindae Officinalis), *xiān máo* (Rhizoma Curculiginis), *xiān líng pí* (Herba Epimedii), *dāng guī* (Radix Angelicae Sinensis), *háng sháo* (Radix Paeoniae Alba), *xiāng fù* (Rhizoma Cyperi), *nǚ zhēn zǐ* (Fructus Ligustri Lucidi), and *sāng shèn* (Fructus Mori),

10g each.

Premenstrual treatment: Medicinals were selected during this period to nourish the Kidney, replenish essence, and tonify qi and blood. They included *yún líng* (Poria), *dāng guī* (Radix Angelicae Sinensis), *dān shēn* (Radix Salviae Miltiorrhizae), *ròu cōng róng* (Herba Cistanches), *tù sī zǐ* (Semen Cuscutae), and *huáng qín* (Radix Scutellariae) 10g each.

In 98 cases, 84 completely regained normal menstruation. 10 cases showed obvious effect. 4 cases showed no response. 87 cases showed normal diphase BBT, 7 cases monophase, and 4 cases were atrophic. [9]

Dr. Yang Xiao-hai treated a group of patients, all of childbearing age. Treatment was applied according to the menstrual stage. The group included 49 subjects with deficiency syndromes and 44 with excess. The basic formula for the excess pattern group included *shēng dì huáng* (Radix Rehmanniae) 30g, *huáng qín* (Radix Scutellariae) 15g, *chì sháo* (Radix Paeoniae Rubra), *mǔ dān pí* (Cortex Moutan), *xiāng fù* (Rhizoma Cyperi) 10g each, and *huáng bǎi* (Cortex Phellodendri Chinensis) 5g. Modifications were made according to pattern differentiation.

With acute flooding due to blood-heat, *guī bǎn* (Testudinis Plastrum) 15g, *hǎi piāo xiāo* (Endoconcha Sepiae) and *guàn zhòng* (Cyrtomii Rhizoma) 10g each were added.

With damp-heat pouring downward, *chūn gēn pí* (Cortex Ailanthi) 30g, *hóng téng* (Caulis Sargentodoxae) and *tǔ fú líng* (Rhizoma Smilacis Glabrae) 15g each were added.

The basic formula for the deficiency group included *lù jiǎo shuāng* (Cornu Cervi Degelatinatum), *tù sī zǐ* (Semen Cuscutae), *shān zhū yú* (Fructus Corni) 15g each, *dān shēn* (Radix Salviae Miltiorrhizae), *jī xuè téng* (Caulis Spatholobi) and *shēng qiàn cǎo* (Raw Radix Rubiae) 10g each. Modifications were made according to pattern differentiation as follows.

With Spleen and Kidney yang deficiency, *huáng qí* (Radix Astragali), *dǎng shēn* (Radix Codonopsis), *bái zhú* (Rhizoma Atractylodis

Macrocephalae), *xù duàn* (Radix Dipsaci), and *bā jǐ tiān* (Radix Morindae Officinalis) 10g each were added.

With Liver and Kidney deficiency, *guī bǎn* (Testudinis Plastrum) 15g, *gǒu qǐ zǐ* (Fructus Lycii), *shēng dì huáng* (Radix Rehmanniae) and *shú dì huáng* (Radix Rehmanniae Praeparata) 10g each, plus *huáng bǎi* (Cortex Phellodendri Chinensis) 5g were added.

The basic formulas both treat the origin and secure the penetrating vessel. Both were modified according to the menstrual period.

The postmenstrual period began on the fourth day of the cycle. With excess patterns, *mǔ dān pí* (Cortex Moutan) and *huáng bǎi* (Cortex Phellodendri Chinensis) were removed. *Hàn lián cǎo* (Herba Ecliptae) and *nǔ zhēn zǐ* (Fructus Ligustri Lucidi) 10g each, with *dì gǔ pí* (Cortex Lycii), and *shā shēn* (Radix Adenophorae seu Glehniae) 15g each, were added. With deficient patterns, *qiàn cǎo* (Radix Rubiae) was removed. *Hàn lián cǎo* (Herba Ecliptae), *nǔ zhēn zǐ* (Fructus Ligustri Lucidi), and *zhì hé shǒu wū* (Radix Polygoni Multiflori Praeparata cum Succo Glycines Sotae) 10g each, were added. 5 doses were prescribed.

The intermenstrual treatment began on the twelfth day of the cycle.

With excess patterns, *shēng dì huáng* (Radix Rehmanniae) was removed and *tù sī zǐ* (Semen Cuscutae) 15g, and *yín yáng huò* (Herba Epimedii) 15g were added with *jī xuè téng* (Caulis Spatholobi) and *dān shēn* (Radix Salviae Miltiorrhizae) 10g.

With deficiency patterns, *shān zhū yú* (Fructus Corni) and *qiàn cǎo* (Radix Rubiae) were removed.

With Spleen and Kidney yang deficiency, *táo rén* (Semen Persicae) and *guì zhī* (Ramulus Cinnamomi) 10g were added.

With Liver and Kidney yin deficiency, *mǔ dān pí* (Cortex Moutan) 10g and *chì sháo* (Radix Paeoniae Rubra) 10g were added.

The premenstrual period began on the 22nd day.

With excess patterns, *tù sī zǐ* (Semen Cuscutae), *yín yáng huò* (Herba

Epimedii) 10g, and *shā shēn* (Radix Adenophorae seu Glehniae) 15g were added.

With deficiency patterns, *zé lán yè* (Herba Lycopi) was removed. Added were *qiàn cǎo* (Radix Rubiae), *huáng qí* (Radix Astragali), and *hé shǒu wū* (Radix Polygoni Multiflori) 15g.

5 doses constituted one course, with treatment continuing for 2 courses. At a three month follow-up, 71 cases showed complete recovery, 20 cases improved, and 2 cases no response. There were no obvious differences among the four treatment groups. [10]

(1) Kidney Yang Deficiency Pattern

1) Bleeding Stage

During the bleeding period, medicinals were selected to nourish Kidney qi and secure the penetrating vessel.

Medicinals included *bái sháo* (Radix Paeoniae Alba) 18g, *xiān hè cǎo* (Herba Agrimoniae) 18g, *chì shí zhī* (Halloysitum Rubrum), *duàn lóng gǔ* (Calcined Fossilia Ossis Mastodi), *duàn mǔ lì* (Calcined Concha Ostreae), *dǎng shēn* (Radix Codonopsis) and *wū zéi gǔ* (Endoconcha Sepiae) 15g each, *ē jiāo* (Colla Corii Asini) 12g, *tù sī zǐ* (Semen Cuscutae) 12g, *bái zhú* (Rhizoma Atractylodis Macrocephalae) 10g, *bǔ gǔ zhī* (Fructus Psoraleae) 10g, *zhì gān cǎo* (Radix et Rhizoma Glycyrrhizae Praeparata cum Melle) 6g, and *ài yè tàn* (Folium Artemisiae Argyi Carbonisata) 6g.

2) Regulating Anovular Menstruation in the Postmenstrual Period

Medicinals were selected to tonify the Kidney, nourish blood, and regulate the penetrating and conception vesssels.

Medicinals included *shú dì huáng* (Radix Rehmanniae Praeparata) 15g, *tài zǐ shēn* (Radix Pseudostellariae) 15g, *xiān líng pí* (Herba Epimedii)15g, *huáng qí* (Radix Astragali) 15g, *shān yào* (Rhizoma Dioscoreae) 15g, *bái sháo* (Radix Paeoniae Alba) 18g, *dāng guī* (Radix Angelicae Sinensis) 10g, *guī jiāo* (Colla Plastri Testudinis) 12g, *fú líng* (Poria) 12g, *gǒu qǐ* (Fructus Lycii) 12g, *xiāng fù* (Rhizoma Cyperi) 6g and *zhì gān cǎo* (Radix et Rhizoma Glycyrrhizae Praeparata cum Melle) 6g.

3) Regulating Anovular Menstruation in the Intermenstrual Period

Medicinals in the intermenstrual period were selected to tonify Kidney qi, warm the channels and harmonize blood.

Medicinals included *dāng guī* (Radix Angelicae Sinensis) 12g, *xiān máo* (Rhizoma Curculiginis) 12g, *dān shēn* (Radix Salviae Miltiorrhizae) 15g, *dǎng shēn* (Radix Codonopsis) 15g, *tù sī zǐ* (Semen Cuscutae) 15g, *xiān líng pí* (Herba Epimedii) 15g, *chuān xiōng* (Rhizoma Chuanxiong) 6g, *zhì gān cǎo* (Radix et Rhizoma Glycyrrhizae Praeparata cum Melle) 6g, *xiāng fù* (Rhizoma Cyperi) 10g, *guì zhī* (Ramulus Cinnamomi) 10g, and *chōng wèi zǐ* (Fructus Leonuri) 10g.

4) Regulating Anovular Menstruation in the Premenstrual Period

Medicinals in the premenstrual period were selected to strengthen the Spleen, tonify qi, nourish the Kidney, and strengthen yang.

Medicinals included *dāng guī* (Radix Angelicae Sinensis) 15g, *shú dì huáng* (Radix Rehmanniae Praeparata) 15g, *huáng qí* (Radix Astragali) 15g, *dǎng shēn* (Radix Codonopsis) 15g, *tù sī zǐ* (Semen Cuscutae) 15g, *gǒu qǐ* (Fructus Lycii) 15g, *lù jiǎo shuāng* (Cornu Cervi Degelatinatum) 15g, *zhì gān cǎo* (Radix et Rhizoma Glycyrrhizae Praeparata cum Melle) 6g, *fú líng* (Poria) 12g and *bā jǐ tiān* (Radix Morindae Officinalis) 10g.

5) Medicinals for Delayed Menstruation

With delayed menstruation, *Cuī Jīng Fāng* (催经方) was selected to invigorate blood and regulate menstruation.

Medicinals included *dāng guī* (Radix Angelicae Sinensis) 15g, *chuān xù duàn* (Radix Dipsaci) 15g, *yì mǔ cǎo* (Herba Leonuri) 15g, *chuān xiōng* (Rhizoma Chuanxiong) 10g, *xiāng fù* (Rhizoma Cyperi) 10g, *zé lán* (Herba Lycopi) 10g, *táo rén* (Semen Persicae) 10g, and *dān shēn* (Radix Salviae Miltiorrhizae) 16g.

(2) Kidney Yin Deficiency Pattern

1) Bleeding Stage

During the bleeding stage, medicinals were selected to nourish blood, clear heat, and secure the penetrating vessel to arrest bleeding.

Medicinals included *shēng dì tàn* (Radix Rehmanniae Carbonisata) and *xiān hè cǎo* (Herba Agrimoniae) 18g each, *ē jiāo* (Colla Corii Asini) and *gǒu qǐ* (Fructus Lycii) 12g each, *bái sháo* (Radix Paeoniae Alba) 20g, *hàn lián cǎo* (Herba Ecliptae) 30g, *shān yào* (Rhizoma Dioscoreae) and *tài zǐ shēn* (Radix Pseudostellariae) 15g each, plus *cè bǎi tàn* (Carbonized Cacumen Platycladi) 10g.

2) Regulating Anovular Menstruation in the Postmenstrual Period

Medicinals were selected to nourish the Liver and Kidney and tonify the penetrating and conception vessels. They included *gān dì huáng* (Radix Rehmanniae) and *bái sháo* (Radix Paeoniae Alba) 20g each, *ē jiāo* (Colla Corii Asini), *sāng shèn zǐ* (Fructus Mori), and *gǒu qǐ* (Fructus Lycii) 12g each, *dāng guī* (Radix Angelicae Sinensis) and *dì gǔ pí* (Cortex Lycii) 10g each, *nǚ zhēn zǐ* (Fructus Ligustri Lucidi) and *shān yào* (Rhizoma Dioscoreae) 15g, plus *gān cǎo* (Radix et Rhizoma Glycyrrhizae) 6g.

3) Regulating Anovular Menstruation in the Intermenstrual Period

During the intermenstrual stage, medicinals were selected to nourish the Kidney, tonify qi, and secure the penetrating vessel.

They included *dāng guī* (Radix Angelicae Sinensis) 12g, *chì sháo* (Radix

Paeoniae Rubra) 10g, *bā jǐ tiān* (Radix Morindae Officinalis) 10g, *xiāng fù* (Rhizoma Cyperi) 10g, *dān shēn* (Radix Salviae Miltiorrhizae) 15g, *dǎng shēn* (Radix Codonopsis) 15g, *tù sī zǐ* (Semen Cuscutae) 15g, *xiān líng pí* (Herba Epimedii) 15g, and *zhì gān cǎo* (Radix et Rhizoma Glycyrrhizae Praeparata cum Melle) 6g.

4) Regulating Anovular Menstruation in the Premenstrual Period

During the premenstrual stage, medicinals were selected to nourish the Kidney, strengthen the Spleen, tonify qi, and nourish blood.

They included *gān dì huáng* (Radix Rehmanniae) 15g, *dǎng shēn* (Radix Codonopsis) 15g, *gǒu qǐ* (Fructus Lycii) 15g, *shān yào* (Rhizoma Dioscoreae) 15g, *tù sī zǐ* (Semen Cuscutae) 15g, *dāng guī* (Radix Angelicae Sinensis) 12g, *yún líng* (Poria) 12g, *lián ròu* (Semen Nelumbinis) 12g, *huáng jīng* (Rhizoma Polygonati) 10g, and *zhì gān cǎo* (Radix et Rhizoma Glycyrrhizae Praeparata cum Melle) 6g.

5) Medicinals for Delayed Menstruation

With delayed menstruation, *Cuī Jīng Tāng* (催经汤) was selected to invigorate blood and regulate menstruation.

The formula included *dāng guī* (Radix Angelicae Sinensis) 15g, *chuān xù duàn* (Radix Dipsaci) 15g, *dān shēn* (Radix Salviae Miltiorrhizae) 15g, *yì mǔ cǎo* (Herba Leonuri) 15g, *chuān xiōng* (Rhizoma Chuanxiong) 10g, *chì sháo* (Radix Paeoniae Rubra) 10g, *xiāng fù* (Rhizoma Cyperi) 10g, *zé lán* (Herba Lycopi) 10g, *táo rén* (Semen Persicae) 10g and *niú xī* (Rhizoma Curcumae) 10g.

147 cases of DUB were treated with these methods, including 49 subjects with Kidney deficiency patterns and 98 with Kidney yang deficiency patterns. Total recovery was seen in 40 and 79 cases, respectively. 7 and 13 cases improved, while 2 and 6 cases showed no response, according to the following criteria.

Total recovery: Menstruation cycles normal, diphase BBT for three cycles, or conception.

Improvement: Two normal regular cycles of normal volume, with either diphase or atypical BBT.

No response: All symptoms unaffected.

Dr. Xing Yu-xia divided 65 cases of adolescent flooding and spotting into two treatment groups. Subjects ranged in age from 11 to 19 years. Protocols were determined according to the bleeding or non-bleeding stages.

(1) Bleeding Stage

During the bleeding period, medicinals were selected to nourish the Kidney and tonify qi. The formula *Zhǐ Xuè Gù Chōng Tāng* (止血固冲汤) was selected.

Medicinals included *huáng qí* (Radix Astragali), *shēng dì tàn* (Radix Rehmanniae Carbonisata), *chǎo dì yú* (Dry-fried Radix Sanguisorbae), *xiān hè cǎo* (Herba Agrimoniae), *duàn lóng gǔ* (Calcined Fossilia Ossis Mastodi) and *duàn mǔ lì* (Calcined Concha Ostreae) 20g each, *dǎng shēn* (Radix Codonopsis), *nǚ zhēn zǐ* (Fructus Ligustri Lucidi) and *chuān xù duàn* (Radix Dipsaci) 15g each, *hàn lián cǎo* (Herba Ecliptae) 30g, *qiàn cǎo* (Radix Rubiae) 12g, *bái zhú* (Rhizoma Atractylodis Macrocephalae) 10g, and *zhì shēng má* (Fried with liquid Rhizoma Cimicifugae) 6g.

With blood-heat, *dǎng shēn* (Radix Codonopsis) and *shēng má* (Rhizoma Cimicifugae) were removed. *Jiāo zhī zǐ* (Scorch-fried Fructus Gardeniae) 9g, *huáng qín* (Radix Scutellariae) 10g, and *chǎo huái huā* (Dry-fried Flos Sophorae) 15g were added.

With hyperactive yang due to yin deficiency, *huáng qí* (Radix Astragali), *dǎng shēn* (Radix Codonopsis), and *shēng má* (Rhizoma Cimicifugae) were removed. *Guī bǎn* (Testudinis Plastrum) and *bái wēi* (Radix et Rhizoma Cynanchi Atrati) 10g each, were added.

With yang deficiency, *dì yú* (Radix Sanguisorbae) was removed and *lù jiǎo shuāng* (Cornu Cervi Degelatinatum), *bǔ gǔ zhī* (Fructus Psoraleae) and *ài yè tàn* (Folium Artemisiae Argyi Carbonisata) 10g each were added.

With profuse bleeding and qi desertion, the doages of *huáng qí* (Radix Astragali) and *dǎng shēn* (Radix Codonopsis) were doubled. Transfusions were indicated in some cases.

(2) Non-bleeding Stage

During the menstruation period, medicinals were selected to nourish the Kidney and regulate menstruation. Medicinals included *shēng dì huáng* (Radix Rehmanniae) 12g, *shú dì huáng* (Radix Rehmanniae Praeparata) 12g, *mò hàn lián* (Herba Ecliptae) 12g, *xù duàn* (Radix Dipsaci) 12g, *huái shān yào* (Rhizoma Dioscoreae) 15g, *hé shǒu wū* (Radix Polygoni Multiflori) 15g, *shān zhū yú* (Fructus Corni) 10g, *gǒu qǐ zǐ* (Fructus Lycii) 10g, *nǔ zhēn zǐ* (Fructus Ligustri Lucidi) 10g, *dāng guī* (Radix Angelicae Sinensis) 10g, *zhì xiāng fù* (Rhizoma Cyperi Praeparata) 10g, *zhì gān cǎo* (Radix et Rhizoma Glycyrrhizae Praeparata cum Melle) 9g, and *chuān xiōng* (Rhizoma Chuanxiong) 5g.

Nearing the midcycle, *hóng huā* (Flos Carthami) 10g, *chuān niú xī* (Rhizoma Curcumae) 12g and *lù lù tōng* (Fructus Liquidambaris) 15g were added to further nourish the Kidney. Following ovulation, the following formula was prescribed. Medicinals included *shú dì huáng* (Radix Rehmanniae Praeparata) 12g, *mò hàn lián* (Herba Ecliptae) 12g, *huái shān yào* (Rhizoma Dioscoreae) 15g, *gǒu qǐ zǐ* (Fructus Lycii) 10g, *dāng guī* (Radix Angelicae Sinensis) 10g, *yín yáng huò* (Herba Epimedii) 10g, *tù sī zǐ* (Semen Cuscutae) 10g, *xiān máo* (Rhizoma Curculiginis) 10g, *nǔ zhēn zǐ* (Fructus Ligustri Lucidi) 10g, and *zhì xiāng fù* (Rhizoma Cyperi Praeparata) 10g.

During the premenstrual period, *shēng shān zhā* (Raw Fructus

Crataegi) 12g, *chǎo wǔ líng zhī* (Dry-fried Faeces Trogopterori) 10g, and *chuān xiōng* (Rhizoma Chuanxiong) 3g were added.

With Spleen and Kidney yang deficiency, yin nourishing medicinals were reduced and *zhì huáng qí* (Radix Astragali Praeparata cum Melle) 15g, *lù jiǎo shuāng* (Cornu Cervi Degelatinatum) 10g, *yín yáng huò* (Herba Epimedii) 10g, and *bǔ gǔ zhī* (Fructus Psoraleae) 10g were added.

With Spleen and Stomach deficiency, *shān zhū yú* (Fructus Corni), *shú dì huáng* (Radix Rehmanniae Praeparata) were removed, and *dǎng shēn* (Radix Codonopsis) 15g, *chǎo bái zhú* (Dry-fried Rhizoma Atractylodis Macrocephalae) 10g, *fú líng* (Poria) 10g and *shā rén* (Fructus Amomi) 6g were added.

With exuberant fire due to yin deficiency, add *guī bǎn* (Testudinis Plastrum) 10g, *dì gǔ pí* (Cortex Lycii), and *xuán shēn* (Radix Scrophulariae) 10g.

Results showed 48 cases in full recovery, 12 cases improved, and 5 cases no response. Short-term results showed 45 cases excellent, 14 cases improved, and 6 cases no response. 38 cases established ovulation, with 90 of 152 total cycles ovulatory. [12]

Dr. Liu Zu-ru treated a group of anovular DUB cases by treating the Kidney according to menstrual stages. During the bleeding period, an empirical formula, *Zī Shèn Gù Chōng Tāng* (滋肾固冲汤) was selected.

Medicinals included *shān zhū yú* (Fructus Corni), *tù sī zǐ* (Semen Cuscutae), *nǚ zhēn zǐ* (Fructus Ligustri Lucidi), *hàn lián cǎo* (Herba Ecliptae), *wǔ wèi zǐ* (Fructus Schisandrae), *ē jiāo* (Colla Corii Asini, dissolved), *wū zéi gǔ* (Endoconcha Sepiae) 15g each, *pú huáng tàn* (Pollen Typhae Carbonisata) 10g, and *sān qī mò* (Radix Notoginseng Powder) 3g (infused). This formula was modified according to symptoms and particular patterns. However, the protocol remained consistent until the cessation of the bleeding pattern.

To regulate the menstruation cycle in both adolescents and mature women, the primary principle was to nourish the Kidney. Methods of invigorating blood, strengthening yang, and rectifying qi were applied according to changes in menstrual cycles, uterine storage and release functions, and the waxing and waning of the uterus.

Postmenstrual treatment began following the 5th-11th day of the cycle, or after the bleeding had been arrested. Medicinals were selected to nourish and invigorating blood promote follicular development.

The formula included *xiān líng pí* (Herba Epimedii), *shān zhū yú* (Fructus Corni), *tù sī zǐ* (Semen Cuscutae), *gǒu qǐ zǐ* (Fructus Lycii), *shú dì huáng* (Radix Rehmanniae Praeparata), *shān yào* (Rhizoma Dioscoreae), and *jī xuè téng* (Caulis Spatholobi) 15g each, with *lù jiǎo jiāo* (Colla Cornus Cervi, dissolved) and *dāng guī* (Radix Angelicae Sinensis) 10g each.

Intermenstrual treatment began on the the 12th-14th day of the cycle. Medicinals were selected to nourish the Kidney and invigorate blood, aiming to benefit the corpus luteum.

Medicinals included *xiān líng pí* (Herba Epimedii), *shān zhū yú* (Fructus Corni), *tù sī zǐ* (Semen Cuscutae), *lù jiǎo jiāo* (Colla Cornus Cervi, dissolved), *dāng guī* (Radix Angelicae Sinensis), *chuān xiōng* (Rhizoma Chuanxiong), *chōng wèi zǐ* (Fructus Leonuri) and *táo rén* (Semen Persicae) 10g each.

Premenstrual treatment began on the the 15th-28th day of the cycle. Medicinals were selected to nourish the Kidney and assist yang.

Medicinals included *xiān líng pí* (Herba Epimedii), *tù sī zǐ* (Semen Cuscutae), *shān zhū yú* (Fructus Corni), *bā jǐ tiān* (Radix Morindae Officinalis), *ròu cōng róng* (Herba Cistanches), *lù jiǎo jiāo* (Colla Cornus Cervi) (dissolved), *gǒu qǐ zǐ* (Fructus Lycii), *xiān máo* (Rhizoma Curculiginis) and *dù zhòng* (Cortex Eucommiae) 10g each.

During the menstrual period, treatment was temporarily discontinued. With a failure to menstruate, medicinals were selected to rectify qi and invigorate blood to promote defluxion of the endometrium.

Medicinals included *chái hú* (Radix Bupleuri), *bái sháo* (Radix Paeoniae Alba), *dāng guī* (Radix Angelicae Sinensis), *chuān xiōng* (Rhizoma Chuanxiong), *zhì xiāng fù* (Rhizoma Cyperi Praeparata), *qiàn cǎo* (Radix Rubiae), *dān shēn* (Radix Salviae Miltiorrhizae) and *suō luó zǐ* (Semen Aesculi) 10g each, plus *yì mǔ cǎo* (Herba Leonuri) 15g.

If bleeding had not ceased by the 5th day of the cycle, *Zī Shèn Gù Chōng Tāng* (滋肾固冲汤) was prescribed to stanch bleeding, followed by the abovementioned treatment plan. BBT was also monitored daily during treatment. Therapeutic effects were evaluated with a one year follow-up exam.

After the cessation of bleeding in menopausal patients, medicianals were selected to nourish the Kidney and tonify both qi and blood.

Medicinals included *xiān líng pí* (Herba Epimedii) 15g, *shān zhū yú* (Fructus Corni) 15g, *tù sī zǐ* (Semen Cuscutae) 15g, *ròu cōng róng* (Herba Cistanches) 15g, *nǔ zhēn zǐ* (Fructus Ligustri Lucidi) 15g, *gǒu qǐ zǐ* (Fructus Lycii) 15g, *shān yào* (Rhizoma Dioscoreae) 15g, *dǎng shēn* (Radix Codonopsis) 15g, *huáng qí* (Radix Astragali) 15g, *bái zhú* (Rhizoma Atractylodis Macrocephalae)10g, *bái sháo* (Radix Paeoniae Alba)10g, and *fú líng* (Poria) 10g.

When menstruation occurred during treatment, *Zī Shèn Gù Chōng Tāng* (滋肾固冲汤) was prescribed on the 5th day of menses. Treatment was restored after the cessation of bleeding.

Results showed 33 cases fully recovered, 28 cases excellent, 16 cases improved, and 3 cases no response. The total effective rate reached 96.3%. [11]

2. SPECIFIC FORMULAS

(1) DUB in Adolescence

Dr. Li Hui-bao and colleagues treated 68 cases of adolescent DUB using the empirical formulas *Zhǐ Xuè Gù Chōng Tāng* (止血固冲汤) and

Yì Shèn Gù Běn Tāng (益肾固本汤).

For the bleeding stage, *Zhǐ Xuè Gù Chōng Tāng* (止血固冲汤) is prescribed.

The formula included *dǎng shēn* (Radix Codonopsis) 10-20g, *bái zhú* (Rhizoma Atractylodis Macrocephalae) 15g, *shēng dì tàn* (Radix Rehmanniae Carbonisata) 15g, *yì mǔ cǎo* (Herba Leonuri) 15g, *chǎo huáng qín* (Dry-fried Radix Scutellariae) 15g, *ē jiāo* (dissolved) (Colla Corii Asini) 15g, *ài yè tàn* (Folium Artemisiae Argyi Carbonisata) 15g, *xiān hè cǎo* (Herba Agrimoniae) 30g, *hàn lián cǎo* (Herba Ecliptae) 30g, *chǎo qiàn cǎo* (Dry-fried Radix Rubiae) 10g, *gān cǎo* (Radix et Rhizoma Glycyrrhizae) 10g, and *sān qī fěn* (Radix Notoginseng Powder) 3g (infused).

With qi deficiency, *shēng huáng qí* (Radix Astragali Cruda) 15-30g, *wǔ wèi zǐ* (Fructus Schisandrae) 10g, and *wū méi tàn* (Fructus Mume Carbonisata) 15g were added.

With blood deficiency, *dāng guī shēn* (Radix Angelicae Sinensis) 10g, *bái sháo* (Radix Paeoniae Alba) 15g, *xuè yú tàn* (Crinis Carbonisatus) 15g, and *zōng lǘ tàn* (Carbonized Petiolus Trachycarpi) 10-20g were added.

With sudden flooding, *gāo lì shēn* (Radix Ginseng) 30g, *shēng shài shēn* (Dry Radix Ginseng) 30g, and *fù piàn* (Radix Aconiti Lateralis Praeparata) 15g were added.

With internal heat due to yin deficiency, *bái zhú* (Rhizoma Atractylodis Macrocephalae) and added *guī bǎn* (Testudinis Plastrum) 10g, *shēng mǔ lì* (Concha Ostreae Cruda) 20g, *ǒu jié tàn* (Nodus Nelumbinis Rhizomatis Carbonisata) 30g, and *lián fáng tàn* (Receptaculum Nelumbinis Carbonisata) 15g were removed.

With blood stasis, *ē jiāo* (Colla Corii Asini), *ài yè tàn* (Folium Artemisiae Argyi Carbonisata) were added and *shēng pú huáng* (Pollen Typhae Crudum) 15g, *chǎo pú huáng* (Dry-fried Pollen Typhae) 15g, *shēng dì huáng* (Radix Rehmanniae) 15g, *chǎo wǔ líng zhī* (Dry-fried Faeces Trogopterori) 15g, *huā ruǐ shí* (Ophicalcitum) 10g, and *dài zhě shí* (Ocherum Rubrum) 10g were removed.

With blood-heat, *dǎng shēn* (Radix Codonopsis) and *bái zhú* (Rhizoma Atractylodis Macrocephalae) were removed. *Cè bǎi tàn* (Carbonized Cacumen Platycladi) 15g and *xiān máo gēn* (Fresh Rhizoma Imperatae) 30g were added.

With Liver and Stomach disharmony, *yù jīn* (Radix Curcumae), *chǎo zǎo rén* (Dry-fried Semen Ziziphi Spinosae), *shān zhā tàn* (Fructus Crataegi Carbonisata) 15g and *xiāng fù* (Rhizoma Cyperi) 10g were added.

3 days following the cessation of bleeding, *Yì Shèn Gù Běn Tāng* (益肾固本汤) was prescribed.

The formula included *xiān líng pí* (Herba Epimedii), *bā jǐ tiān* (Radix Morindae Officinalis), *guī bǎn* (Testudinis Plastrum), *shēng dì huáng* (Radix Rehmanniae), *shú dì huáng* (Radix Rehmanniae Praeparata), *shān yào* (Rhizoma Dioscoreae), *chuān xù duàn* (Radix Dipsaci), *bái sháo* (Radix Paeoniae Alba) 15g each, *xiān máo* (Rhizoma Curculiginis), *dān pí* (Cotex Moutan), *dāng guī* (Radix Angelicae Sinensis) and *zhì gān cǎo* (Radix et Rhizoma Glycyrrhizae Praeparata cum Melle) 10g each, plus *shā rén* (Fructus Amomi) 16g.

After three courses of treatment, results showed 48 cases fully recovered, 13 cases excellent response, 4 cases improved, and 3 cases no response.

Cui Lin randomly divided 84 adolescents into treatment and control groups of 48 and 36 subjects respectively. The formula selected was *Èr Zhì Wán* (二至丸) modified with *Guī Pí Tāng* (归脾汤).

Medicinals included *nǚ zhēn zǐ* (Fructus Ligustri Lucidi) 15g, *hàn lián cǎo* (Herba Ecliptae) 15g, *dǎng shēn* (Radix Codonopsis) 15g, *huáng qí* (Radix Astragali) 15g, and *zhì yuǎn zhì* (Fried with liquid Radix Polygalae) 6g.

With profuse bleeding, added *xiān hè cǎo* (Herba Agrimoniae) 30g and *lù xián cǎo* (Herba Pyrolae) 30g.

With blood-heat, added *dān pī* (Cortex Moutan) 10g, *mǎ chǐ xiàn* (Herba

Portulacae) 30g, and *shēng dì yú* (Raw Radix Sanguisorbae) 30g.

With loose stools, added *bái zhú* (Rhizoma Atractylodis Macrocephalae) 10g and *shān yào* (Rhizoma Dioscoreae) 15g.

5 days constituted one course.

The control group was administered cefradine injections 14g, aminomethylbenzoic acid injections 0.4g, and oxytocin injections 10g for 5 days. The respective results in the treatment and control groups were 22 and 11 cases fully recovered, 16 and 10 cases improved, with 10 and 15 cases no response. [13]

Dr.Yang Wen treated adolescents using medicinals that nourish yin, tonify the Kidney, and secure the penetrating vessel to stanch bleeding. The empirical formula *Zī Yīn Zhǐ Bēng Tāng* (滋阴止崩汤) was selected.

Medicinals included *shēng dì huáng* (Radix Rehmanniae), *shú dì huáng* (Radix Rehmanniae Praeparata), *shān yú ròu* (Fructus Corni), *bái sháo* (Radix Paeoniae Alba), *shān yào* (Rhizoma Dioscoreae), *chuān xù duàn* (Radix Dipsaci), and *dù zhòng* (Cortex Eucommiae) 12g each. Also *hǎi piāo xiāo* (Endoconcha Sepiae) 20g, *duàn mǔ lì* (Calcined Concha Ostreae) 30g, *sāng jì shēng* (Herba Taxilli) 12g, *ē jiāo* (Colla Corii Asini) 12g, *chǎo dì yú* (Dry-fried Radix Sanguisorbae) 15g, and *pú huáng tàn* (Pollen Typhae Carbonisata) 15g.

With profuse bleeding, the dosage of *chǎo dì yú* (Dry-fried Radix Sanguisorbae) was doubled with *chén zōng tàn* (Carbonized Petiolus Trachycarpi) and *cè bǎi* (Cacumen Platycladi) 15g each added.

With feverish dysphoria, added *mài dōng* (Radix Ophiopogonis) 12g, *dì gǔ pí* (Cortex Lycii) 15g, *huáng bǎi* (Coxtex Phellodendri Chinensis) 12g, and *zhī mǔ* (Rhizoma Anemarrhenae) 12g.

With profuse light-colored bleeding, lassitude and shortness of breath, *tài zǐ shēn* (Radix Pseudostellariae) 20g and *bái zhú* (Rhizoma Atractylodis Macrocephalae) 12g were added.

A single menstrual cycle constituted one course of treatment.

Treatment ranged from 1-6 courses. Results showed 15 cases fully recovered, 14 cases improved, and 3 with no response. The total effective rate reached 90.6%. [14]

Dr. Yi Qin-hua treats flooding and spotting according to the following method of pattern differentiation.

Blood-heat: Nourish yin and cool blood to stop bleeding. Select *Qín Zhú Sì Wù Tāng* (芩术四物汤), *Yì Yīn Jiān* (一阴煎) and *Liǎng Dì Tāng* (两 地汤). With profuse bleeding or chronic spotting, add *cè bǎi yè* (Cacumen Platycladi), *dì yú* (Radix Sanguisorbae), and *zhī zǐ* (Fructus Gardeniae).

Spleen qi deficiency: Tonify qi to contain blood. Select *Bǔ Zhōng Yì Qì Tāng* (补中益气汤) with added *ài yè* (Folium Artemisiae Argyi), *jīng jiè tàn* (Herba Schizonepetae Carbonisatum), and *mò hàn lián* (Herba Ecliptae).

Spleen and Kidney deficiency: Strengthen the Spleen, tonify the Kidney, and astringe to stanch bleeding. Select *Ān Chōng Tāng* (安冲汤) with added *ài yè* (Folium Artemisiae Argyi), and *zōng lǔ tàn* (Carbonized Petiolus Trachycarpi).

Medicinals that nourish Kidney yin should be added to the main formula after the cessation of bleeding, according to the presenting pattern. Select *mò hàn lián* (Herba Ecliptae), *nǚ zhēn zǐ* (Fructus Ligustri Lucidi), *hàn lián cǎo* (Herba Ecliptae), and *shú dì huáng* (Radix Rehmanniae Praeparata).

In a study, 5 doses were prescribed before and after menstruation, 1 dose every 2 days. 36 cases were treated for 2-3 menstruation cycles. 2 cases were treated for 6 cycles. 2 subjects discontinued treatment after bleeding had ceased.

Results showed 38 cases showing normal menstruation with symptomatic relief and improvement of anemia. 6 cases showed recurrence, one after 4 months and one after 6 months. All patients recovered after returning for subsequent treatment. [15]

Dr. Xie Bo divided 90 subjects into a treatment group of 60 cases with a control group of 30. Formulas were selected to tonify qi, nourish yin, nourish the Kidney, and secure the penetrating vessel. *Fù Fāng Shú Dì Huáng Jiāo Náng* (复方熟地胶囊) was prescribed.

Medicinals included *shú dì huáng* (Radix Rehmanniae Praeparata) 15g, *tù sī zǐ* (Semen Cuscutae) 15g, *shān yú ròu* (Fructus Corni) 10g, *shān yào* (Rhizoma Dioscoreae) 10g, *bái sháo* (Radix Paeoniae Alba) 10g, *yǐ rén* (Semen Coicis) 15g, *chuān xù duàn* (Radix Dipsaci) 15g, *hàn lián cǎo* (Herba Ecliptae) 15g, *nǚ zhēn zǐ* (Fructus Ligustri Lucidi) 15g, *xiān líng pí* (Herba Epimedii) 10g, *yì mǔ cǎo* (Herba Leonuri) 30g, *chǎo pú huáng* (Dry-fried Pollen Typhae) 12g, *chǎo wǔ líng zhī* (Dry-fried Faeces Trogopterori) 15g, and *zǐ cǎo* (Radix Arnebiae) 15g. These medicinals were processed as *Shú dì Jiāo Náng Yī Hào* (熟地胶囊一号) and *Shú Dì Jiāo Náng Èr Hào* (熟地胶囊二号) tablets, each containing 0.5g.

The first formula was prescribed outside the menstrual period, while the latter during menstruation. The control group was administered estrogen and progestogen. Three menstrual cycles constituted one course.

Results showed a total effective rate of 85.0% in the treatment group and 84.6% in the control showing similar effect (P>0.05). 19 subjects in the treatment group stopped bleeding after 2 days, with 6 in the control after 3 days. Comparison shows no shows no significant difference (P>0.05). After 6 month follow-up recurrence in treatment group was 9.7%, where the control reached 52.9%. Recurrence in the control group was significantly higher than that of the treatment group (P<0.05). This indicates that medicinals which tonify the Kidney show considerable advantage in the treatment of adolescent DUB. [16]

Dr. He Gui-xiang and colleagues find that *Yì Shèn Jiàn Pí Kē Lì* (益肾健脾颗粒) may give symptomatic relief as well as improving hormone, blood, and BBT levels in the later stages of adolescent DUB. The total effective rate reached 96.7% with statistical significance (P<0.01). [17]

(2) DUB during the Childbearing Period

The main function of the formula *Gōng Xuè Yǐn* (功血饮) is to secure the penetrating vessel and contain blood Medicinals include *jīn yīng zǐ* (Fructus Rosae Laevigatae) 15g, *zhì shǒu wū* (Radix Polygoni Multiflori Praeparata cum Succo Glycines Sotae) 15g, *zǐ zhū cǎo* (Folium Callicarpae Pedunculatae) 15g, *chì dì lì* (Polygonum Chinensis) 15g, *lì zhī ké* (Litchi Chinensis Sonn) 15g and *xiān hè cǎo* (Herba Agrimoniae) 9g.

With blood-heat, include *shēng dì huáng* (Radix Rehmanniae), *mài dōng* (Radix Ophiopogonis), *dì gǔ pí* (Cortex Lycii), *shā shēn* (Radix Adenophorae seu Glehniae), and *hēi zhī* (Carbonized Fructus Gardeniae).

With blood stasis, include *dān shēn* (Radix Salviae Miltiorrhizae) and *tǔ niú xī* (Radix et Rhizome Achyranthes).

With Spleen deficiency, include *dǎng shēn* (Radix Codonopsis), *huáng qí* (Radix Astragali) and *bái zhú* (Rhizoma Atractylodis Macrocephalae).

With Kidney yang deficiency, include *xiān máo* (Rhizoma Curculiginis), *xiān líng pí* (Herba Epimedii), and *pào jiāng tàn* (Rhizoma Zingiberis Carbonisata).

With Kidney yin deficiency, include *nǚ zhēn zǐ* (Fructus Ligustri Lucidi), *hàn lián cǎo* (Herba Ecliptae), and *zhì huáng jīng* (Rhizoma Polygonati Praeparata).

In this study, there were 19 subjects with blood-heat, 7 cases with blood stasis, 9 with Kidney yang deficiency, and 11 cases of Kidney yin deficiency. After 2-36 doses, the result showed 33 cases fully recovered, 29 cases excellent response, 11 cases responsive, 10 cases with no response. The total effective rate reached 87.9% . The criteria are as follows.

Full recovery: Normal menstruation with relief of sudden flooding, spotting, lower abdominal coldness and pain, cold limbs, and dizziness. No recurrence for one year.

Excellent response: The main clinical symptoms show obvious

improvement with no reccurence for 6 months.

Responsive: Symptomatic relief with intermittent or profuse bleeding within 2-3 months.

No response: No change in symptoms or abnormal uterine bleeding patterns. [18]

(3) DUB in the Menopausal Period

The main treatment principle for menopausal period DUB is to strengthen the Spleen, tonify qi, secure the penetrating vessel, and arrest bleeding. Dr. Liang Bing treats menopausal patients with an empircal formula, *Jiàn Pí Yì Qì Tāng* (健脾益气汤).

The formula included *huáng qí* (Radix Astragali) 15g, *tài zǐ shēn* (Radix Pseudostellariae) 12g, *bái zhú* (Rhizoma Atractylodis Macrocephalae) 12g, *fú líng* (Poria) 12g, *dāng guī* (Radix Angelicae Sinensis) 3g, *yuǎn zhì* (Radix Polygalae) 12g, *chǎo zǎo rén* (Dry-fried Semen Ziziphi Spinosae) 15g, *mù xiāng* (Radix Aucklandiae) 9g, *chǎo dù zhòng* (Dry-fried Cortex Eucommiae) 15g, *chǎo shān yào* (Dry-fried Rhizoma Dioscoreae) 15g, *wū zéi gǔ* (Endoconcha Sepiae), *duàn lóng gǔ* (Calcined Fossilia Ossis Mastodi) and *duàn mǔ lì* (Calcined Concha Ostreae) 20g each, and *chǎo pú huáng* (Dry-fried Pollen Typhae) 15g.

With lumbar weakness, add *nǚ zhēn zǐ* (Fructus Ligustri Lucidi) 15g, and *hàn lián cǎo* (Herba Ecliptae) 15g.

With a dry mouth and a feverish sensation, add *mài dōng* (Radix Ophiopogonis) 12g, *dì gǔ pí* (Cortex Lycii) 15g, and *zhī mǔ* (Rhizoma Anemarrhenae) 12g. One menstrual cycle constitutes one course of treatment.

A study of 36 cases was performed, with treatments ranging from two to 6 courses. 18 cases fully recovered, 15 cases improved, with 3 cases no response. The total effective rate reached 91.7%. [19]

Dr. Xin Li-jia treats menopausal DUB with *Huà Yū Tāng* (化瘀汤). The formula included *wǔ líng zhī* (Faeces Trogopterori) 15g, *pú huáng* (Pollen Typhae) 10g (wrapped), *zǐ cǎo* (Radix Arnebiae), *chóng lóu* (Rhizoma Paridis), *yì mǔ cǎo* (Herba Leonuri) 30g each, *sān qī fěn* (Radix Notoginseng Powder) 3g (infused), *shú dà huáng* (Prepared Radix et Rhizoma Rhei) 5g, *shēng dì yú* (Raw Radix Sanguisorbae) 40g, and *shēng dì huáng* (Radix Rehmanniae) 20g.

With predominate yin deficiency, add *chǎo zhī mǔ* (Dry-fried Rhizoma Anemarrhenae), *dì gǔ pí* (Cortex Lycii) 15g each, and *chǎo huáng bǎi* (Dry-fried Cortex Phellodendri Chinensis) 20g.

With qi deficiency, add *huáng qí* (Radix Astragali) 30g, *ē jiāo* (Colla Corii Asini) 10g (dissolved), and *shú dì huáng* (Radix Rehmanniae Praeparata) 40g.

Prescribe one divided dose, taken once daily and once nightly. 7 doses constitute one course.

Yin deficiency and blood stasis patterns are treated with *Zhī Bǎi Dì Huáng Wán* (知柏地黄丸) and *Rén Shēn Guī Pí Wán* (人参归脾丸) for two weeks after the abnormal bleeding ceases.

Qi deficiency and blood stasis patterns are treated with *Bǔ Zhōng Yì Qì Wán* (补中益气丸) and *Dà Huáng Zhè Chóng Wán* (大黄蛰虫丸) for two weeks.

In a study of 60 cases, results showed 34 cases excellent response, 24 cases responsive, with 2 cases no response. The total effective rate reached 96.67%. [20]

Dr. Wu Min treated 48 cases of premenopausal period flooding and spotting with modified *Sì Cǎo Tāng* (四草汤). Medicinals included *mǎ biān cǎo* (Herba Verbanae) 30g, *lù xián cǎo* (Herba Pyrolae) 30g, *qiàn cǎo gēn* (Radix et Rhizoma Rubiae) 15-30g, and *yì mǔ cǎo* (Herba Leonuri) 15-30g.

Results showed 31 cases fully recoverd, 14 cases responsive, with 3 cases no response. The total effective rate reached 93.7%. [21]

Dr. Liu Ying-jie and colleagues treated subjects with menopausal

DUB using an empirical formula, *Xuè Níng Tāng* (血宁汤). The formula included *dǎng shēn* (Radix Codonopsis) 15g, *huáng qí* (Radix Astragali) 20g, *shān yú ròu* (Fructus Corni) 10g, *zhì bái zhú* (Dry-fried Rhizoma Atractylodis Macrocephalae) 15g, *shēng má* (Rhizoma CimicWithugae) 10g, *bái sháo* (Radix Paeoniae Alba) 15g, *chén zōng tàn* (Carbonized Petiolus Trachycarpi) 10g, *duàn lóng gǔ* (Calcined Fossilia Ossis Mastodi) and *duàn mǔ lì* (Calcined Concha Ostreae) 30g each, *shēng pú huáng* (Pollen Typhae Crudum) 15g (wrapped), *shú dì huáng* (Radix Rehmanniae Praeparata) 12g, *wǔ wèi zǐ* (Fructus Schisandrae) 10g and *gān cǎo* (Radix et Rhizoma Glycyrrhizae) 6g.

With qi deficiency, remove *dǎng shēn* (Radix Codonopsis) and add *rén shēn* (Radix et Rhizoma Ginseng) 10g.

With yin deficiency and heat, add *nǚ zhēn zǐ* (Fructus Ligustri Lucidi) 15g and *dì gǔ pí* (Cortex Lycii) 15g.

With yang deficiency, add *xiān líng pí* (Herba Epimedii) 10g and *ròu cōng róng* (Herba Cistanches) 10g.

With blood stasis, add *shēng pú huáng* (Pollen Typhae Crudum) 18-20g and *sān qī fěn* (Radix Notoginseng Powder) 3g (infused).

For Liver qi stagnation, add *cù chái hú* (Fried with vinegar Radix Bupleuri) 6g.

One decocted dose daily during the bleeding period. Cheng Yuan and Gu Ben may be added after bleeding ceases, which may shorten course the course of treatment. These medicinals nourish the Kidney, regulate the Liver, strengthen the Spleen, and secure the penetrating vessel. *Liù Wèi Dì Huáng Wán* (六味地黃丸) and *Nǚ Jīn Dān* (女金丹) may be used together.

In a study of 95 cases, results showed 83 cases fully recovered (87.4%), 7 cases excellent response (6.84%), 5 cases responsive (4.74%), and 3 cases no response. The total effective rate reached 98%. There were no toxic side effects and adverse reactions in all cases. [22]

Dr. Yu Gui-fen and colleagues randomly divided 115 cases of peri-menopausal DUB into a Chinese medicinal treatment group (60 cases) and a biomedicine control group (55 cases). The formula administered during the bleeding stage was an empirical formula, *Gù Běn Zhǐ Bēng Tāng.* (固本止崩汤)

This formula included *dǎng shēn* (Radix Codonopsis), *huáng qí* (Radix Astragali) 30g each, *dān shēn* (Radix Salviae Miltiorrhizae), *mǔ dān pí* (Cortex Moutan), *yì mǔ cǎo* (Herba Leonuri), *mǎ chǐ xiàn* (Herba Portulacae), *xiāng fù* (Rhizoma Cyperi), *hàn lián cǎo* (Herba Ecliptae) 15g each, *chì sháo* (Radix Paeoniae Rubra), *táo rén* (Semen Persicae), *chǎo pú huáng* (Dry-fried Pollen Typhae), *huā ruǐ shí* (Ophicalcitum) 10g each, and *tián sān qī* (Radix et Rhizoma Notoginseng) 3g.

With qi stagnation, add *chái hú* (Radix Bupleuri), *chuān liàn zǐ* (Fructus Toosendan), and *wū yào* (Radix Linderae).

With yin deficiency and blood-heat, remove *chì sháo* (Radix Paeoniae Rubra), *táo rén* (Semen Persicae) and add *shú dì huáng* (Radix Rehmanniae Praeparata) 20g, *shān zhū yú* (Fructus Corni) 20g, and *nǚ zhēn zǐ* (Fructus Ligustri Lucidi) 15g.

With Liver qi stagnation and excessive heat, add *dà huáng tàn* (Carbonized Radix et Rhizoma Rhei) 8g, *guàn zhòng tàn* (Carbonized Cyrtomii Rhizoma) 15g, and *chǎo shān zhī* (Dry-fried Fructus Garderniae) 15g.

With Kidney yang deficiency, add *yín yáng huò* (Herba Epimedii) and *bǔ gǔ zhī* (Fructus Psoraleae), 15g each.

Modifications during the non-bleeding period are as follows.

Remove *chǎo pú huáng* (Dry-fried Pollen Typhae), *táo rén* (Semen Persicae), *hóng huā* (Flos Carthami), *chì sháo* (Radix Paeoniae Rubra), *huā ruǐ shí* (Ophicalcitum), and *tián sān qī* (Radix et Rhizoma Notoginseng). Add *shān zhū yú* (Fructus Corni)20g, *shān yào* (Rhizoma Dioscoreae) 20g, *tù sī zǐ* (Semen Cuscutae)20, *gǒu qǐ zǐ* (Fructus Lycii) 20g, *nǚ zhēn zǐ* (Fructus Ligustri Lucidi) 15g, *huáng jīng* (Rhizoma Polygonati) 15g, *dāng guī* (Radix

Angelicae Sinensis) 15g, and *chái hú* (Radix Bupleuri) 15g.

The treatment principles here are to strengthen the Spleen, nourish the Kidney, regulate Liver qi, and regulate the penetrating and conception vessels in order to reinforce and secure the origin and generate new blood.

The control group received norethisterone 5-7.5mg, once every 6 hours during the bleeding period, and once every 8 hours after a significant decrease in volume. The dosage was then reduced daily by 1/3 for 3 days reaching a 5mg maintenance dose. Norethisterone was not withdrawn until 20 days after bleeding ceases, due to potential withdrawal symptoms. Medroxyprogesterone was prescribed to regulate menstruation at the second half of the cycle for 10 days. Three menstruation cycles constituted one course.

Results showed a total effective rate of 91.7% in the Chinese medicinal group, and 72.7% in the biomedicine group (P<0.025). After follow-up, the rate of recurrence in the treatment group reached 27.3% (15/55) and 47.5% in the control (19/40). These results indicate that the effective response to Chinese medicinals remain stable over time. [23]

Dr. Ran Qing-zhen treats menopausal period DUB patients with *Chì Shí Zhī Zhǐ Bēng Tāng* (赤石脂止崩汤).

The formula included *chì shí zhī* (Halloysitum Rubrum) 30g (decocted first) 15g, *wū zéi gǔ* (Endoconcha Sepiae) 15g, *guàn zhòng tàn* (Carbonized Cyrtomii Rhizoma) 15g, *ē jiāo* (Colla Corii Asini) 15g (dissolved), *bǔ gǔ zhī* (Fructus Psoraleae) 15g, *dǎng shēn* (Radix Codonopsis) 15g, *qiàn cǎo* (Radix Rubiae) 10g, *yì zhì rén* (Amomi Amari) 10g, *bái zhú* (Rhizoma Atractylodis Macrocephalae) 10g, *xuè yú tàn* (Crinis Carbonisatus) 10g, *yuǎn zhì* (Radix Polygalae) 6g, and *gān cǎo* (Radix et Rhizoma Glycyrrhizae) 6g.

The results of a study treating 58 cases showed 9 cases fully recovered, 21 cases responsive, 22 cases improved, and 6 cases no response. The total effective rate reached 88%. [24]

(4) DUB in Different Age Groups

Dr. Li Yan-ling treated 80 cases of flooding and spotting with an empirical formula, *Gōng Xuè Jìng* (宫血净).

The formula included *huáng qí* (Radix Astragali) 30g, *wū zéi gǔ* (Endoconcha Sepiae) 25g, *shān yú ròu* (Fructus Corni) 12g, *dān pí tàn* (Cotex Moutan Carbonisata) 12g, *jiǔ chǎo dà huáng* (Fried with wine Radix et Rhizoma Rhei) (decocted later) 12g, *qiàn cǎo tàn* (Radix Rubiae Carbonisata) 12g, *ē jiāo* (Colla Corii Asini) 12g (dissolved), *dì yú tàn* (Radix Sanguisorbae Carbonisata) 15g, *zōng tàn* (Carbonized Petiolus Trachycarpi) 15g, *sān qī fěn* (Radix Notoginseng Powder) 5g, and *gān cǎo* (Radix et Rhizoma Glycyrrhizae) 6g.

Results showed 35 cases fully recovered, 18 cases excellent response, 4 cases improved with 3 cases no response. The total effective rate reached 95%. [25]

Dr. Wang Jian-ling divided 70 DUB cases into a treatment and control group of 40 and 30 subjects respectively. All patients presented Spleen qi or blood deficient patterns and ranged in age from into 19-52 years. The treatment group received a decoction of *Yì Qì Yǎng Xuè Tāng* (益气养血汤), and the control a patent medicine, *Gōng Xuè Níng* (宫血宁).

Yì Qì Yǎng Xuè Tāng (益气养血汤) containd *shēng huáng qí* (Radix Astragali Cruda) 24g, *lù dǎng shēn* (Radix Codonopisis Pilosulae) 15g, *shú dì huáng* (Radix Rehmanniae Praeparata) 15g, *shān yú ròu* (Fructus Corni) 15g, *jī xuè téng* (Caulis Spatholobi) 15g, *hàn lián cǎo* (Herba Ecliptae) 15g, *zǐ dān shēn* (Radix Saltiae Miltiorrhizae) 15g, *dāng guī shēn* (Radix Angelicae Sinensis) 10g, *jiāo bái zhú* (Scorch-fried Rhizoma Atractylodis Macrocephalae) 10g, *zhēn ē jiāo* (Colla Corii Asini) 10g, *hēi jīng jiè* (Herba Schizonepetae Carbonisatum) 6g, *pào jiāng tàn* (Rhizoma Zingiberis Praeparata Carbonisata) 6g, *shēng má tàn* (Rhizoma Cimicifugae Carbonisata) 6g, and *sān qī fěn* (Radix Notoginseng Powder) 1.5g.

Treatment groups results showed 8 cases fully recovered, 15 cases excellent response, 15 cases improved, and 2 cases no response. The control group showed 2 cases fully recovered, 6 with excellent response, 13 subjects improved, and 13 with no response. The curative effect in the treatment group is significantly higher than that of the control (P<0.05). [26]

Dr. Yang Yu-you treated 269 subjects ranging in age from 11-50 years with modified Bao Yin Decoction.

The basic formula included *shēng dì huáng* (Radix Rehmanniae) 12g, *shú dì huáng* (Radix Rehmanniae Praeparata) 12g, *shēng bái sháo* (Raw Radix Paeoniae Alba) 12g, *huái shān yào* (Rhizoma Dioscoreae) 30g, *chuān xù duàn* (Radix Dipsaci) 10g, *chǎo kū qín* (Dry-fried Radix Scutellariae) 10g, *chǎo huáng bǎi* (Dry-fried Cortex Phellodendri Chinensis) 10g, and *shēng gān cǎo* (Raw Radix et Rhizoma Glycyrrhizae) 5g. The following modifcations were applied.

With yin deficiency due to external heat, added *dì gǔ pí* (Cortex Lycii), *dān pí* (Cotex Moutan) and *shān zhī* (Fructus Gardeniae).

With dry mouth and insomnia, added *mài dōng* (Radix Ophiopogonis), *fú shén* (Poriae Sclerotium Pararadicis), and *suān zǎo rén* (Semen Ziziphi Spinosae).

With yin and blood deficiency, added *ē jiāo* (Colla Corii Asini), *hàn lián cǎo* (Herba Ecliptae), and *nǚ zhēn zǐ* (Fructus Ligustri Lucidi).

With profuse bleeding, added *dì yú tàn* (Radix Sanguisorbae Carbonisata), *wū méi tàn* (Fructus Mume Carbonisata), *huái huā tàn* (Flos Sophorae Carbonisata), *cè bǎi tàn* (Carbonized Cacumen Platycladi), and *guàn zhòng tàn* (Carbonized Cyrtomii Rhizoma).

With blood stasis, added *qiàn cǎo* (Radix Rubiae), *pú huáng tàn* (Pollen Typhae Carbonisata) and *yì mǔ cǎo* (Herba Leonuri).

With qi stagnation, removed *shú dì huáng* (Radix Rehmanniae Praeparata) and added *qīng pí* (Pericarpium Citri Reticulatae Viride), *chén pí* (Pericarpium Citri Reticulatae), *dāng guī* (Radix Angelicae Sinensis), and *xiāng fù* (Rhizoma Cyperi).

With Kidney deficiency, added *sāng jì shēng* (Herba Taxilli), *tù sī zǐ* (Semen Cuscutae), *shā yuàn jí lí* (Semen Astragali Complanati), *dù zhòng* (Cortex Eucommiae), and *gǒu qǐ* (Fructus Lycii).

5 doses constituted one course of treatment. Results showed 183 cases fully recovered, 49 cases excellent response, 23 cases improved, with 14 cases no response. [27]

Dr. Chen Xia treated 43 DUB subjects all presenting Liver and Kidney yin deficiency patterns. The selected formula for the treatment group was *Gōng Xuè Yǐn Chōng Jì* (功血饮冲剂).

Medicinals included *shú dì huáng* (Radix Rehmanniae Praeparata), *ē jiāo* (Colla Corii Asini), *huáng qí* (Radix Astragali), and *xuè yú tàn* (Crinis Carbonisatus).

Wū Jī Bái Fèng Kǒu Fú Yè (乌鸡白凤口服液) was prescribed for 20 subjects in the control group.

Results showed 26 cases fully recovered, and 2 cases improved. Among 26 cases with prolonged menstruation, 24 cases fully recovered, 1 case improved and 1 case no response. In 26 cases of irregular menstruation, 25 cases fully recovered and 1 case with no response. The total effective rate reached 92.24% .

In the control group results showed 4 cases fully recovered, 3 cases improved and 2 cases no response among 9 cases presenting profuse bleeding. Among the 11 subjects presenting prolonged menstruation, 5 cases fully recovered and 6 cases improved. In 10 subjects with irregular menstruation, 5 cases fully recovered, 3 cases improved and 2 cases no response. The curative effect of treatment group is obvious higher than that of control group ($P < 0.01$) The total effective rate reached 46% .

Gōng Xuè Yǐn (功 血 饮) may significantly increase E_2, and P levels in adolescent and childbearing period patients. This was determined by monitoring estrogen and progestin in the 38 subjects in the treatment group. However, no response was found in menopausal subjects. [28]

Dr. Chen Yun treated subjects presenting flooding and spotting with the formula *Gōng Xuè Tāng* (宫血汤).

The basic formula included *dǎng shēn* (Radix Codonopsis), *shēng huáng qí* (Radix Astragali Cruda), *dāng guī* (Radix Angelicae Sinensis), *shú dì huáng* (Radix Rehmanniae Praeparata), *xiān hè cǎo* (Herba Agrimoniae), *wū zéi gǔ* (Endoconcha Sepiae), *ē jiāo* (Colla Corii Asini), *ài yè* (Folium Artemisiae Argyi), *cè bǎi yè* (Cacumen Platycladi), *hàn lián cǎo* (Herba Ecliptae), *shān yú ròu* (Fructus Corni), and *sān qī* (Radix Notoginseng).

Modifications were as follows.

With qi deficiency, the dosages of *huáng qí* (Radix Astragali) and *dǎng shēn* (Radix Codonopsis) were doubled, and *chǎo bái zhú* (Dry-fried Rhizoma Atractylodis Macrocephalae) added.

With blood deficiency, *chǎo bái sháo* (Dry-fried Radix Paeoniae Alba), *shēng dì huáng* (Radix Rehmanniae) added.

With blood-heat, *dì gǔ pí* (Cortex Lycii) and *yú xīng cǎo* (Herba Houttuyniae) added.

With Kidney deficiency, *gǒu qǐ* (Fructus Lycii) and *nǚ zhēn zǐ* (Fructus Ligustri Lucidi) added.

With blood stasis, *shēng pú huáng* (Pollen Typhae Crudum) and *yì mǔ cǎo* (Herba Leonuri) added.

Results among 120 cases showed 89 cases excellent response (74.17%), 28 cases improved (23.33%) and 3 cases no response. The total effective rate reached 97.50%. [29]

Dr. Pan Wen treated flooding and spotting subjects with the formula *Gōng Xuè Yǐn* (宫血饮). The basic formula contained *zhì huáng qí* (Radix Astragali Praeparata cum Melle) 24g, *chǎo bái zhú* (Dry-fried Rhizoma Atractylodis Macrocephalae) 18g, *xù duàn* (Radix Dipsaci)12g, *bǔ gǔ zhī* (Fructus Psoraleae) 12g, *bái sháo* (Radix Paeoniae Alba) 6g, *wū zéi gǔ* (Endoconcha Sepiae) 6g, *qiàn cǎo* (Radix Rubiae) 6g, *pú huáng* (Pollen

Typhae) 6g, *shēn sān qī* (Radix Notoginseng) 3g (infused), and *zhì gān cǎo* (Radix et Rhizoma Glycyrrhizae Praeparata cum Melle) 6g.

Results showed 28 cases fully recovered, 12 cases improved and 2 cases no response. The total effective rate reached 95%. In 16 subjects bleeding ceased after 1-3 doses, in 20 subjects after 4-6 doses, and in 4 subjects after 9 doses. [30]

Dr. Shan Jing-wen and colleagues treated DUB with *Gōng Xuè Tíng Kē Lì* (宫血停颗粒).

The basic formula in the treatment group contained *huáng qí* (Radix Astragali), *shēng má* (Rhizoma Cimicifugae), *dǎng shēn* (Radix Codonopsis), *yì mǔ cǎo* (Herba Leonuri), *pú huáng* (Pollen Typhae), *zhǐ qiào* (Fructus Aurantii), *duàn lóng gǔ* (Calcined Fossilia Ossis Mastodi), *duàn mǔ lì* (Calcined Concha Ostreae), *dāng guī* (Radix Angelicae Sinensis), *nǚ zhēn zǐ* (Fructus Ligustri Lucidi) and *hàn lián cǎo* (Herba Ecliptae).

The control group was administered *Gōng Xuè Níng* (宫血宁) 0.26g three times daily, during the bleeding stage, with *Yún Nán Bái Yào* (云南白药) 0.25g, twice daily until cessation of bleeding. Subjects received diethylstilbestrol 0.5mg beginning on the 5th day of menstruation, once nightly for 20 days. Control also received 5 daily intramuscular injections of progesterone 10mg, beginning at day 16.

Results in the treatment group showed 29 cases fully recovered, including 11 cases with Kidney yin deficiency, 10 cases Kidney yang deficiency pattern and 8 cases with blood stasis. 15 subjects improved, including 6 cases with Kidney yin deficiency, 7 cases Kidney yang deficiency with blood stasis, and 2 cases with blood stasis. 3 cases no response with 2 cases Kidney yin deficiency and 1 case Kidney yang deficiency with blood stasis. The course of treatment ranged from 5 to 30 days.

Control group results showed 17 cases fully recovered, including 7 cases of Kidney yin deficiency, 5 cases Kidney yang deficiency with blood stasis, and 5 cases with blood stasis. 9 cases showed no response, with 3 subjects presenting Kidney yin deficiency, Kidney yang deficiency with blood stasis, and blood stasis patterns respectively. [31]

Dr. Peng Zhen-sheng treated 80 cases of DUB with an empirical formula, *Cán Shā Gù Jīng Tāng* (蚕砂固经汤).

The basic formula contained *cán shā* (Faeces Bombycis) 6g (carbonized and swallowed), *lù jiǎo shuāng* (Cornu Cervi Degelatinatum) 12g, *guì zhī* (Ramulus Cinnamomi) 6g, *dù zhòng* (Cortex Eucommiae) 12g, *dāng guī* (Radix Angelicae Sinensis) 10g, *shā yuàn zǐ* (Semen Astragali complanati) 12g, *fú shén* (Poriae Sclerotium Pararadicis) 12g, *ē jiāo* (Colla Corii Asini) 10g (dissolved), *huáng qí* (Radix Astragali) 20g, and *hǎi piāo xiāo* (Endoconcha Sepiae) 15g.

Patients were prescribed 200ml twice daily, decocted. A minimum of 6-12 doses per week were recommended during the premenstrual period, with three months as one course of treatment. The control group of 20 subjects received norethisterone or megestrol acetate, 8 tablets, 3 times daily.

The treatment group results showed 30 cases fully recovered, 10 cases excellent response, 8 cases improved, and 2 cases no response. The total effective rate reached 97.5%; The results in the control group showed 10 cases fully recovered, 2 cases excellent response, 2 cases improved, 6 cases no response. The total effective rate reached 70%. The curative effect in the treatment group was significantly higher than that of the control. [32]

Dr. Xing Cui-ling treated subjects with DUB using an empirical formula, *Tiáo Jīng Tāng* (调经汤).

The basic formula contained *huáng qí* (Radix Astragali) 50g, *dǎng shēn* (Radix Codonopsis), *duàn lóng gǔ* (Calcined Fossilia Ossis Mastodi), *duàn mǔ lì* (Calcined Concha Ostreae), *fú líng* (Poria), *shān yú ròu* (Fructus Corni), *ē jiāo* (Colla Corii Asini), *bái zhú* (Rhizoma Atractylodis Macrocephalae) 20g each, *dù zhòng*(Cortex Eucommiae), *wǔ bèi zǐ* (Galla Chinensis), *hǎi piāo xiāo* (Endoconcha Sepiae) 15g each, and *yì mǔ cǎo* (Herba Leonuri) 10g.

Modifications to the formula were as follows.

With qi deficiency, *dǎng shēn* (Radix Codonopsis) was replaced with *rén shēn* (Radix et Rhizoma Ginseng) 10g.

With internal heat due to yin deficiency, added *shēng dì huáng* (Radix Rehmanniae) 15g.

With blood stasis, added *táo rén* (Semen Persicae) and *hóng huā* (Flos Carthami), 10g each.

With qi and blood deficiency, added *tāi pán fěn* (Placenta Hominis Powder) 10g.

One decocted dose was administered daily. 5-10 days in a menstruation cycle constitutes one course of treatment.

In a total of 160 cases, results showed 104 cases fully recovered, 35 cases excellent response, 15 cases improved, and 6 cases no response. The recovery rate reached 65% with a total effective rate reaching 96.2%. [33]

Dr. Liu Gui-shu treated 68 DUB cases with *Tiáo Jīng Zhǐ Xuè Tāng* (调 经止血汤).

The formula included *shú dì huáng* (Radix Rehmanniae Praeparata) 20g, *dāng guī* (Radix Angelicae Sinensis) 15g, *bái sháo* (Radix Paeoniae Alba) 15g, *pú huáng* (Pollen Typhae) 10g, *wǔ líng zhī* (Faeces Trogopterori) 10g, *hǎi piāo xiāo* (Endoconcha Sepiae) 10g, *xù duàn* (Radix Dipsaci) 10g, *lóng gǔ* (Fossilia Ossis Mastodi) 20g, *mǔ lì* (Concha Ostreae) 20g, *qiàn cǎo* (Radix Rubiae) 10g, and *dà huáng* (Carbonized with vinegar Radix et Rhizoma Rhei) 15g.

Modifications were as follows.

With qi deficiency, *huáng qí* (Radix Astragali) and *rén shēn* (Radix et Rhizoma Ginseng) added.

With the middle qi sinking, *chái hú* (Radix Bupleuri), *shēng má* (Rhizoma Cimicugae), and *jié gěng* (Radix Platycodonis) added.

With blood-heat, *shēng dì huáng* (Radix Rehmanniae), *dì yú* (Radix Sanguisorbae), *huáng qín* (Radix Scutellariae), and *huáng bǎi* (Cortex

Phellodendri Chinensis) added.

With Liver and Kidney deficiency, *tù sī zǐ* (Semen Cuscutae) and *dù zhòng* (Cortex Eucommiae) added.

Results showed 25 cases fully recovered, 40 cases improved, and 3 cases no response. The total effective rate reached 95.6%. 12 cases showed improvement with the first course of treatment, 21 cases improved with the second, and 32 cases improved by the third. [34]

Dr. Shen Rong treated 232 cases of DUB using an integrative medicine approach. Biomedicines included injections of 10% G.S. 500ml, vitamin K 30mg, etamsylate 3g, aminomethylbenzoic acid 0.3g, once daily for 3-5 days. Blood transfusion used for cases of severe anemia. In cases of hormone abuse, medications should be adjusted or discontinued. Estradiol benzoate was administered to adolescents, norethisterone or complex progesterone to those of childbearing age, while testosterone was given to menopausal subjects.

The formula *Bǔ Shèn Zhǐ Xuè Tāng* (补肾止血汤) included *huáng qí* (Radix Astragali) 15g, *chǎo bái zhú* (Dry-fried Rhizoma Atractylodis Macrocephalae) 15g, *shú dì huáng* (Radix Rehmanniae Praeparata) 15g, *gǒu qǐ zǐ* (Fructus Lycii) 15g, *chuān xù duàn* (Radix Dipsaci) 15g, *bǔ gǔ zhī* (Fructus Psoraleae) 10g, *chǎo pú huáng* (Dry-fried Pollen Typhae) 10g, *xuè yú tàn* (Crinis Carbonisatus) 15g, *mò hàn lián* (Herba Ecliptae) 15g, *duàn lóng gǔ* (Calcined Fossilia Ossis Mastodi) and *duàn mǔ lì* (Calcined Concha Ostreae) 20g each.

With yin deficiency, *nǚ zhēn zǐ* (Fructus Ligustri Lucidi) added and *shú dì huáng* (Radix Rehmanniae Praeparata) replaced with *shēng dì huáng* (Radix Rehmanniae) 20g.

With profuse bleeding due to overwork, *dǎng shēn* (Radix Codonopsis) 20g added.

With Liver qi stagnation, *chái hú* (Radix Bupleuri) 10g and *xiāng fù* (Rhizoma Cyperi) 10g added.

With blood deficiency, *ē jiāo* (Colla Corii Asini) 15g (dissolved) added.

Yì Huáng Tiáo Zhōu Fāng (益黄调周方) was prescribed after the bleeding period. The Formula included *shú dì huáng* (Radix Rehmanniae Praeparata), *chuān xù duàn* (Radix Dipsaci), *dù zhòng* (Cortex Eucommiae), *chǎo bái zhú* (Dry-fried Rhizoma Atractylodis Macrocephalae), *tù sī zǐ* (Semen Cuscutae), *bā jǐ tiān* (Radix Morindae Officinalis), *gǒu qǐ zǐ* (Fructus Lycii), *ròu cōng róng* (Herba Cistanches), *chén pí* (Pericarpium Citri Reticulatae) 10g each, and *dāng guī* (Radix Angelicae Sinensis) 6g.

In order to promote ovulation, one decocted dose taken twice daily was prescribed until the onset of menstruation.

Results showed 214 cases fully recovered (92.2%), 12 cases excellent response (5.2%), 6 cases improved (2.6%). The criteria used are as follows. Full recovery: symptomatic relief with the cessation of bleeding in 7 days. Excellent response: symptomatic relief with the cessation of bleeding in 8-10 days. Improvement: symptomatic relief with the cessation of bleeding in 11-15 days. The total effective rate reached 100%. [35]

Dr. Song Su-ying treated 316 DUB cases with *Huí Chūn Zhǐ Xuè Sǎn* (回春止血散). The basic formula included *dǎng shēn* (Radix Codonopsis) 20g, *bái zhú* (Rhizoma Atractylodis Macrocephalae) 15g, *fú líng* (Poria) 12g, *huáng qí* (Radix Astragali) 30g, *ē jiāo* (dissolved) (Colla Corii Asini) 18g, *yì mǔ cǎo* (Herba Leonuri) 15g, *mò hàn lián* (Herba Ecliptae) 15g, *xiān hè cǎo* (Herba Agrimoniae) 15g, and *sān qī fěn* (Radix Notoginseng Powder) 3g (infused).

Medicinals were administered in the following forms.

(1) One decocted dose, taken twice daily.

(2) 4 to 6 powdered capsules 0.43g, taken with warm water 2-3 times daily.

Modifications were as follows.

With lassitude, a pale complexion, and a downbearing sensation in the lower abdomen, *shēng má* (Rhizoma Cimicifugae) 6g was added and the dosage of *huáng qí* (Radix Astragali) increased.

With chest and flank swelling, vexation and poor appetite, *chái hú* (Radix Bupleuri) 10g and *zhǐ qiào* (Fructus Aurantii) 12g were added.

With purple clotting, distending abdominal pain, and a deep red tongue with stasis spots on the tip, *pào jiāng* (Rhizoma Zingiberis Praeparata) 10g and *pú huáng* (Pollen Typhae) 15g were added.

With profuse and bright red bleeding, *fú líng* (Poria) was removed, and *duàn lóng gǔ* (Calcined Fossilia Ossis Mastodi), *duàn mǔ lì* (Calcined Concha Ostreae), and *shēng dì yú* (Raw Radix Sanguisorbae) added, 30g each. All other medicines were withdrawn during treatment. This formula was continued until the complete cessation of bleeding, after which *Guī Pí Wán* (归脾丸), or *Liù Wèi Dì Huáng Wán* (六味地黄丸) with *Xiāo Yáo Wán* (逍遥丸) were prescribed to regulate menses and secure the origin.

Results showed 207 cases fully recovered (65.51%), 56 cases excellent response (17.72%), 41 cases improved (12.97%), 12 cases no response (3.80%). The total effective rate reached 96.21%. Bleeding completely ceased in 216 cases after 1-3 doses (68.35%), in 66 cases after 4-8 (20.89%), and 22 cases after dose 9 (6.96%). Both menstrual volume and cycles returned to normal after 2-8 decocted doses, where those who took capsules showed effect after 2-3 days with normal menstruation occurring after 5 days of treatment. [36]

Dr. Wang Yun-yi treated 86 cases with *Liǔ Zhī Tāng* (柳枝汤).

50g *Liǔ Zhī Tāng* (柳枝汤) was initially administered to all subjects, where bleeding generally ceased after 3 doses. Then subjects were treated according to age and presenting patterns. For subjects over 35 years, *Dì Huáng Tāng* (地黄汤), *Xiāo Yáo Wán* (逍遥丸) and *Guī Pí Wán* (归脾丸) were used to relieve Liver qi constraint and balance both Kidney yin and yang. For those displaying uterine hypoplasia, vitamins E and B, plus thyroxine were prescribed as well. Menstrual volume was also monitered. With recurrent and profuse bleeding, *Liǔ Zhī Tāng* (柳枝汤) was re-administered until cessation. In the course of the study, one subject was administered medicines to induce artificial cycles. Three cases were prescribed methyltestosterone. *Liǔ Zhī Tāng* (柳枝汤) formula containd *liǔ zhī* (Salix Babylonica), *bái sháo* (Radix Paeoniae Alba), *shú dì huáng* (Radix Rehmanniae Praeparata), and *dāng guī* (Radix Angelicae Sinensis).

Results showed 71 cases with excellent response (82.5%), 11 cases improved (13.3%), and 4 cases no response 4.4%. [37]

Dr. Chen Xia treated Liver and Kidney yin deficiency patterns associated with adolescent DUB using *Gōng Xuè Yǐn* (功血饮). The formula contained *shēng dì huáng* (Radix Rehmanniae) 15g, *ē jiāo* (Colla Corii Asini) 6g, *xù duàn* (Radix Dipsaci) 10g, *huáng qí* (Radix Astragali) 15g, *dì gǔ pí* (Cortex Lycii) 10g, *nǚ zhēn zǐ* (Fructus Ligustri Lucidi) 12g and *hàn lián cǎo* (Herba Ecliptae) 12g.

The decoction was prepared as granules, where each 10g packet contained 2.36g crude drugs. The dosages prescribed were 2 packets 3 times daily during the bleeding stage, and one packet 3 times daily in non-bleeding stage. The prescription for the control group was a prepared medicine, *Wū Jī Bái Fèng Kǒu Fú Yè* (乌鸡白凤口服液). Ingredients included *wū jī* (Gallus Domesticus Brisson), *shēng dì huáng* (Radix Rehmanniae), *bái sháo* (Radix Paeoniae Alba), *zhī mǔ* (Rhizoma Anemarrhenae), *chái hú* (Radix Bupleuri), *dān pí* (Cotex Moutan), and *huáng qí* (Radix Astragali). Subjects were prescribed 2 bottles, three times daily. 30 days constituted one course of treatment, with 3 courses recommended.

Treatment group results showed 19 subjects fully recovered (52.8%), 14 with excellent response (38.9%), and 3 improved (8.3%). The total effective rate reached 100%. Control group results showed 1 subject fully recovered (5.9%), 5 cases excellent response (29.4%), 9 cases improved (52.9%), and 2 with no response (11.8%). The total effective rate reached 88.2%. The differences in the total effective rates were significant (u=4.1546, P<0.01). [38]

Dr. Ou Zhong-bo treated 105 flooding and spotting cases with modified *Wēn Qīng Yǐn* (温清饮). The decoction contained *dāng guī* (Radix Angelicae Sinensis) 3g, *bái sháo* (Radix Paeoniae Alba) 4g, *shēng dì huáng* (Radix Rehmanniae) 4g, *chuān xiōng* (Rhizoma Chuanxiong) 3g, *huáng lián* (Rhizoma Coptidis) 3g, *huáng qín* (Radix Scutellariae) 3g, *huáng bǎi* (Cortex Phellodendri Chinensis) 3g, *shēng zhī zǐ* (Raw Fructus Gardeniae) 3g, *duàn lóng gǔ* (Calcined Fossilia Ossis Mastodi) 20g (decocted first), *duàn mǔ lì* (Calcined Concha Ostreae) 20g (decocted first), *qiàn gēn* (Radix et Rhizoma Rubiae) 6g, and *hǎi piāo xiāo* (Endoconcha Sepiae) 6g. Decocted with 600-800ml water and divided into two parts, taken daily for 3-6 days.

Results showed 85 cases fully recovered, 12 cases improved and 8 cases no response. The total effective rate reached 92.4%. [39]

Dr. Yin Yue-hui and Dr. Fan Ji-xiang treated 40 cases of flooding and spotting with *Guī Pí Tāng* (归脾汤).

The decoction included *dǎng shēn* (Radix Codonopsis) 30g, *huáng qí* (Radix Astragali) 30g, *bái zhú* (Rhizoma Atractylodis Macrocephalae) 10g, *fú líng* (Poria) 15g, *lóng yǎn ròu* (Arillus Longan) 15g, *suān zǎo rén* (Semen Ziziphi Spinosae) 12g, *mù xiāng* (Radix Aucklandiae) 6g, *dāng guī* (Radix Angelicae Sinensis) 12g, and *yuǎn zhì* (Radix Polygalae) 10g. One divided dose was taken daily for up to 30 days.

Modifications were as follows.

With urgent bleeding *xuè yú tàn* (Crinis Carbonisatus) 10g, *zōng lǘ tàn* (Carbonized Petiolus Trachycarpi) 10g, and *qiàn cǎo gēn* (Radix et Rhizoma Rubiae) 10g were added.

With flooding with cold, *ài yè* (Folium Artemisiae Argyi) 10g and *pào jiāng* (Rhizoma Zingiberis Praeparata) 3g were added.

Results showed 30 cases fully recovered (75%), 8 cases improved (20%), and 2 cases no response (5%). The total effective rate reached 95%. [40]

Dr. Ding Xiu-ying treated 100 DUB cases with *Gù Bēng Tāng* (固崩汤).
The basic formula contained *hé shǒu wū* (Radix Polygoni Multiflori)
20g, *ē jiāo* (Colla Corii Asini) 20g, *wū zéi gǔ* (Endoconcha Sepiae) 30g,
chǎo dì yú (Dry-fried Radix Sanguisorbae) 60g, *xiān hè cǎo* (Herba
Agrimoniae) 60g, *duàn lóng gǔ* (Calcined Fossilia Ossis Mastodi) 40g,
duàn mǔ lì (Calcined Concha Ostreae) 40g, *xiāng fù* (Rhizoma Cyperi) 10g,
yì mǔ cǎo (Herba Leonuri) 10g, and *bái sháo* (Radix Paeoniae Alba) 15g.
Modifications were applied according to pattern differentiation.

Results showed 87 cases with excellent response (87%) and 13 cases
improved (13%). The total effective rate reached 100%. In 56 subjects,
bleeding ceased after 1-2 doses (56%), 8 cases after 2-3 doses (38%), and
6 after 3-4 doses (6%). Herbs to regulate menses were continued for 2
to 6 months. This group included 39 menopausal subjects. In 26 cases,
menstruation ceased after three cycles and in 13 cases, after one year.
There were 36 adolescent subjects, all with excellent response. 25 subjects
were in the childbearing period, all with improvement or excellent
response. [41]

Dr. Xing Jin-xia treated 125 flooding and spotting cases with an
empirical formula, *Èr Cǎo Wǔ Tàn Tāng* (二草五炭汤). Medicinals included
xiān hè cǎo (Herba Agrimoniae) 45g, *bái jí tàn* (Carbonized Rhizoma
Bletillae) and *jīng jiè tàn* (Herba Schizonepetae Carbonisatum) 20g each,
yì mǔ cǎo (Herba Leonuri) 30g, *zǐ huā dì dīng* (Herba Violae) 30g, *dì yú tàn*
(Carbonized Radix Sanguisorbae) 30g, *zōng lǚ tàn* (Trachycarpi Petiolus
Carbonisatus) 10g, *pú huáng tàn* (Carbonized Pollen Typhae) 10g and *dāng
guī* (Radix Angelicae Sinensis) 15g.

With Spleen and Kidney yang deficiency, added *ròu guì tàn*
(Carbonized Cortex Cinnamomi) 3g, *pú huáng tàn* (Carbonized Pollen
Typhae) 10g and *dāng guī* (Radix Angelicae Sinensis) 15g.

With Spleen and Kidney yang deficiency, added *ròu guì* (Cortex
Cinnamomi) 3g, and *dì gǔ pí* (Cortex Lycii) 15g.

With Liver qi stagnation, added *xiāng fù* (Rhizoma Cyperi) 12g, and *cù zhì chái hú* (prepared with vinegar Radix Bupleuri) 15g.

With qi deficiency, added *tài zǐ shēn* (Radix Pseudostellariae) 30g, *huáng qí* (Radix Astragali) 30g, *fú líng* (Poria) 15g, and *bái zhú* (Rhizoma Atractylodis Macrocephalae) 15g.

With blood deficiency, added *ē jiāo* (Colla Corii Asini, dissolved) and *xuè yú tàn* (Crinis Carbonisatus) 30g each.

With clotting and abdominal pain, added *táo rén* (Semen Persicae) 12g and *hóng huā* (Flos Carthami) 12g.

Results showed all 125 cases fully recovered. 90 cases recovered fully after 3 doses, 28 cases after 6 doses, and 9 cases after 7 doses. After 3 courses of treatment, the total effective rate reached 100%. [42]

Dr. Tang Chun-qiong treated 64 cases of flooding and spotting with *Gù Chōng Tāng* (固冲汤) and *Dēng Xīn Zhǐ Xuè Táng Jiāng* (灯心止血糖浆). *Gù Chōng Tāng* (固冲汤) containd *zhì huáng qí* (Radix Astragali Praeparata cum Melle) 20g, *dǎng shēn* (Radix Codonopsis) 18g, *bái zhú* (Rhizoma Atractylodis Macrocephalae), *shān yào* (Rhizoma Dioscoreae), *shān yú ròu* (Fructus Corni), *bái sháo* (Radix Paeoniae Alba), *zhì shǒu wū* (Radix Polygoni Multiflori Praeparata cum Succo Glycines Sotae), *ē jiāo* (Colla Corii Asini, dissolved), *qiàn cǎo* (Radix Rubiae) and *wǔ wèi zǐ* (Fructus Schisandrae) 10g each, *wū zéi gǔ* (Endoconcha Sepiae) 10-15g, *zōng lǚ tàn* (Trachycarpus) 10-15g, *yì mǔ cǎo* (Herba Leonuri) 10-15g, *duàn lóng gǔ* (Calcined Fossilia Ossis Mastodi) and *duàn mǔ lì* (Calcined Concha Ostreae) 24-30g each, and *zhì gān cǎo* (Radix et Rhizoma Glycyrrhizae Praeparata cum Melle) 6g.

Results showed 45 cases fully recovered, 14 cases improved, and 5 cases no response. The maximum dosage of *Gù Chōng Tāng* (固冲汤) was 5 doses and the minimum 2 doses. The maximum dosage of *Dēng Xīn Zhǐ Xuè Táng Jiāng* (灯心止血糖浆) was 3 bottles and the minimum 1 bottle. The total effective rate reached 92.2%. [43]

Dr. Zhao Wen-yan and colleagues treated one 31 year old patient with *Guì Zhī Tāng* (桂枝汤). The abnormal bleeding pattern was initially caused by wading in water and exposure to rain. Porridge was taken with the decoction as part of treatment, and all symptoms were alleviated with 3 doses. Normal menstruation was maintained at a one year follow-up exam. [44]

Dr. Chen Yong-pu and colleagues treated one case of menstrual disorder with *Huáng Lián Ē Jiāo Tāng* (黄连阿胶汤). Her condition was associated with dilatation and curettage. The formula contained *huáng lián* (Rhizoma Coptidis) 5g, *ē jiāo* (Colla Corii Asini, dissolved), *bái sháo* (Radix Paeoniae Alba) 12g, *huáng qín* (Radix Scutellariae) 12g, *shēng dì huáng* (Radix Rehmanniae) 12g, *guī bǎn* (Testudinis Plastrum) 12g, and *dì gǔ pí* (Cortex Lycii) 15g.

Bleeding significantly reduced after 2 doses, with some symptomatic relief. The condition resolved completely after dose 6. To reinforce the effect, *nǚ zhēn zǐ* (Fructus Ligustri Lucidito) 15g was added, and 5 doses prescribed. [45]

Dr. Liu Jin-xing studied 60 cases of DUB associated with qi deficiency and blood stasis. Subjects were evenly divided at random into a treatment group and a control group. The formula administered to the treatment group was *Gù Chōng Zhǐ Xuè Tāng* (固冲止血汤).

Medicinals included *zhì huáng qí* (Radix Astragali Praeparata cum Melle), *chǎo bái zhú* (Dry-fried Rhizoma Atractylodis Macrocephalae), *chǎo shēng má* (Dry-fried Rhizoma Cimicifugae), *jiè suì tàn* (Spica Schizonepetae Carbonisata), *guàn zhòng tàn* (Carbonized Cyrtomii Rhizoma), *yuǎn zhì* (Radix Polygalae), *wū zéi gǔ* (Endoconcha Sepiae), *qiàn cǎo tàn* (Carbonized Radix Rubiae), *sān qī* (Radix Notoginseng), *pú huáng tàn* (Carbonized Pollen Typhae) and *wǔ wèi zǐ* (Fructus Schisandrae).

For the control group, *Yì Gōng Zhǐ Xuè Kóu Fú Yè* (益宫止血口服液) was prescribed.

Blood stanching effects, clinical symptoms, endometrial thickness, prothrombin and partial thromboplastin rates, Ca^{2+} levels, endocrine hormone levels, prostaglandin E_2 (PGE_2) and $F_{2\alpha}$ ($PGF_{2\alpha}$) levels, endometrial estrogen (ER) and progesterone receptors (PR) receptors were all monitored.

Results showed the total effective rate of stanching bleeding with *Gù Chōng Zhǐ Xuè Tāng* (固冲止血汤) was 93.3%, significantly higher that that of control (70.0%, P<0.05). There was a significant difference in all measurements as compared to control (P<0.05). [46]

Dr. Xia Tian and colleagues randomly divided 50 patients into treatment and control groups of 35 and 15 subjects respectively. The treatment group recieved *Kūn Níng Huó Xuè Tāng* (坤宁活血汤).

The medicinals included *sān qī* (Radix Notoginseng, infused) 3g, *táo rén* (Semen Persicae) 9g, *chì sháo yào* (Radix Paeoniae Rubra) 9g, *dān pí* (Cortex Moutan) 9g, *huáng qí* (Radix Astragali) 18g, *guì zhī* (Ramulus Cinnamomi) 6g, *jiǔ dà huáng* (Prepared with wine Radix et Rhizoma Rhei) 6g, and *gān cǎo* (Radix et Rhizoma Glycyrrhizae) 6g.

One divided dose was taken twice daily for 6 days, as one course of treatment. Subjects were observed for up to 2 courses.

The medicinal for the control was *Sān Qī Piàn* (三七片), 4 pills, 3 times daily. 6 days constituted one course of treatment. Blood stanching effects, clinical symptoms, and endometrial thickness was monitored. In addition, animal experiments were performed to observe influences on uterine contraction, bleeding and clotting times, blood flow, hormone levels, and the estrogen and progesterone receptors. 2 menstruation cycles constituted one course of treatment. Clinical manifestations and endometrial thickness of both groups showed significant differences after treatment (P<0.05-0.01). The total effective rate in the treatment group reached 91.4%, while that of control reached 66.7% (P<0.05). Empirical studies indicate that *Kūn Níng Huó Xuè Tāng* (坤宁活血汤) promotes uterine contraction, shortens bleeding and clotting time, improves blood flow, and reduces endometrial ER and PR levels. [47]

(5) The Application of Carbonized Medicinals

In Fu Dong-ming's opinion, the use of carbonized medicinals in the treatment of flooding and spotting effectively treats both the abnormal bleeding symptoms and the underlying cause of the disorder. Carbonized medicinals do not contain charcoal, and these processed medicinals in fact retain their original therapeutic properties. They may be effectively used to tonify deficiency, clear heat and even dispel blood stasis. The pathomechanisms of flooding and spotting are addressed by the natures of the medicinals which have been carbonized. There are a variety of factors which create blood stasis in the course of treatment. Despite the saying, "bleeding may be stanched with black (carbonized madicinals)", we should not consider carbonized medicinals to be completely responsible for the appearance of blood stasis patterns. In clinic, we should always follow the principles of pattern differentiation and thus bring the effect of carbonized medicinals fully into play. [48]

(6) Frequently Reported Medicinals in the Treatment of DUB

The most commonly used medicinals for DUB in reports from over the last 10 years include *huáng qí* (Radix Astragali), *bái zhú* (Rhizoma Atractylodis Macrocephalae), *dāng guī* (Radix Angelicae Sinensis), *bái sháo* (Radix Paeoniae Alba), *shēng dì huáng* (Radix Rehmanniae), *rén shēn* (Radix et Rhizoma Ginseng), *ē jiāo* (Colla Corii Asini), *qiàn cǎo* (Radix Rubiae), *shú dì huáng* (Radix Rehmanniae Praeparata), *xù duàn* (Radix Dipsaci), *duàn mǔ lì* (Calcined Concha Ostreae), *shān zhū yú* (Fructus Corni), *gān cǎo* (Radix et Rhizoma Glycyrrhizae), *shān yào* (Rhizoma Dioscoreae), *lóng gǔ* (Fossilia Ossis Mastodi), *dì yú* (Radix Sanguisorbae), *hǎi piāo xiāo* (Endoconcha Sepiae), *wū zéi gǔ* (Endoconcha Sepiae), *yì mǔ cǎo*

(Herba Leonuri), *chuān xiōng* (Rhizoma Chuanxiong), *xiāng fù* (Rhizoma Cyperi), *jīng jiè tàn* (Herba Schizonepetae Carbonisatum), *nǚ zhēn zǐ* (Fructus Ligustri Lucidi), *pú huáng* (Pollen Typhae), *shēng má* (Rhizoma Cimicifugae), *xiān hè cǎo* (Herba Agrimoniae), *dān pí* (Cortex Moutan), *lù jiǎo shuāng* (Cornu Cervi Degelatinatum), *sān qī* (Radix Notoginseng), *fú líng* (Poria), *wǔ wèi zǐ* (Fructus Schisandrae), *hé shǒu wū* (Radix Polygoni Multiflori), *guī bǎn* (Testudinis Plastrum), *tù sī zǐ* (Semen Cuscutae), *gǒu qǐ* (Fructus Lycii), *ài yè* (Folium Artemisiae Argyi), *zōng lǘ tàn* (Trachycarpus), *chái hú* (Radix Bupleuri), *dà huáng* (Radix et Rhizoma Rhei), *pào jiāng* (Rhizoma Zingiberis Praeparata), *hóng huā* (Flos Carthami), *mài dōng* (Radix Ophiopogonis), *wǔ líng zhī* (Faeces Trogopterori), *xiān máo* (Rhizoma Curculiginis), *xiān líng pí* (Herba Epimedii), *jī xuè téng* (Caulis Spatholobi), *sāng jì shēng* (Herba Taxilli) and *huā ruǐ shí* (Ophicalcitum).

3. ACUPUNCTURE AND MOXIBUSTION

(1) Arresting Bleeding

Dr. Yu Shan-tang and colleagues treated 38 cases of flooding and spotting, ages 14-46, by combining acupuncture with supplementary Chinese medicinal treatment. 23 subjects presented bleeding for 6-15 days, 11 cases for 16-30 days, and 4 for more than 30 days.

The principle selected points were SP 1 (*yǐn bǎi*), KI 7 (*fù liu*) and RN 4 (*guān yuán*).

Supplementary points:

With excessive heat, added SP 10 (*xuè hǎi*).

With Spleen qi deficiency, added ST 36 (*zú sān lǐ*).

With yin deficiency, added PC 6 (*nèi guān*).

Using the flicking needle insertion method, needles were retained for 30 minutes, scraping the needles every 10 minutes. Ideal effects occurred with the needling sensation radiating to the inner thigh. With deficiency signs, the reinforcing method was applied, and with excess, the reducing method. 10 days constituted one course of treatment. The main points were alternated bilaterally such as needling KI 7 on the left and SP 1 on the right. Supplementary points were selected according to pattern differentiation. In cases of persistent bleeding following acupuncture treatment, Chinese medicinals were also prescribed.

Medicinals included *dāng guī* (Radix Angelicae Sinensis) 20g, *jiǔ bái sháo* (Prepared with wine Radix Paeoniae Alba) 20g, *shēng dì huáng* (Radix Rehmanniae) 20g, *dǎng shēn* (Radix Codonopsis) 15g, *huáng qí* (Radix Astragali) 30g, *chǎo bái zhú* (Dry-fried Rhizoma Atractylodis Macrocephalae) 25g, *chǎo dì yú* (Dry-fried Radix Sanguisorbae) 20g, *bái tóu wēng* (Radix Pulsatillae) 20g, and *yì mǔ cǎo tàn* (Carbonized Herba Leonuri) 20g. One daily dose decocted, 5-10 days per course.

The criteria and results of the study are as follows:

Excellent response: cessation of bleeding within 7 days using acupuncture alone.

Improved: the cessation of bleeding within 10 days, using both acupuncture and medicinals.

No response: failure to completely stanch bleeding.

Results showed 26 cases excellent response (68.4%), 10 cases improved (26.3%), 2 cases no response (5.3%). [49]

Dr. Xue Di-cheng and colleagues used auricular therapy to treat DUB in 54 subjects, aged 14-52, who previously showed no response to Chinese medicinals, or biomedicine for more than one month.

Primary selected points included uterus, ovary, endocrine, Spleen, Liver and Kidney. Supplementary points: subcortex, shenmen and sanjiao.

Method: auricular points were pressed in sequence every 2 hours, both ears alternately. Seeds were reapplied every 2 days, with 18 days constituting one course of treatment.

Results showed cessation of bleeding in 32 cases after 1 course (59.3%), 20 cases after 2 courses (37%). In 2 cases, bleeding was significantly reduced. The curative effect seems to be related to age, course of treatment, and the amount of daily ear pressing applied. [50]

Dr. Xu Tian and colleagues treated DUB in 49 subjects, aged 20-46, with a combination of acupuncture, moxibustion, and infrared radiation.

The points selected were PC 6 (*nèi guān*), ST 25 (*tiān shū*), RN 6 (*qì hǎi*), RN 4, ST 36, and SP 6 (*sān yīn jiāo*).

The insertion method used for RN 6 and RN 4 induced a strong sensation with tendinomuscular spasm. Ideal effects occurred with the needling sensation radiating to the dorsum of the foot. Needles were retained for 30 minutes following the arrival of qi, and no further manipulation was applied. Infrared radiation was applied with mild moxibustion on points RN 8 (*shén quē*) and RN 4 after needling. 6 daily treatments constituted one course.

The criteria and results of the study are as follows:

Full recovery: menstruation normal with 3-7 day cycles. No recurrence at 3 month followup exams.

Improved: menstruation normal, with light bleeding. Cycles longer than 7 days.

Results showed 41 cases fully recovered (84%), 6 cases improved (12%), and 2 cases no response (4%). [51]

Dr. Zhang Yong-luo and colleagues treated 142 cases of DUB, aged 14-49. Subjects were divided at random into four treatment groups: acupuncture (35 cases), moxibustion (33 cases), Chinese medicinals (40 cases), and acupuncture with medicinals (34 cases).

The following points were applied in both the acupuncture and moxibustion groups:

RN 4, *zǐ gōng* (EX-CA1), SP 6, and BL 32 (*cì liáo*).

With profuse bleeding, added LI 4 (*hé gǔ*) and SP 1.

With excessive heat, added SP 10 and LV 3 (*tài chōng*).

With Spleen deficiency, added ST 36.

With Kidney deficiency, added DU 3 (*yáng guān*).

Both acupuncture and moxibusion were applied once every 3 days. 5 days constituted one course of treatment.

The formula applied to stanch bleeding included:

Dăng shēn (Radix Codonopsis) 20g, *hàn lián căo* (Herba Ecliptae) 20g, *cè băi tàn* (Carbonized Cacumen Platycladi) 15g, *shēng dì huáng* (Radix Rehmanniae) 30g, *yì mŭ căo* (Herba Leonuri) 20g, *huáng qín* (Radix Scutellariae) 10g, *jiāo dì yú* (Scorch-fried Radix Sanguisorbae) 30g, *chăo pú huáng* (Dry-fried Pollen Typhae) 10g, *dà jì* (Herba Cirsii Japonici) 15g, *xiăo jì* (Herba Cirsii) 15g, and *mù zéi* (Herba Equiseti Hiemalis), 10g.

The formula applied to regulate menses included:

With Kidney deficiency, *shú dì huáng* (Radix Rehmanniae Praeparata) 30g, *dāng guī* (Radix Angelicae Sinensis) 12g, *xiān líng pí* (Herba Epimedii) 15g, *gŏu qĭ zĭ* (Fructus Lycii) 15g, *tù sī zĭ* (Semen Cuscutae) 15g, *fù pén zĭ* (Fructus Rubi) 15g, *bā jĭ tiān* (Radix Morindae Officinalis) 10g, *shān yú ròu* (Fructus Corni) 15g, and *lù jiăo jiāo* (Colla Cornus Cervi) 10g were added.

With Spleen deficiency, *dăng shēn* (Radix Codonopsis) 15g, and *huáng qí* (Radix Astragali) 20g were added.

With excess patterns, *huáng qín* (Radix Scutellariae) and *huáng băi* (Cortex Phellodendri Chinensis) 10g each were added.

30 doses of this formula constitute one course. Curative effects were determined following 2 courses of treatment.

In the acupuncture with medicinals group, RN 4, *zĭ gōng* (EX-CA1), SP 6, and BL 32 were added, beginning on the 15-17th day of menstruation. Needles were retained for 15 minutes daily, and treatments continued until cessation of bleeding occurred. Complete cessation of bleeding for 7 days constituted full recovery.

Results showed recovery in the acupuncture, moxibustion, Chinese medicinal, and groups of 12, 17, 13, and 22 subjects respectively. The effective rates of the both the acupuncture and combined therapy groups were significantly higher than those of the other two groups (P < 0.05). [52]

Dr. Chen Jian-ping treated 26 cases of flooding and spotting with scalp acupuncture points. Points selected were reproductive area, foot motor and sensation area, bilaterally. Daily treatment began 3 days before menstruation and continued until the cessation of bleeding. Subjects were treated for 1-3 courses, with one menstrual constituting one course of treatment.

Results showed 26 cases fully recovered with full cessation of abnormal bleeding and normal menstruation occurring in non-menopausal subjects. 10 cases improved, with a significant reduction of bleeding. 2 cases showed no response, noting that these subjects displayed hysteromyoma. The effective rate reached 94.17%. [53]

Dr. Cao Wen-zhong and his colleagues treated DUB in a group of subjects all displaying cystic and glandular hyperplasia. Subjects were divided with acupuncture treatment group of 110 cases and a biomedicine group of 120 as control.

The primary selected points included DU 20 (*bǎi huì*), RN 4, LI 4, and SP 6.

The control group was administered hormonal therapy.

After treatment, significant differences in the total effective rates of the two groups were recorded, including the incidence of endometrial pathology. The therapeutic effect in the acupuncture group was significantly higher than the control group (P<0.05 or P<0.01). [54]

(2) Inducing Ovulation

Dr. Tu Guo-chun studied 62 anovular cases to compare the ovulation-inducing effect of HMG intramuscular injection with the effects of acupuncture point injection. Subjects were divided into two treatment groups.

Prior to treatment, 42 subjects displayed proliferative endometrium, 11 cases showing hyperplasia, 9 cases secretory phase dysfunction, 50 cases presenting monophasic BBT, and 12 cases diphase BBT. All were diagnosed as anovlatory due to disturbances of the pituitary-hypothalamus complex, and had been prescribed clomifene and HCG to induce ovulation.

The treatment group was administered daily clomifene 50mg, for 5 days, followed with acupuncture point injections of HMG beginning on day 6.

Point selection included RN 4, RN 3 (*zhōng jí*), RN 6, *zǐ gōng* (EX-CA1), SP 6, BL 23 (*shèn shù*), BL 32, and BL 33 (*zhōng liáo*).One point was selected for each treatment.

Patients were asked to void the bladder prior to the use of abdominal points. Insertion and injection was accompanied by a distending sensation, radiating to either the genitalia or sole of the foot.

With CMS increases (≥10) and ovarian follicle growth (≥18mm), intramuscular injections of antophysin 5 000-10 000IU were administered the following day. After 24 hours, in the absence of rising BBT, additional injections of 5 000IU were given. With no reaction, HMG was also administered on day 14. HCG injections were then continued.

In the control group, intramuscular injections of clomifene were given on day one, followed by HGM once daily for 7 days. With no response, 2 daily injections were given. With no reaction after 7 days, HMG was withdrawn and treatment continued following the treatment group protocol.

Results showed 64 subjects ovulatory in the treatment group, with 1-2 dominant follicles developing within 52 total cycles. Follicular diameter within 45 total cycles exceeded 18mm with ovulation before day 14. In the control group, 39 subjects achieved ovulation, with 1-3 dominant follicles developing within 30 total cycles. The follicular diameter within 27 total cycles exceeded 18mm with ovulation before day 14. The ovulation rates reached 70.3% and 69.2% respectively. Research results show that intramuscular injection in control group used 9-19 HMG, with some side effects presenting. The follicular development and ovulation rates of both groups were similar. However in the treatment group, the quantity of medicines administered were reduced from 15.31 to 6.22, which indicates that acupuncture point injection is more cost effective. [55]

Dr. Liu Gang and colleagues studied 85 cases presenting ovulatory dysfunction. Subjects were divided into a Chinese medicinal treatment group of 40 cases, with 45 subjects in a group combining medicinal therapy with moxibustion. Chinese medicinal group was differentiated into four patterns: Kidney yang patterns, Kidney yin patterns, Liver qi stagnation patterns and internal accumulation of phlegm-damp. Chinese medicinal protocol was the same in both groups.

Basic point selection included RN 4, *zǐ gōng* (EX-CA1) and SP 6.

With Kidney deficiency patterns, BL 23 was added.

With Liver qi stagnation patterns, BL 18 (*gān shù*) was added.

With internal accumulation of phlegm-damp, BL 20 (*pí shù*) and ST 40 (*fēng lóng*) were added.

Alternating moxibustion was the main treatment method. Treatments were applied with 20 minutes for each main point, 15 minutes for the supplementary points, daily or every other day. On 12th-16th days of the cycle, daily treatments continued until the cessation of menses. One month constituted one course of treatment, with evaluation performed after 3 courses. Effective treatment of both groups included 30 and 41 subjects, with an effective rate reaching 75.1% and 91.9% respectively. The comparison of these two groups reached statistical significance (P < 0.05). [56]

4. INTEGRATIVE APPROACHES TO TREATMENT

(1) Chinese Medicinals and Anti-inflammatory Biomedicines

Dr. Luo Zhan-jun reports from the following DUB study.

During the bleeding period, the principles of treatment included clearing heat, cooling blood and dispelling blood stasis.

Treatment included an empirical formula which contained *dāng guī* (Radix Angelicae Sinensis), *bái sháo* (Radix Paeoniae Alba), *shēng dì huáng* (Radix Rehmanniae), *dì yú tàn* (Carbonized Radix Sanguisorbae), *duàn lóng gǔ* (Calcined Fossilia Ossis Mastodi), *duàn mǔ lì* (Calcined Concha Ostreae), *qiàn cǎo* (Radix Rubiae), *yì mǔ cǎo* (Herba Leonuri) and *xiān hè cǎo* (Herba Agrimoniae).

With deficient heat, *shā shēn* (Radix Adenophorae seu Glehniae), *mài dōng* (Radix Ophiopogonis), *wǔ wèi zǐ* (Fructus Schisandrae), *ē jiāo* (Colla Corii Asini) and *dì gǔ pí* (Cortex Lycii) were added.

With excessive heat, *huáng qín* (Radix Scutellariae), *jiāo shān zhī* (Scorch-fried Fructus Gardeniae), and *ǒu jié* (Nodus Nelumbinis Rhizomatis) were added.

With Kidney yang deficiency, *shān yào* (Rhizoma Dioscoreae), *gǒu qǐ zǐ* (Fructus Lycii), *tù sī zǐ* (Semen Cuscutae), and *nǚ zhēn zǐ* (Fructus Ligustri Lucidi) added.

With Spleen deficiency, *shān yào* (Rhizoma Dioscoreae), *dà zǎo* (Fructus Jujubae), *bái zhú* (Rhizoma Atractylodis Macrocephalae), *fú líng* (Poria), and *huáng qí* (Radix Astragali) were added.

With blood stasis, *sān qī* (Radix Notoginseng), *hóng huā* (Flos Carthami), *chuān xiōng* (Rhizoma Chuanxiong), and *táo rén* (Semen Persicae) were added.

Also prescribed was sulfamethoxazole 1g, twice daily.

During the non-bleeding period, the principles of treatment included strengthening the Spleen, rectifying qi, invigorating blood and dispelling blood stasis.

Rén Shēn Guī Pí Wán (人参归脾丸) or *Chái Hú Shū Gān Sǎn* (柴胡疏肝散) were administered by Ⅳ drip, as well as the complex prescription *Dān Shēn Zhù Shè Yè* (丹参注射液). Additionally, *Yě Jú Huā Shuān* (野菊花栓) suppositories and hot abdominal compresses were prescribed. [57]

With bleeding stage treatments, cessation generally occurred after 3-14 days of treatment. Results showed 65 cases with full recovery, 5 cases improved, and 3 cases no response.

(2) Chinese Medicinals and Endocrine Therapy

The treatment of adolescent DUB emphasizes the establishment of regular ovulatory menstrual cycles. When the blood stanching and ovulation promoting effects of Chinese medicinals are not satisfactory, an integrative approach to treatment may increase therapeutic effectiveness.

Dr. Huang Gang and colleagues treated a group of adolescents with hemorrhaging DUB by administering Chinese medicinals combined with of intramuscular injections of estradiol benzoate 1mg, 3-4 times daily. Dosage was reduced to reduce to 0.5mg after the cessation of bleeding. Treatment continued for a total of 20 days, with added progesterone 10mg daily. During the final 5 days subjects received supplemental aminocaproic acid, ethamsylate, and Vitamin K_3. Blood transfusions were performed in severe cases, or experience point *duàn hóng* was needled. With no ovulation after 3 artificially induced cycles, clomifene and HCG were prescribed to induce ovulation. [58]

Dr. Wu Xin-hua and colleagues treated a group presenting with anovular DUB:

During the bleeding stage, modified *Yì Qì Zhǐ Xuè Tāng* (益气止血汤) was prescribed. Medicinals included *dǎng shēn* (Radix Codonopsis) 30g, *huáng qí* (Radix Astragali) 30g, *mǎ chǐ xiàn* (Herba Portulacae) 30g, *yì mǔ cǎo* (Herba Leonuri) 30g, *shēng pú huáng* (Pollen Typhae Crudum)

30g, *xiān hè cǎo* (Herba Agrimoniae) 30g, *dì yú* (Radix Sanguisorbae) 30g, *jiāo bái zhú* (Scorch-fried Rhizoma Atractylodis Macrocephalae) 12g, *qiàn cǎo* (Radix Rubiae) 12g, and *zhì gān cǎo* (Radix et Rhizoma Glycyrrhizae Praeparata cum Melle) 6g. Modified *Guī Pí Tāng* (归脾汤) was prescribed beginning 3 days after the cessation of bleeding.

With total blood pigment levels were lower than 80g/L, blood transfusions were performed. When bleeding failed to cease following 6-10 doses of *Yì Qì Zhǐ Xuè Tāng* (益气止血汤), progestogin and clomifene were added due to the limitations of Chinese medicinals in promoting ovulation. After general symptoms have improved, nourishing the Kidney and regulating menses are effective methods to improve the physical constitution, especially in anemic patients. [59]

Dr. Zhang Hua and colleagues treated 2 100 cases of DUB with an empirical formula, modified *Pí Shèn Gù Chōng Tāng* (脾肾固冲汤). Hormone therapy was applied concurrently for symptomatic relief. A control group of 890 subjects received biomedical treatments only.

The basic decoction included *shú dì huáng* (Radix Rehmanniae Praeparata) 12g, *chuān xù duàn* (Radix Dipsaci) 12g, *bái sháo* (Radix Paeoniae Alba) 12g, *chǎo jīng jiè suì* (Dry-fried Spica Schizonepetae) 6g, *cè bǎi tàn* (Carbonized Cacumen Platycladi) 6g, *yì mǔ cǎo* (Herba Leonuri) 6g, *chái hú* (Radix Bupleuri) 4.5g, *huáng qín* (Radix Scutellariae) 9g, *dān pí* (Cortex Moutan) 9g, *duàn mǔ lì* (Calcined Concha Ostreae) 24g, and *ē jiāo kuài* (Colla Corii Asini) 15g. Subjects were prescribed one dose daily, with 3-6 doses constituting one course of treatment. Modifications made to the formula are as follows.

With Spleen and Kidney deficiency, and exuberant Liver qi with blood-heat, medicinals were prescribed to strengthen the Spleen, tonify the Kidney, cool blood, and course the Liver.

Removed were *duàn mǔ lì* (Calcined Concha Ostreae), *ē jiāo kuài* (Colla Corii Asini), *cè bǎi tàn* (Carbonized Cacumen Platycladi). Added were *shān yào* (Rhizoma Dioscoreae) 15g, *shí lián* (Semen Nelumbinis), *tù sī zǐ* (Semen Cuscutae) and *shēng dì huáng* (Radix Rehmanniae) 9g each.

With Spleen and Kidney deficiency accompanied by instability of the penetrating and conception vessels, treatment was applied to strengthen the Spleen, nourish the Kidney, tonifying qi, and secure the penetrating vessel.

Removed were *chǎo jīng jiè suì* (Dry-fried Spica Schizonepetae), *chái hú* (Radix Bupleuri), *huáng qín* (Radix Scutellariae), *dān pí* (Cortex Moutan), *yì mǔ cǎo* (Herba Leonuri) and *bái sháo* (Radix Paeoniae Alba).

Added were *huáng qí* (Radix Astragali) 24g, *dǎng shēn* (Radix Codonopsis) 12g, *jiāo bái zhú* (Scorch-fried Rhizoma Atractylodis Macrocephalae) 12g, *zhì gān cǎo* (Radix et Rhizoma Glycyrrhizae Praeparata cum Melle) 9g, *yuǎn zhì* (Radix Polygalae) 9g, *guì yuán ròu* (Arillus Longan) 9g, *chǎo zǎo rén* (Dry-fried Semen Ziziphi Spinosae) 9g, *dì yú tàn* (Carbonized Radix Sanguisorbae) 9g, *wū zéi gǔ* (Endoconcha Sepiae) 12g, *zōng lǘ tàn* (Carbonized Petiolus Trachycarpi) 12g, and *sān qī miàn* (Radix Notoginseng Powder) 1.5g (infused).

With blood deficiency, blood stasis, and disorder of the penetrating and conception vessels, the treatment principle applied was to nourish and invigorate blood, dispel stasis and regulate menses.

Removed were *shú dì huáng* (Radix Rehmanniae Praeparata), *chuān xù duàn* (Radix Dipsaci), *huáng qín* (Radix Scutellariae), *dān pí* (Cortex Moutan), *duàn mǔ lì* (Calcined Concha Ostreae), and *ē jiāo* (Colla Corii Asini).

Added were *cè bǎi tàn* (Carbonized Cacumen Platycladi) with *pú huáng tàn* (Carbonized Pollen Typhae) 6g each.

Added were *bái sháo* (Radix Paeoniae Alba) with *chì sháo* (Radix Paeoniae Rubra) 6g each, *dāng guī* (Radix Angelicae Sinensis) 9g, *chuān xiōng* (Rhizoma Chuanxiong) 4.5g, *mò yào* (Myrrha) 4.5g, *táo rén* (Semen Persicae) 3g, *hóng huā* (Flos Carthami) 3g, *zé lán* (Herba Lycopi) 6g and *dān shēn* (Radix Salviae Miltiorrhizae) 6g.

With blood-heat due to yin deficiency, and instability of the penetrating and conception vessels, the treatment should nourish yin, clear heat, calm the penetrating vessel, and regulate menses.

Removed were *shú dì huáng* (Radix Rehmanniae Praeparata), *chuān xù duàn* (Radix Dipsaci), *chǎo jīng jiè suì* (Dry-fried Spica Schizonepetae), *chái hú* (Radix Bupleuri), and *yì mǔ cǎo* (Herba Leonuri). Added were *qīng hāo* (Herba Artemisiae Annuae) 9g, *dì gǔ pí* (Cortex Lycii), *hàn lián cǎo* (Herba Ecliptae) 9g, and *chūn gēn bái pí* (Cortex Ailanthi) 9g.

The age of the patient is a determining factor in the application of biomedicines. The principle treatment for adolescent women is to stanch bleeding and regulate menstruation in order to promote ovulation. The main treatment for peri-menopausal women is to regulate menstruation and reduce menstrual volume after the cessation of the bleeding pattern. The most effective treatment for women in the childbearing period is the use of progestogen and HCG. Dilatation and curettage is also commonly indicated. Electrical coagulation and laser surgery may also be used to for removal of the endometrium or in recent years, to perform a complete uterectomy. The total effective rate in the integrative medicine group reached 94.5%, where the total effective rate in the control reached 55.9%. An integrative treatment approach to DUB may be more effective in treating both symptoms and the underlying cause. [60]

(3) Chinese Medicinals with Endocrine Therapy and Anti-inflammatory Drugs

Dr. Zhu Shi-long and colleague showed the effectiveness of using the formula, *Yì Xiān Hé Jì* (益仙合剂), when accompanied with intramuscular injection of testosterone and gentamicin.

The decoction included *yì mǔ cǎo* (Herba Leonuri) 15g and *xiān hè cǎo* (Herba Agrimoniae) 15g, decocted with brown sugar, for 3-5 minutes.

One divided dose, prescribed 3 times daily. Injections included 50mg testosterone and 80 000u gentamicin. 3-5 days constituted one course of treatment.

In 500 cases, results showed 453 cases totally recovered, 45 cases greatly improved, and 2 cases improved. [61]

Dr. Tao Hua studied adolescent DUB by first ruling out structural disease in all subjects with ultrasonic examination. The selected Chinese medicinals included *dǎng shēn* (Radix Codonopsis) 9g, *wū méi* (Fructus Mume) 9g and *shí liú pí* (Pericarpium Granati) 9g, prescribed once daily. 3 doses constituted one course of treatment. In subjects reporting abnormal bleeding for over 30 days, metronidazole 0.2g, was administered 3 times daily for 3 days. With anemia iron supplements were prescribed. The formula was prescribed to to mature subjects with an endometrial thickness (0.8cm). With a thickness (>0.8cm), diagnostic curettage was performed, and to prevent infection, the antibiotic metronidazole was prescribed, in addition to Chinese medicinals.

Results showed 44 cases fully recovered, with 38 cases recovering after 1 course of treatment, and 6 cases after 2 courses. 9 cases improved, including 2 cases adolescent DUB, 1 case childbearing period DUB and 6 cases menopause period DUB, but with some recurrence. 3 cases showed no response. The total effective rate reached 94%. [62]

Experimental Studies

1. RESEARCH ON THE EFFICACY OF SINGLE CHINESE MEDICINALS

Medicinals that have been shown to stimulate uterine smooth muscle contraction include *gǒu qǐ* (Fructus Lycii), *guī bǎn* (Testudinis Plastrum) and *dǎng shēn* (Radix Codonopsis).

Medicinals with anti-inflammatory properties include *nǚ zhēn zǐ* (Fructus Ligustri Lucidi), *shān zhū yú* (Fructus Corni), *rén shēn* (Radix et

Rhizoma Ginseng) and *dǎng shēn* (Radix Codonopsis).

Medicinals demonstrating antibacterial actions in vitro include *nǔ zhēn zǐ* (Fructus Ligustri Lucidi), *mài dōng* (Radix Ophiopogonis), *shān zhū yú* (Fructus Corni), *rén shēn* (Radix et Rhizoma Ginseng) and *dǎng shēn* (Radix Codonopsis).

Medicinals which act on the hypothalmic-pituitary-adrenal axis include *nǔ zhēn zǐ* (Fructus Ligustri Lucidi) and *rén shēn* (Radix et Rhizoma Ginseng).

Lù xián cǎo (Herba Pyrolae) demonstrates inhibitory actions which have been shown to cause uterine and ovarian atrophy in rats. [63]

2. Research on the Efficacy of Herbal Prescriptions

(1) Tonifying Qi, Engendering Blood and Blood Stanching Effects of *Tài Zǐ Chǎn Níng* (太子产宁)

Dr. Ding Ding and colleagues observed the effects of *Tài Zǐ Chǎn Níng* (太子产宁) on fatigue levels in a group of swimming mice. In another group, the blood stanching and tonifying effects were evaluated.

This formula was normally indicated for symptoms of profuse menstruation. The formula containd *tài zǐ shēn* (Radix Pseudostellariae), *shān zhā* (Fructus Crataegi), and *xiāng fù* (Rhizoma Cyperi).

One group was administered *Tài Zǐ Chǎn Níng* (太子产宁) and the effects were compared with a distilled water control group. Swimming rates and blood levels in both groups were observed.

Results showed the swimming rates of the control group and the *Tài Zǐ Chǎn Níng* (太子产宁) group at 5.04 ± 3.38 and 11.58 ± 7.53 minutes, respectively.

Significant differences were found in RBC and hemoglobin levels when measured following 192 hours of bleeding. Levels reached 6.888 ± 0.825, 8.073 ± 0.571, 117.2 ± 19.1, and 141.5 ± 12.1 respectively ($P < 0.05$).

Study concludes that the formula, *Tài Zǐ Chǎn Níng* (太子产宁) effectively shortens bleeding time by tonifying qi to engender blood and promote fluids. [64]

(2) Research on the Estrogen-like Action of *Yù Yīn Líng* (育阴灵)

Dr. Xiao Donghong and colleagues studied the effects of the Kidney tonifying and yin nourishing formula *Yù Yīn Líng* (育阴灵) in mice with surgically removed ovaries. Uterine weight and density, protein levels, and measurements of the estrogen and progesterone receptors were evaluated.

Medicinals included *shú dì huáng* (Radix Rehmanniae Praeparata), *guī jiǎ* (Caraoax et Plastrum Testudinis), *shān yú ròu* (Fructus Corni), *huái shān yào* (Rhizoma Dioscoreae), *dù zhòng* (Cortex Eucommiae), *chuān niú xī* (Radix Cyathulae), *sāng jì shēng* (Herba Taxilli), *xù duàn* (Radix Dipsaci), *bái sháo* (Radix Paeoniae Alba), *ē jiāo* (Colla Corii Asini), *hǎi piāo xiāo* (Endoconcha Sepiae), *duàn mǔ lì* (Calcined Concha Ostreae) and *tù sī zǐ* (Semen Cuscutae).

Results showed that *Yù Yīn Líng* (育阴灵) may increase uterine weight (P < 0.01), promote the synthesis of uteroglobin (P < 0.05), and increase the content of estrogen and progesterone receptors. Study concludes that *Yù Yīn Líng* (育阴灵) has estrogenic actions on the uterus, further supporting the theory that the Kidney is responsible for reproduction. This study also provides evidence that the application of a single method may effectively treat a variety of gynecological diseases, such as DUB, amenorrhea, or infertility. [65]

(3) Efficacy of Formulas that Invigorate Yang

Dr. Lin You-yu and colleagues compared a Chinese medicinal formula with the effects of dexamethasone on the blood hydrocortisone, estradiol and estrogen receptors with inhibited function of the hypothalamic-pituitary-adrenal axis.

The formula contained *fù zǐ* (Radix Aconiti Lateralis Praeparata) 20g, *ròu guì* (Cortex Cinnamomi) 15g, *ròu cōng róng* (Herba Cistanches) 45g, *xiān líng pí* (Herba Epimedii) 45g, *bǔ gǔ zhī* (Fructus Psoraleae) 45g and *lù jiǎo piàn* (Sliced Cornu Cervi) 20g.

Results indicated formulas that invigorate yang may significantly increase the affinity of estradiol and E-R, as well as increasing the levels of both. [66]

(4) Dosages and Forms of New Medicinals

Research in the blood stanching mechanism of *Gōng Bēng Kǒu Fú Yè* (宫崩口服液):

Dr. Xie Ke-rong and colleagues found that *Gōng Bēng Kǒu Fú Yè* (宫崩口服液) is effective in shortening clotting time in mice, increasing uterine and ovarian weight, promoting follicular development, and stimulating the contraction of uterine smooth muscle. Estrogenic effects were also observed. The blood stanching mechanism may be related to the regulation of the adrenal axis. [67]

(5) Integrative Treatment

Dr. Shao Shou-jin summarized the clinical diagnosis and treatment of DUB in 161 hospitalized patients from 1966 to 2001. Subjects were divided into two groups, according to the age of onset, and the corresponding treatment principle.

Group one included 12 cases of adolescent DUB with an average age of 14.9 years. The average hemoglobin levels were measured at 5.2 ± 1.6g. Group two included 149 mature subjects with an average age of 39.9 years. Hemoglobin levels averaged 9.3 ± 2.5g.

The treatment approach in the adolescent cases was to address anemia while promoting endometrial repair with relatively large doses of estrogen. This was followed by the administration of the hormone chloramiphene, to both induce artificial cycles and promote ovulation. In this group, 7 subjects conceived, 9 received follow-up treatments, with 2 reporting normal menstruation.

The approach for the menopausal subjects focused on promoting denudation through the application of progestogen treatments. With severe symptoms and no response to medication, hysterectomy was typically performed in patients over 40 years of age. Diagnostic curettage also plays an important role in the differential diagnosis and treatment of menopausal DUB patients. In menopausal and childbearing age patients, both cancer and atypical hyperplasia of the endometrium should be ruled out prior to treatment. [68]

REFERENCES

[1] Liu Zheng-jian, Huang Li-guang. Treatment in Adolescent DUB with Hua Rui Shi and Da Huang according to Pattern Differentiation (擅用花蕊石大黄辨治青春期崩漏). *Liaoning Journal of Traditional Chinese Medicine* (辽宁中医杂志). 1997, 24(4)：172.

[2] Han Zheng, Song Li-feng. Four Empirical Principles in the Treatment of Flooding and Spotting (崩漏治验四则). *Shandong Journal of Traditonal Chinese Medicine* (山东中医杂志). 2005, 24(12)：753-754.

[3] Bi Hua, Zhang Dan-hua. Treatment Adolescent DUB with the Nourishing Yin and Purging Yang Method (补阴泻阳法治疗青春期功血). *Shanghai Journal of Traditional Chinese Medicine* (上海中医药杂志). 2004, 38(4)：140-141.

[4] Shi Heng-min. Spleen and Kidney Treatment in 45 Cases of Adolescent DUB (从脾肾论治青春期功血 45 例). *Shanxi Journal of Traditonal Chinese Medicine* (陕西中医). 2004, 25(11)：972.

[5] Zhu Pei-yan. Gui Pi Tang and Liu Wei Di Huang Wan in the Cyclic Treatment of 129 Cases of Adolescent DUB (归脾六味周期分时用药治疗青春期功血 129 例). *Sichuan Journal of Traditional Chinese Medicine* (四川中医). 2004, 22(5)：61-62.

[6] Gao Li-ping, Chen Min. Treatment in 223 Cases of DUB According to Pattern

Differentiation (辨证分型治疗功能失调性子宫出血症 223 例). *Hubei Journal of Traditional Chinese Medicine* (湖北中医杂志). 1996, 18(1)：42-43.

[7] Sheng Wen-yan, Yang Wen-lan. Clinical Observations of 147 Cases of DUB with Artificial Cycles Induced by Chinese Medicinals (中药人工周期治疗功能性子宫出血 147 例临床观察). *Hubei Journal of Journal Chinese Medicine* (湖北中医杂志). 1994, 16(2)：12-13.

[8] Feng Shi-song. Treatment in 81 Cases of DUB with Tai Pan Wu Bei San (胎盘乌贝散治疗功能性子宫出血 81 例). *Sichuan Journal of Traditional Chinese Medicine* (四川中医). 1999, 17(3)：40.

[9] Dong Su-qin, Liu Gui-hua. Treatment in 98 Cases of DUB with Artificial Cycles Induced by Chinese Medicinals (中药周期疗法治疗功能性子宫出血 98 例). *Tianjin Journal of Traditional Chinese Medicine* (天津中医). 1997, 14(5)：216-217.

[10] Yang Xiao-hai. Differentiation and Treatment of Flooding and Spotting in the Childbearing Period (生育期崩漏的辨治). *Guangxi Journal of Traditional Chinese Medicine* (广西中医药). 2001, 24(2)：31.

[11] Xing Yu-xia. Treatment in 65 Cases of Adolescent Flooding and Spotting by Arresting Bleeding, Tonifying the Kidney, and Regulating Menstruation (塞流止血补肾调经法治疗室女崩漏 65 例). *Liaoning Journal of Traditional Chinese Medicine Journal* (辽宁中医杂志). 1998, 25(11)：520.

[12] Li Hui-bao, Wang Hui, Wang Bao-shu. Clinical Report on Treatment of 68 Cases of Adolescent DUB by Arresting Bleeding and Securing the Origin (塞流固本法治疗青春期子宫出血 68 例临床报道). *China Journal of Traditional Chinese Medicine and Pharmacy* (中国医药学报). 1995, 10(4)：20-21.

[13] Cui Lin. Treatment in 48 Cases of Adolescent DUB with Er Zhi Wan and Gui Pi Tang (二至丸合归脾汤治疗青春期功血 48 例). *Journal of Zhejiang College of Traditional Chinese Medicine* (浙江中医学院学报). 1999, 23(3)：44.

[14] Yang Wen. Treatment in 32 Cases of Adolescent DUB with the Empirical Formula Zi Yin Zhi Beng Tang (自拟滋阴止崩汤治疗青春期功能失调性子宫出血 32 例). *Research of Traditional Chinese Medicine* (中医药研究). 2001, 17(1)：15.

[15] Yi Qin-hua. Treatment in 40 Cases of Adolescent DUB based on Pattern Differentiation (辨证治疗室女崩漏 40 例). *Hebei Journal of Traditional Chinese Medicine* (河

北中医). 2001, 23(10)：753-754.

[16] Xie Bo. Treatment in 60 Cases of Adolescent DUB with Fu Fang Shu Di Jiao Nang (复方熟地胶囊治疗青春期功血 60 例). *Journal of Shanghai Uniuverity of Traditional Chinese Medicine* (上海中医药大学学报), 2003, 17(1)：25-26.

[17] He Gui-xiang, Zheng Xiang-yin, Zhu Xuan-xuan. Clinical Research on Yi Shen Jian Pi Ke Li in the Treatment of Adolescent DUB (益肾健脾颗粒治疗青春期功能性出血的临床研究). *Journal of Nanjing University of Traditional Chinese Medicine* (南京中医药大学学报). 2003, 19(1)：21-23.

[18] Wu Xi. Clinical Observations of Gong Xue Yin Formula in the Treatment of 83 Cases of Flooding and Spotting ("功血饮" 治疗崩漏 83 例疗效观察). *A Review of Wu Xi's Gynecology (Volume One)* (吴熙妇科朔洄第一集). Xiamen: Xiamen University Publishing House (厦门大学出版社). 1994, 181-182.

[19] Liang Bing. Treatment in 36 Cases of, Menopausal DUB with Jian Pi Yi Qi Tang (健脾益气汤治疗更年期功能失调性子宫出血 36 例). *Journal of Shanxi Medical College for Continuing Education* (山西职工医学院学报). 2001, 11(1)：24.

[20] Xin Li-jia, Dai Li-hui, Hu Xiu-lan. Treatment in 60 Cases of Menopausal DUB with Hua Yu Tang. (化瘀汤治疗更年期功能失调性子宫出血 60 例). ACMP. 2001, 29(2)：28.

[21] Wu Min. Treatment in 48 Cases of Peri-menopausal Flooding and Spotting with Modified Si Cao Tang (四草汤化裁治疗围绝经期崩漏 48 例). *Shanxi Journal of Traditonal Chinese Medicine* (陕西中医). 2005, 26(5)：388-389.

[22] Liu Ying-jie, Li Jun. Treatment in 95 Cases of Menopausal DUB with the Empirical Formula Xue Ning Tang (自拟血宁汤治疗更年期功血 95 例). *China Journal of Basic Medicine In Traditional Chinese Medicine* (中国中医基础医学杂志). 2002, 8(9)：72.

[23] Yu Gui-fen, You Xue-mei, Xu Guan-bing. Clinical Observation in the Treatment of 60 Cases of Perimenopausal DUB with Chinese Medicinals (中药治疗围绝经期功血 60 例临床观察). *Journal of Traditional Chinese Medicine* (中医药学报). 2003, 31(2)：43.

[24] Ran Qing-zhen. Treatment in 58 Cases of Senile Flooding with Chi Shi Zhi Zhi Beng Tang (赤石脂止崩汤治疗老年血崩 58 例). *Shanxi Journal of Traditional Chinese Medicine* (陕西中医). 2004, 25(11)：971-972.

[25] Li Yan-ling, Lei Qing-li. Treatment in 60 Cases of Flooding and Spotting with

Gong Xue Jing (宫血净治崩漏 60 例). *Shanxi Journal of Traditional Chinese Medicine* (陕西中医). 2005, 26(10)：1013-1014.

[26] Wang Jian-ling, Dong Lian-ling. Treatment in 40 Cases of DUB with Yi Qi Yang Xue Tang (益气养血汤治疗功能性子宫出血 40 例). *Shanxi Journal of Traditional Chinese Medicine* (山西中医). 1999, 15(1)：15.

[27] Yang Yu-xiu. Treatment in 269 Cases of DUB with Bao Yin Jian (保阴煎治疗功能性子宫出血 269 例). *Shanxi Journal of Traditional Chinese Medicine* (陕西中医). 1999, 20(5)：195-196.

[28] Chen Xia. Clinical Observation of Gong Xue Yin Formula. (功血饮临床观察). *China Journal of Traditional Chinese Medicine and Pharmacy* (中国医药学报). 1998, 13(3)：79-80.

[29] Chen Yun. Clinical observation in the Treatment of 120 Cases of Flooding and Spotting with Gong Xue Tang (宫血汤治疗崩漏 120 例疗效观察). *Journal of Zhenjiang Medical College* (镇江医学院学报) 2001.11(1)：127-128.

[30] Pan Wen. Observation in the Treatment of 42 Cases of Flooding and Spotting with Gong Xue Yin (宫血饮治疗崩漏 42 例疗效观察). *Jilin Journal of Traditional Chinese Medicine* (吉林中医药). 2000, (3)：26.

[31] Shan Jing-wen, Ma Fu-wei, Wang Dian-xiang. Clinical Research on DUB Treatment with Gong Xue Ting Ke Li (宫血停颗粒治疗功能性子宫出血的临床研究). *Journal of Traditional Chinese Medicine* (中医药学报). 2000, 3：33-34.

[32] Peng Zhen-sheng. Observation in the Treatment of 80 Cases of DUB with Can Sha Gu Jing Tang (蚕砂固经汤治疗功能失调性子宫出血 80 例疗效观察). *Chinese Journal of Information on TCM* (中国中医药信息杂志). 2001, 8(6)：66.

[33] Xing Cui-ling, Kang Qun-ye, He Yan. Treatment in 160 Cases of DUB with the Empirical Formula Tiao Jing Tang (自拟调经汤治疗功能失调性子宫出血 160 例). *Forum on Traditional Chinese Medicine* (国医论坛). 2000, 15(5)：37.

[34] Liu Gui-shu, Wang Jing. Treatment in 68 Cases of DUB with Tiao Jing Zhi Xue Tang (调经止血汤治疗功能失调性子宫出血病 68 例). *Hebei Journal of Chinese Medicine* (河北中医). 2000, 22(4)：270.

[35] Shen Rong, Zhao Cui-ying. Treatment in 232 Cases of DUB with Integrative Medicine (中西医结合治疗功能失调性子宫出血 232 例). *Jiangsu Journal of Chinese Medicine*

（江苏中医）. 2000, 21(12)：28.

[36] Song Su-Ying. Observation in Teatment of 316 Cases of DUB with Hui Chun Zhi Xue San（回春止血散治疗功能失调性子宫出血 316 例疗效观察）. *Clinical Medicine of China*（中国综合临床）. 2000, 16(12)：939.

[37] Wang Yun-yi. Observation in the Treatment of 86 Cases of DUB with Liu Zhi Tang（柳枝汤治疗功能失调性子宫出血 86 例疗效观察）. *Modern Journal of Integrated Traditional Chinese and Western Medicine*（现代中西医结合杂志）. 2000, 9(18)：1808.

[38] Chen Xia, Yu Hong-juan. Clinical Observation in the Treatment of Liver and Kidney Deficiency Pattern DUB in Adolescents with Gong Xue Yin（功血饮治疗肝肾阴虚型青春期功能失调性子宫出血的临床观察）. *China Journal of Integrated Traditional Chinese and Western Medicine*（中国中西医结合杂志）. 2000, 20(12)：936-937.

[39] Ou Zhong-bo. Treatment in 105 Cases of Flooding and Spotting with Modified Wen Qing Yin（加味温清饮治疗崩漏 105 例）. *Hunan Journal of Traditional Chinese Medicine*（湖南中医杂志）. 2001, 17(2)：47-48.

[40] Yin Yue-hui, Fan Ji-xiang. Treatment in 40 Cases of Flooding and Spotting with Gui Pi Tang（归脾汤治疗崩漏 40 例）. *Hunan Journal of Traditional Chinese Medicine*（湖南中医杂志）. 2001, 17(3)：43.

[41] Ding Xiu-ying. Treatment in 100 Cases of DUB with Gu Beng Tang（固崩汤治疗功能性子宫出血 100 例）. *Sichuan Journal of Traditional Chinese Medicine*（四川中医）. 2002, 20(8)：50-51.

[42] Xing Jin-xia. Treatment in 125 Cases of Flooding and Spotting with Er Cao Wu Tan Tang（二草五炭汤治疗崩漏 125 例）. *Shanxi Journal of Traditional Chinese Medicine*（陕西中医）. 2005, 26(10)：1012-1013.

[43] Tang Chun-qiong, Huang Zhi-lan. Treatment in 64 Cases of Flooding and Spotting with Modified Gu Chong Tang and Deng Xin Zhi Xue Tang Jiang（固冲汤加味配合灯心止血糖浆治疗崩漏 64 例）. *Shanxi Journal of Traditional Chinese Medicine*（陕西中医）. 2004, 25(11)：968.

[44] Zhai Wen-yan. New Uses of Gui Zhi Tang in Gynecology（桂枝汤妇科新用）. *New Journal of Traditional Chinese Medicine*（新中医）. 2004, 36(8)：66-67.

[45] Chen Yong-pu, Tang Shi-hui. New Uses of Huang Lian E Jiao Tang according to

Pattern Differentiation (黄连阿胶汤辨证新用). *Sichuan Journal of Trditional Chinese Medicine* (四川中医). 2004, 22(8)：140-141.

[46] Liu Jin-xing. Clinical Observation in the Treatment of Anovular DUB with Gu Chong Zhi Xue Tang (固冲止血汤治疗无排卵型功能失调性子宫出血的临床观察). *China Journal of Integrated Traditional Chinese and Western Medicine* (中国中西医结合杂志). 2006, 26(2)：159-162.

[47] Xia Tian, Ye Qing. Experimental and Clinical Research in the Treatment of Menopausal DUB with Kun Ning Huo Xue Tang (坤宁活血汤治疗更年期功血的临床及实验研究). *Shanghai Journal of Traditional Chinese Medicine* (上海中医药杂志). 2004, 38(9)：32-34.

[48] Fu Dong-ming. Discussion on the Usages of Carbonized Medicinals in the Treatment of Flooding and Spotting (崩漏治疗中炭药应用问题的探讨). *Journal of Traditional Chinese Medicine* (中医杂志). 1993, 34(10)：585-587.

[49] Yu Shan-tang, Dong Qing-hua. Using Acupuncture in the Treatment of 38 Cases of Flooding and Spotting (针刺为主治疗崩漏38例). *China Acupuncture and Moxibustion* (中国针灸). 1999, (1)：37.

[50] Xue Di-cheng, Xue Hong-peng, Wang Shen-yu. Treatment in 54 Cases of DUB with Ear Acupoint Pressing (耳穴贴压治疗功能性子宫出血54例). *China Acupuncture and Moxibustion* (中国针灸). 1994, (2)：20.

[51] Xu Tian, Xu Chun-yi. Acupuncture, Moxibustion and Infrared Radiation in the Treatment of 49 Cases of DUB (针刺配合红外线、艾条灸治疗功能性子宫出血49例). *Journal of Clinical Acupuncture and Moxibustion* (针灸临床杂志). 1999, 15(9)：29.

[52] Zhang Yong-luo, Guo Jin-feng, Wen guang-yun. Observations in the Treatment of DUB with Acupuncture and Chinese Medicinals (针灸中药治疗功能性子宫出血的疗效观察). *China Acupuncture and Moxibustion* (中国针灸). 1995, (3)：19-20.

[53] Chen Jian-ping. Treatment in 38 Cases of DUB with Scalp Acupuncture. (头针治疗崩漏38例). *China Acupuncture and Moxibustion* (中国针灸). 2004, 24(9)：595.

[54] Cao Wen-zhong, Zhang li, Han Zhen-kun, Li Zhao-hui, Song Shu-bang, Bai Xiu-mei. Observation in the Treatment of 110 DUB Cases with Endometrial Cystic and Glandular Hyperplasia Using Acupuncture (针灸治疗子宫内膜囊腺型增生性功血110例疗

效观察). *China Acupuncture and Moxibustion* (中国针灸). 2004, 24(2)：93-96.

[55] Tu Guo-chun. Clinical Observation in the Treatment of Ovulatory Dysfunctional Infertility with Acupuncture Injection (穴位注射治疗排卵障碍性不孕症临床观察). *China Acupuncture and Moxibustion* (中国针灸). 1999, (6)：333-334.

[56] Liu Gang, Shi Xiao-lin. Observation in the Treatment of 45 Cases of Ovulatory Dysfunction with Chinese Medicinals and Moxibustion (中药加艾灸治疗排卵障碍 45 例疗效观察). *China Acupuncture and Moxibustion* (中国针灸). 1999, (2)：91-92.

[57] Luo Zhan-jun. Observations in the Treatment of 73 Cases of DUB (功能性子宫出血 73 例疗效观察). *Correspondence Journal of Traditional Chinese Medicine* (中医函授通讯). 1994, (5)：30.

[58] Fang Xiao-dong, Xu Yi-zhen, Lu Jian-ying. Clinical Observation in the Treatment of DUB by Invigorating the Spleen, Tonifying the Kidney and Regulating the Penetrating Vessel (健脾补肾调冲法治疗功能性子宫出血的临床观察). *Shanghai Journal of Traditional Chinese Medicine* (上海中医药杂志). 2002, 3：31-32.

[59] Wu Xin-hua, Liu Jing-jun. Treatment in 150 Cases of Anovular DUB with Integrative Medicine (中西医结合治疗无排卵功血 150 例). *Journal of Shandong University of Traditional Chinese Medicine* (山东中医学院学报), 1994, (6)：391-392.

[60] Zhang Hua, Shen Li-fang, Ge Hua-xiang, Zun Chao-qun. Treatment in 2 100 cases of DUB with Integrative Medicine (中西医结合治疗功能性子宫出血 2 100 例). *Journal of Integrated Traditional Chinese and Western Medicine* (中西医结合杂志). 2004, 32(2)： 513-514.

[61] Zhu Shi-long, Pan Yu-lan. Observation in the treatment of 500 Cases of DUB with Integrative Medicine (中西医结合治疗功血 500 例疗效观察). *Sichuan Journal of Traditional Chinese Medicine* (四川中医). 2004, 32(2)：513-514.

[62] Tao Hua. Treatment in 56 Cases of Anovular DUB with Integrative Medicine (中西医结合治疗无排卵性功血 56 例). *Sichuan Journal of Traditional Chinese Medicine* (四川中医). 2004, 22(1)：72.

[63] Li Yong-sheng. Treatment in 68 Cases of Menopausal DUB with the Purging the Liver, Strengthening the Spleen and Dispelling Blood Stasis Methods (清肝健脾化瘀法治疗更年期功能性子宫出血 68 例). *Zhejiang Journal of Traditional Chinese Medicine* (浙江中医杂志). 1999, 34(1)：8.

[64] Ding Ding, Hao Xian-ping, Sun Cui-hua. Clinical and Experimental Research in the Treatment of Menorrhagia with Tai Zi Chan Ning (太子产宁治疗月经过多的临床及实验研究). *Practical Integrative Medicine* (实用中西医结合杂志). 1996, 9(4)：195-196.

[65] Xiao Dong-hong, Yang Shou-fan. Experimental Research on Estrogen and Progesterone Receptors of Yu Yin Ling (育阴灵与雌孕激素受体的实验研究). *Tianjin Journal of Traditional Chinese Medicine* (天津中医). 1996, 13(1)：33-34.

[66] Lin You-yu, Chen Yu-sheng, Han Xin-min. Yang-warming Medicinals Effect on Uterine Estrogen Receptors and HPA Inhibition in Rats (温阳药对下丘脑—垂体—肾上腺皮质轴受抑大鼠模型的子宫雌激素受体的作用). *Journal of Integrated Traditional Chinese and Western Medicine* (中西医结合杂志), 1985, 5(3)：175-177.

[67] Xie Ke-rong, Liu Min-ru, Tang Yong-shu. Clinical and Experimental Observation of the Mechanism of the Blood Stanching Effect of Gong Beng Kou Fu Ye (宫崩口服液止血作用的临床与实验观察及机理初探). *New Journal of Traditional Chinese Medicine* (新中医). 1993, (4)：53-54.

[68] Shao shou-jin, Wu Yi-yong, Gong Hua-fen. Clinical Diagnosis in the Treatment of 161 Cases of DUB (子宫功能性出血的诊断和治疗 161 例临床分析). *Journal of Chinese Physician* (中国临床医生). 2002, 30(9)：29-30.

Amenorrhea

by **Si-tu Yi**, Professor of Chinese Medical Gynecology
Wang Xiao-yun, Professor of Chinese Medical Gynecology
Lu Hua, Ph.D. TCM
Ran Qing-zhen, Ph.D. TCM
Wen Ming-hua, M.S. TCM

OVERVIEW

Rather than a diagnosis, amenorrhea is a symptom that frequently presents in a number of gynecological diseases. Its clinical manifestation is the absence of menstruation. There are two types of amenorrhea, primary and secondary. Primary amenorrhea is defined either as absence of menses by the age of 16 with normal development of secondary sexual characteristics, or the absence of menses by 14 years of age without secondary sexual characteristics. Secondary amenorrhea is defined as a cessation of menstruation for at least 3 or 6 months after the establishment of menarche.

Primary amenorrhea is commonly caused by congenital disease, anatomic defects of the genital tract, and functional or secondary diseases taking place before puberty. Secondary amenorrhea may result from secondary tumors or an acquired dysfunction of particular organs. Psychological stress, malnourishment, anorexia nervosa, excessive exercise and certain drugs all may induce functional disorders, or restraint of GnRH secreted by the hypothalamus, which indicates a central nervous system-hypothalamic type amenorrhea. In addition, hypophyseal tumors, empty sella syndrome, and Sheehan syndrome due to postpartum hemorrhage and shock can all cause hypogonadism, which may indicate pituitary amenorrhea. Furthermore, Turner's syndrome, retrogression or secondary ovarian diseases may lead to ovarian-type amenorrhea. Finally, uterine amenorrhea may be associated with either a congenital defect of the uterus, or an acquired pathology of the endometria. Since structural disorders and genital dysplasia are not generally treated with medication, they will not be discussed in this section.

The diagnosis of amenorrhea is clearly based on a history of the absence of menstruation. However, in sexually active patients, pregnancy must first be ruled out. Distinguishing the specific etiology is the key to proper diagnosis and treatment of amenorrhea. Patients with amenorrhea always present particular symptoms and signs that are clearly related to the cause. For example, patients with Asherman syndrome may present periodic pain of the lower abdomen, while galactorrhea is often associated with hypophyseal tumors. Empty sella syndrome may result in cephalalgia, while Sheehan syndrome often shows signs of general debilitation, drowsiness, an aversion to cold, poor appetite, hair loss, or myxedema. Amenorrhea due to pathology of the thalamencephalon and central nervous system may lead to weight loss and anosphresia, while polycystic ovarian syndrome may induce acne and hypertrichiasis. In addition, amenorrhea produced by premature ovarian failure often has the same symptoms of perimenopausal syndrome, such as anxiety and hyperidrosis.

To evaluate the condition of the internal and external genitalia, and to identify the possible existence of a structural condition, a gynecologic examination is needed. A series of diagnostic steps are required to correctly identify the specific location and etiology of the pathology.

(1) Hysteroscopy, endometrial biopsy and estrogen-progesterone testing to evaluate uterine function.

(2) Measurement of basal body temperature and hormone levels to evaluate ovarian function.

(3) Gonadotropin and pituitary function testing are indicated in order to determine the functional capacity of the gland. Rule out hypophyseal tumors using sella turcica X-ray or CT scan.

The effective treatment of amenorrhea may include both mind-body therapies as well as treatment of the endocrine system. Psychological treatment is indicated for stress-related conditions, which should also include dietary recommendations especially in cases caused by excessive dieting. For exercise-related amenorrhea, nutritional advice should be provided and exercise should be reduced to a reasonable level. In cases of amenorrhea due to systemic disease, the associated disease should be treated. Endocrine treatments are selected based on the etiology and pathogenesis of the disease

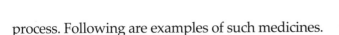

process. Following are examples of such medicines.

(1) Pharmaceutical drugs that regulate the secretion of pituitary lactogenic hormone such as bromocriptine and thyreoidin. The former has a direct effect on prolactin secretion, while the latter can be applied to hyperprolactinemia due to hypothyroidism.

(2) Drugs that induce ovulation such as clomiphene, gonadorelin, and HCG.

(3) Estrogen and progestin as used in hormone replacement therapy.

Furthermore, amenorrhea associated with structural disorders may require surgical treatment.

In Chinese medicine gynecology, an absence of menstruation for over 3 months constitutes a diagnosis of amenorrhea. Such a definition can help to meet the patients' immediate need, and also may prevent untimely delays in treatment.

CHINESE MEDICAL ETIOLOGY AND PATHOMECHANISM

In Chinese medical theory, the causes of amenorrhea can be divided into two general categories: deficiency and excess. The ancient doctors of Chinese medicine held that there were two principal causes of amenorrhea, blood exhaustion and blood obstruction. One refers to an extreme depletion of blood that is not seen in the other, which is a condition of excess. Blood obstruction occurs due to qi stagnation, accumulation of evils, or as a result of congealing cold.

1. ETIOLOGY

(1) Deficiency

1) Kidney Deficiency

In Chinese medicine, the Kidney plays a highly significant role in the production of menstruation. Congenital insufficiency of Kidney qi and essence, or any acquired dysfunction of the Kidney may later result in amenorrhea. Acquired conditions are often caused by overindulgence in sexual activities, abortion, excessive pregnancy, or as a result of chronic disease.

2) Enduring Depletion of the Spleen and Stomach

This pattern is often caused by an improper diet, overexertion, anxiety and overthinking, excessive dieting and weight loss, prolonged lactation, or any depletion of blood related to abortion, parasitosis, hematemesis or hemafecia. All of the above may lead to the cessation of menstruation.

3) Insufficiency of Nutrient-blood

This may result from a longstanding blood deficiency, or depletion of blood and yin due to bleeding or chronic disease. Both may lead to the onset of amenorrhea.

(2) Excess

1) Qi Stagnation and Blood Stasis

Melancholy disposition, or anxiety and depression related to any longstanding illness may lead to qi stagnation and blood stasis. Binding constraint of Liver qi due to suppression of the seven affects is also a common cause of amenorrhea.

2) Stagnation of Phlegm-damp

Such patients may present phlegm-damp as a constitutional factor, often associated with obesity. However, the appearance of phlegm-damp is usually due to excessive consumption of greasy or sugary foods.

Spleen deficiency with failure to transport and transform also results in the production of phlegm-damp. The stagnation of phlegm-damp often obstructs the free movement of blood, leading to amenorrhea.

3) Blood Stasis due to Congealing Cold

The presence of internal cold may congeal blood, leading to menstrual block. Patients presenting this pattern may have had a longstanding yang deficiency, or a history of eating an excessive amount of cold or raw foods. Exposure to the elements may lead to an invasion of pathogenic cold. Eating an excessive amount of cold-natured food, being caught in the rain, or wading during the menstrual or post-partum periods may also lead to this condition, because at that time the uterus is more vulnerable to exterior pathogenic factors.

2. PATHOGENESIS

(1) Deficiency

Amenorrhea may result from deficiencies of the Kidney, Liver, or Spleen, which eventually lead to an insufficiency of essence, qi or blood.

The Kidney is considered to be the source of essence and blood, therefore Kidney deficiency leads to an insufficiency of these vital substances and dysfunction of the penetrating vessel. Patients with deficiency typically present late menarche, or delayed menstruation with scant menstrual flow. Over time, the menses may cease completely. A deficient Kidney may be unable to properly nourish the brain and lumbar region. Soreness and weakness of the lower back and knees result, along with other possible symptoms such as dizziness and tinnitus.

Kidney deficiency cases can then be divided into two subcategories: yang deficiency and yin deficiency. The former may experience coldness of the trunk and limbs with a lack of sexual desire, while the latter may show a particular redness of the cheeks and lips, which are signs of internal heat due to deficient yin.

The Spleen is responsible for the transformation and transportation of qi and blood. Spleen deficiency may lead to an insufficiency of qi and blood in the penetrating and conception vessels, causing the dysfunction of the penetrating vessel. Therefore, a patient with Spleen deficiency is likely to have poor appetite and loose stools, as well as a history of late or absent periods for several months.

For those cases with a deficiency of nutrient-blood, there may also be symptoms such as palpitations due to blood failing to nourish the Heart and the spirit. Deficient blood may also fail to nourish the skin, resulting in a withered appearance.

(2) Excess

Amenorrhea of the excess type is typically a result of an obstruction of blood circulation in the penetrating and conception vessels. Possible causative factors are qi and blood stagnation, stagnation of phlegm-damp, or congealing cold. Menstrual blood becomes blocked, leading to dysfunction of the penetrating vessel.

Qi stagnation amenorrhea may be accompanied by lower abdominal pain that is aggravated by pressure. Patients with qi constraint may present emotional states such as depression, anxiety or irritability.

Amenorrhea may be associated with phlegm-damp obstruction. Symptoms then include obesity due to internal excessive phlegm-damp, lassitude, and swollen face and limbs due to phlegm-damp retention in the Spleen.

Pathogenic cold may congeal blood of the penetrating and conception vessels, obstructing circulation. Blood stasis and yang depletion due to congealing cold have symptoms such as coldness of the trunk and limbs, a pale complexion, and cold pain of the lower abdomen that are caused by obstruction and aggravated by pressure.

CHINESE MEDICAL TREATMENT

The primary objective in the treatment of amenorrhea is to restore normal ovulatory endocrine function and to re-establish regular and predictable menstrual cycles. In Chinese medicine, the general treatment principle is based on proper assessment of the patient's condition. For deficiency conditions, tonification is the correct therapeutic method. For those presenting with an excess condition, the draining method is the appropriate treatment. When deficiency and excess are combined, both tonifying and draining methods must be applied together. Furthermore, when amenorrhea occurs as a result of another disease, menstruation can be restored only after the associated disease has been successfully treated.

For deficiency cases, specific treatment principles may include tonification of the Liver and Kidney, nourishing essence and blood, invigorating the Spleen and Stomach, and replenishing qi and blood.

For excess patterns, treatment may involve warming the vessels to dispel cold, invigorating blood, regulating the movement of qi, and eliminating phlegm and dampness.

There are three important points to consider.

(1) Purely excess patterns are seldom seen in cases of amenorrhea. Excess patterns are most commonly accompanied by some degree of deficiency. Therefore, the use of strong purgatives and stasis-dispelling medicinals are generally inappropriate for this condition.

(2) The objective is to establish regular menstrual cycles of normal color, texture, and amount. To accomplish this, it is important to continue treatment for some period of time after menstruation initially resumes.

(3) In patients of reproductive age who wish to conceive, the final objective is to induce ovulation and promote follicular development. Both Chinese medicine and integrative medical approaches are effective.

For those patients who are not planning for pregnancy, contraceptive methods must be used during treatment.

Pattern Differentiation and Treatment

The key to pattern differentiation is to first differentiate deficiency from excess according to local and constitutional symptoms, the etiology and progression of the disorder, and patient history. After this, differentiate the viscera patterns, and finally, determine the condition of qi and blood.

1. DEFICIENCY

(1) Deficiency of Both Spleen and Kidney

【Syndrome Characteristics】

These patients present irregular or frequently absent periods, and their histories often show menarche of late onset. Menstrual irregularities may have progressed gradually, eventually resulting in amenorrhea. Additional symptoms include dizziness and tinnitus, soreness and weakness of the lumbar region and knees, lassitude, reluctance to speak, palpitation and shortness of breath, and insomnia or dream-disturbed sleep. Patients may also exhibit a sallow or pale complexion, a pale tongue and deficient, thready pulses.

【Treatment Principle】

Tonify the Kidney and invigorate the Spleen, nourish blood and regulate menstruation.

【Commonly Used Medicinals】

To tonify the Kidney and invigorate the Spleen, the following medicinals are generally indicated.

Shú dì huáng (Radix Rehmanniae Praeparata), *gǒu qǐ zǐ* (Fructus Lycii), *dù zhòng* (Cortex Eucommiae), *shú fù zǐ* (Prepared Radix Aconiti Lateralis

Praeparata), *bái zhú* (Rhizoma Atractylodis Macrocephalae) and *shān yào* (Rhizoma Dioscoreae).

To nourish blood and regulate menstruation, choose *dāng guī* (Radix Angelicae Sinensis), *bái zhú* (Rhizoma Atractylodis Macrocephalae), *huáng qí* (Radix Astragali), *xiāng fù* (Rhizoma Cyperi), and *jī xuè téng* (Caulis Spatholobi).

【Representative Formula】

Modified *Dà Yíng Jiān* (大营煎加减)

【Ingredients】

当归	dāng guī	15g	Radix Angelicae Sinensis
熟地黄	shú dì huáng	20g	Radix Rehmanniae Praeparata
枸杞子	gǒu qǐ zǐ	12g	Fructus Lycii
炙甘草	zhì gān cǎo	6g	Radix et Rhizoma Glycyrrhizae Praeparata cum Melle
杜仲	dù zhòng	15g	Cortex Eucommiae
熟附子	shú fù zǐ	9g	Radix Aconiti Lateralis Praeparata
白术	bái zhú	15g	Rhizoma Atractylodis Macrocephalae
黄芪	huáng qí	15g	Radix Astragali seu Hedysari
香附	xiāng fù	9g	Rhizoma Cyperi

Decoct in 500ml of water until 200ml remains. Take one-half of the decoction warm, twice daily.

【Formula Analysis】

Shú dì huáng (Radix Rehmanniae Praeparata) and *gǒu qǐ zǐ* (Fructus Lycii) both tonify the Kidney and nourish the essence and blood. *Dù zhòng* (Cortex Eucommiae) and *shú fù zǐ* (Prepared Radix Aconiti Lateralis Praeparata) warm the Kidney yang. *Bái zhú* (Rhizoma Atractylodis Macrocephalae) and *huáng qí* (Radix Astragali) both strengthen the Spleen and tonify qi. *Dāng guī* (Radix Angelicae Sinensis) and *xiāng fù* (Rhizoma Cyperi) both nourish and invigorate blood, as well as acting to regulate menstruation. *Zhì gān cǎo* (Radix et Rhizoma Glycyrrhizae Praeparata cum Melle) moderates and harmonizes the formula.

【Modifications】

Severe cases may present signs such as an aversion to cold, apathy, dryness or roughness of the vagina, hair loss, lack of libido, and atrophy of the generative organs. Modifications are then indicated to increase the supply of qi and blood by adding medicinals that tonify both the Kidney and Spleen.

Shèng Yù Tāng (圣愈汤)[1] combined with *Wŭ Zĭ Yăn Zōng Wán* (五子衍宗丸)[2] is effective for such cases. Modify with *lù jiǎo shuāng* (Cornu Cervi Degelatinatum) 10g, and *zĭ hé chē* (Placenta Hominis) 10g.

[1] Recorded in *Secrets from the Orchid Chamber* (兰室秘藏 , *Lán Shì Mì Cáng*).

[2] Recorded in *Introduction to Medicine* (医学入门 , *Yī Xué Rù Mén*).

(2) Yin Deficiency of the Liver and Kidney

【Syndrome Characteristics】

A sudden or gradual cessation of menses may occur as a result of miscarriage, abortion, childbirth, or any serious and longstanding disease. The patient may present with soreness and weakness of the lumbus and knees, heel pain, scant leucorrhea, and dryness or roughness of the vagina. Other symptoms include feverish sensations in palms and soles, vexation, insomnia, emaciation, a pale complexion, general debilitation and hair loss. The tongue may be red, with little or no coating. Pulses may be deep and weak, or rapid, thready and weak.

【Treatment Principle】

Tonify the Liver and Kidney, nourish blood and promote menstruation.

【Commonly Used Medicinals】

To tonify the Liver and Kidney, the following medicinals are generally indicated.

Shú dì huáng (Radix Rehmanniae Praeparata), *huáng jīng* (Rhizoma Polygonati), *zǐ hé chē* (Placenta Hominis), *guī bǎn* (Carapax et Plastrum Testudinis), *nǚ zhēn zǐ* (Fructus Ligustri Lucidi), *hàn lián cǎo* (Ecliptae Herba), *gǒu qǐ zǐ* (Fructus Lycii), *hé shǒu wū* (Radix Polygoni Multiflori) and *shān zhū yú* (Fructus Corni).

Dāng guī (Radix Angelicae Sinensis), *ē jiāo* (Colla Corii Asini) and *bái sháo* (Radix Paeoniae Alba) both nourish blood and promote menstruation.

【Representative Formula】

Yù Yīn Tāng (育阴汤)

【Ingredients】

熟地黄	shú dì huáng	12g	Radix Rehmanniae Praeparata
山药	shān yào	12g	Rhizoma Dioscoreae
川续断	chuān xù duàn	12g	Radix Dipsaci
桑寄生	sāng jì shēng	12g	Herba Taxilli
杜仲	dù zhòng	12g	Cortex Eucommiae
菟丝子	tù sī zǐ	12g	Semen Cuscutae
龟板	guī bǎn	10g	Carapax et Plastrum Testudinis
怀牛膝	huái niú xī	12g	Radix Achyranthis Bidentatae
山萸肉	shān yú ròu	12g	Fructus Corni
海螵蛸	hǎi piāo xiāo	10g	Endoconcha Sepiae
白芍	bái sháo	12g	Radix Paeoniae Alba
牡蛎	mǔ lì	12g	Concha Ostreae

Decoct in 500ml of water until 200ml of liquid remains. Take once daily.

【Formula Analysis】

This prescription tonifies the Liver and Kidney, while nourishing blood and promoting menstruation.

To tonify the Kidney, select *shú dì huáng* (Radix Rehmanniae

Praeparata), *shān yào* (Rhizoma Dioscoreae), *chuān xù duàn* (Radix Dipsaci), *sāng jì shēng* (Herba Taxilli), *dù zhòng* (Cortex Eucommiae), *tù sī zǐ* (Semen Cuscutae) and *huái niú xī* (Radix Achyranthis Bidentatae).

To nourish the Liver, select *shān zhū yú* (Fructus Corni) and *bái sháo* (Radix Paeoniae Alba). *Guī bǎn* (Carapax et Plastrum Testudinis) and *mǔ lì* (Concha Ostreae) both soothe the Liver and subdue yang.

【Modifications】

If the patient has hemorrhaged during delivery, or if the endometrium has been damaged by abortion or diagnostic curettage, add powdered *zǐ hé chē* (Placenta Hominis) 3g, *ròu cōng róng* (Herba Cistanches) 12g, *lù jiǎo piàn* (Cornu Cervi) 10g, and *lù róng* (Cornu Cervi Pantotrichum) 6g.

(3) Dryness due to Deficient Yin and Blood

【Syndrome Characteristics】

This pattern is often found in patients with a history of late periods with scant menstrual flow. Menses may be viscous in quality and dark in color. Other symptoms include tidal fever or feverish sensations in the chest, palms and soles, and dryness of the pharynx and mouth. Severe cases may present additional symptoms such as night sweats, steaming bone disorder, emaciation, and cough with expectoration of blood. The tongue is often red with little coating and pulses both rapid and thready.

【Treatment Principle】

Nourish yin and blood, regulate the penetrating and conception vessels, promote menstruation.

【Commonly Used Medicinals】

A great number of medicinals are effective in the treatment of deficient yin and blood conditions.

Select *bái sháo* (Radix Paeoniae Alba), *shēng dì huáng* (Radix Rehmanniae), *bái wēi* (Radix et Rhizoma Cynanchi Atrati), *yù zhú* (Rhizoma Polygonati

Odorati), *mài dōng* (Radix Ophiopogonis), *shā shēn* (Radix Adenophorae seu Glehniae), *huáng jīng* (Rhizoma Polygonati), *hé shǒu wū* (Radix Polygoni Multiflori), *nǚ zhēn zǐ* (Fructus Ligustri Lucidi), *zǐ hé chē* (Placenta Hominis), *dāng guī* (Radix Angelicae Sinensis), *gǒu qǐ zǐ* (Fructus Lycii), *zhī mǔ* (Rhizoma Anemarrhenae), *guī bǎn* (Carapax et Plastrum Testudinis), *ē jiāo* (Colla Corii Asini), *wǔ wèi zǐ* (Fructus Schisandrae Chinensis), *yè jiāo téng* (Caulis Polygoni Multiflori), *yuǎn zhì* (Radix Polygalae), *lóng gǔ* (Fossilia Ossis Mastodi) and *mǔ lì* (Concha Ostreae).

Medicinals created from animals have a particular ability to act on the penetrating and conception vessels. Some medicinals of this type are *zǐ hé chē* (Placenta Hominis), *guī bǎn* (Carapax et Plastrum Testudinis), and *ē jiāo* (Colla Corii Asini).

【Representative Formula】

Modified *Yī Yīn Jiān* (加减一阴煎) with added *gǒu qǐ zǐ* (Fructus Lycii), *nǚ zhēn zǐ* (Fructus Ligustri Lucidi) and *tù sī zǐ* (Semen Cuscutae).

【Ingredients】

生地黄	shēng dì huáng	12g	Radix Rehmanniae
熟地黄	shú dì huáng	12g	Radix Rehmanniae Praeparata
白芍	bái sháo	12g	Radix Paeoniae Alba
知母	zhī mǔ	10g	Rhizoma Anemarrhenae
麦冬	mài dōng	12g	Radix Ophiopogonis
地骨皮	dì gǔ pí	12g	Cortex Lycii
枸杞	gǒu qǐ zǐ	12g	Fructus Lycii
菟丝子	tù sī zǐ	12g	Semen Cuscutae
女贞子	nǚ zhēn zǐ	20g	Fructus Ligustri Lucidi
甘草	gān cǎo	6g	Radix et Rhizoma Glycyrrhizae

Decoct in 500ml of water until 200ml of liquid remains. Take one-half of the decoction warm, twice daily.

【Formula Analysis】

In this prescription, *shēng dì huáng* (Radix Rehmanniae), *mài dōng*

(Radix Ophiopogonis), *zhī mǔ* (Rhizoma Anemarrhenae), *nǔ zhēn zǐ* (Fructus Ligustri Lucidi) and *gǒu qǐ zǐ* (Fructus Lycii) have the functions of tonifying yin and clearing heat, while *shú dì huáng* (Radix Rehmanniae Praeparata) and *bái sháo* (Radix Paeoniae Alba) are responsible for nourishing blood and essence. *Dì gǔ pí* (Cortex Lycii) is used to cool blood and relieve steaming bone disorder, while *tù sī zǐ* (Semen Cuscutae) tonifies both the yin and yang of Kidney. This combination promotes menstruation by nourishing yin and blood, as well as regulating both the penetrating and conception vessels.

【Modifications】

➤ With Lung dryness and cough due to yin deficiency, add *chuān bèi mǔ* (Bulbus Fritillariae Cirrhosae) 12g.

➤ With expectoration of blood, add *ē jiāo* (Colla Corii Asini) 10g, *bái máo gēn* (Rhizoma Imperatae) 30g, *bǎi hé* (Bulbus Lilii) 12g, and *bái jí* (Rhizoma Bletillae) 12g. If tuberculosis is present, it is important to treat this condition concurrently.

➤ With ascendant hyperactivity of Liver yang, symptoms such as headache, insomnia and vexation may be present. Add *guī bǎn* (Carapax et Plastrum Testudinis) 12g, *mǔ lì* (Concha Ostreae) 10g, *wǔ wèi zǐ* (Fructus Schisandrae Chinensis) 10g and *yè jiāo téng* (Caulis Polygoni Multiflori) 30g.

➤ With vaginal heat or dryness, the formula may be decocted again and applied externally. Other medicinals to add for external use are *dà huáng* (Radix et Rhizoma Rhei) 30g, *gān cǎo* (Radix et Rhizoma Glycyrrhizae) 10g, and *qīng hāo* (Herba Artemisiae Annuae) 10g.

(4) Deficiency of Both Qi and Blood

【Syndrome Characteristics】

Patients in this category usually show a history of late periods with scant menstruation. Menses may have ceased gradually, eventually resulting in amenorrhea. Menses are thin and of a light color. Other symptoms include dizziness, blurry vision, palpitation with shortness of breath, lack of appetite, fatigue, and dream-disturbed sleep. We may find visible signs such as a sallow or pale complexion, withered hair and skin, and graying hair at a young age. The tongue appears pale with a thin, white, or absent coating. Pulses may be deep and slow, or weak and rapid.

【Treatment Principle】

Tonify qi and nourish blood, tonify and regulate the penetrating and conception vessels.

【Commonly Used Medicinals】

Medicinals such as *huáng qí* (Radix Astragali), *rén shēn* (Radix et Rhizoma Ginseng), *dǎng shēn* (Radix Codonopsis), *bái zhú* (Rhizoma Atractylodis Macrocephalae) and *shān yào* (Rhizoma Dioscoreae) tonify qi and invigorate the Spleen.

To nourish blood and yin, select *dāng guī* (Radix Angelicae Sinensis), *chuān xiōng* (Rhizoma Chuanxiong), *gǒu qǐ zǐ* (Fructus Lycii), *shú dì huáng* (Radix Rehmanniae Praeparata), *hé shǒu wū* (Radix Polygoni Multiflori), *ē jiāo* (Colla Corii Asini), *bái sháo* (Radix Paeoniae Alba) and *nǚ zhēn zǐ* (Fructus Ligustri Lucidi).

In addition, *zǐ hé chē* (Placenta Hominis) is selected to tonify and regulate the penetrating and conception vessels.

【Representative Formula】

Zī Xuè Tāng (滋血汤) with powdered *zǐ hé chē* (Placenta Hominis).

【Ingredients】

人参	rén shēn	12g	Radix Ginseng
山药	shān yào	20g	Rhizoma Dioscoreae
黄芪	huáng qí	20g	Radix Astragali seu Hedysari
茯苓	fú líng	12g	Poria
川芎	chuān xiōng	9g	Rhizoma Chuanxiong

当归	dāng guī	12g	Radix Angelicae Sinensis
白芍	bái sháo	12g	Radix Paeoniae Alba
熟地黄	shú dì huáng	12g	Radix Rehmanniae Praeparata
紫河车粉	zǐ hé chē fěn	3g	Placenta Hominis Powder

Decoct in 500ml of water until 200ml of liquid remains. Take one-half of the decoction warm, twice daily.

【Formula Analysis】

Rén shēn (Radix et Rhizoma Ginseng) strongly tonifies the original qi. *Huáng qí* (Radix Astragali), *shān yào* (Rhizoma Dioscoreae) and *fú líng* (Poria) strengthen the Spleen and tonify qi. *Dāng guī* (Radix Angelicae Sinensis), *chuān xiōng* (Rhizoma Chuanxiong), *bái sháo* (Radix Paeoniae Alba) and *shú dì huáng* (Radix Rehmanniae Praeparata) nourish blood and regulate menstruation, while powdered *zǐ hé chē* (Placenta Hominis) benefits and regulates the penetrating and conception vessels. This formula nourishes both qi and blood. Its particular ability to supplement yin and yang while nourishing both essence and blood makes it an effective formula to restore menstruation.

【Modifications】

For patients with insomnia or dream-disturbed sleep, calm the spirit by adding *wǔ wèi zǐ* (Fructus Schisandrae Chinensis) 6g, and *yè jiāo téng* (Caulis Polygoni Multiflori) 15g.

2. Excess

(1) Qi Stagnation with Blood Stasis

【Syndrome Characteristics】

Patients with this pattern often report regular menstrual cycles followed by amenorrhea of sudden onset. They often suffer from depression or anxiety, hypochondriac pain, or distending pain of the lower abdomen that are aggravated by pressure. The tongue body may be normal, possibly dusky in color or with dark spots, indicating stasis. The tongue coating may be normal, or thin and yellow. Pulses qualities are typically wiry or tight.

【Treatment Principle】

Activate qi and invigorate blood, dispel blood stasis and promote menstruation.

【Commonly Used Medicinals】

To invigorate blood and dispel stasis select *chuān xiōng* (Rhizoma Chuanxiong), *dān shēn* (Radix Salviae Miltiorrhizae), *chuān shān jiǎ* (Squama Manis), *shuǐ zhì* (Hirudo), *méng chóng* (Tabanus), *dāng guī* (Radix Angelicae Sinensis), *chì sháo* (Radix Paeoniae Rubra), *táo rén* (Semen Persicae), *hóng huā* (Flos Carthami), *jī xuè téng* (Caulis Spatholobi), *mǔ dān pí* (Cortex Moutan), and *chuān niú xī* (Radix Cyathulae).

Yù jīn (Radix Curcumae), *é zhú* (Rhizoma Curcumae), *xiāng fù* (Rhizoma Cyperi) and *méi guī huā* (Flos Rosae Rugosae) also activate the movement of qi.

【Representative Formula】

Gé Xià Zhú Yū Tāng (膈下逐瘀汤) with *chuān niú xī* (Radix Cyathulae).

【Ingredients】

当归	dāng guī	12g	Radix Angelicae Sinensis
川芎	chuān xiōng	9g	Rhizoma Chuanxiong
赤芍	chì sháo	12g	Radix Paeoniae Rubra
桃仁	táo rén	12g	Semen Persicae
红花	hóng huā	8g	Flos Carthami
枳壳	zhǐ qiào	12g	Fructus Aurantii
延胡索	yán hú suǒ	12g	Rhizoma Corydalis
五灵脂	wǔ líng zhī	12g	Faeces Togopteri
丹皮	dān pí	10g	Cortex Moutan
乌药	wū yào	12g	Radix Linderae
制香附	zhì xiāng fù	12g	Rhizoma Cyperi Praeparata
川牛膝	chuān niú xī	15g	Radix Cyathulae

甘草	gān cǎo	6g	Radix et Rhizoma Glycyrrhizae

Decoct in 500ml of water until 200ml of liquid remains. Take one-half of the decoction warm, twice daily.

【Formula Analysis】

In this prescription, *zhǐ qiào* (Fructus Aurantii), *wū yào* (Radix Linderae), *zhì xiāng fù* (Rhizoma Cyperi Praeparata) and *yán hú suǒ* (Rhizoma Corydalis) are used to activate the movement of qi and blood, while *chì sháo* (Radix Paeoniae Rubra), *táo rén* (Semen Persicae), *hóng huā* (Flos Carthami), *mǔ dān pí* (Cortex Moutan) and *wǔ líng zhī* (Faeces Togopteri) invigorate blood and dispel stasis. Both groups of medicinals help to relieve pain. *Dāng guī* (Radix Angelicae Sinensis) and *chuān xiōng* (Rhizoma Chuanxiong), nourish blood and promote circulation, and *gān cǎo* (Radix et Rhizoma Glycyrrhizae) moderates and harmonizes the formula.

【Modifications】

➤ With symptoms of restlessness and hypochondriac pain, add *chái hú* (Radix Bupleuri) 9g, *yù jīn* (Radix Curcumae) 12g, and *zhī zǐ* (Fructus Gardeniae Praeparatus) 9g.

➤ With internal heat signs such as a dry mouth or constipation, add *huáng bǎi* (Cortex Phellodendri Chinensis) 9g, and *zhī mǔ* (Rhizoma Anemarrhenae) 12g.

(2) Stagnation of Phlegm-damp

【Syndrome Characteristics】

A history of late periods with scant menstrual flow that becomes gradually absent over time. It is always accompanied by weight gain, acne, or profuse white and thin leucorrea, fullness and discomfort of the chest and hypochondrium, vomiting with excessive phlegm, and lassitude. The tongue is likely to be pale, swollen, and tender, with a white and greasy coating. Pulse qualities in this pattern are usually slippery and deep.

【Treatment Principle】

Dispel dampness and transform phlegm, regulate the penetrating and conception vessels.

【Commonly Used Medicinals】

Medicinals such as *fǎ bàn xià* (Rhizoma Pinelliae Praeparatum), *zào jiǎo cì* (Spina Gleditsiae), *cāng zhú* (Rhizoma Atractylodis), *fú líng* (Poria), *chén pí* (Pericarpium Citri Reticulatae), *hòu pò* (Cortex Magnoliae Officinalis), *zhè bèi mǔ* (Bulbus Fritillariae Thunbergii), *zhú rú* (Caulis Bambusae in Taenia), *bái zhú* (Rhizoma Atractylodis Macrocephalae) and *dǎn nán xīng* (Arisaema cum Bile) transform phlegm and dispel dampness, while *tù sī zǐ* (Semen Cuscutae) and *xù duàn* (Radix Dipsaci) act to regulate the penetrating and conception vessels.

【Representative Formula】

Cāng Fù Dǎo Tán Wán (苍附导痰丸) with *zào jiǎo cì* (Spina Gleditsiae) and *tù sī zǐ* (Semen Cuscutae).

【Ingredients】

苍术	cāng zhú	9g	Rhizoma Atractylodis
香附	xiāng fù	12g	Rhizoma Cyperi
茯苓	fú líng	12g	Poria
法半夏	fǎ bàn xià	12g	Rhizoma Pinelliae Praeparatum
陈皮	chén pí	9g	Pericarpium Citri Reticulatae
甘草	gān cǎo	6g	Radix et Rhizoma Glycyrrhizae
胆南星	dǎn nán xīng	10g	Arisaema Cum Bile
枳壳	zhǐ qiào	12g	Fructus Aurantii
生姜	shēng jiāng	3slices	Rhizoma Zingiberis Recens
神曲	shén qū	12g	Massa Medicata Fermentata
皂刺	zào jiǎo cì	10g	Spina Gleditsiae
菟丝子	tù sī zǐ	15g	Semen Cuscutae

Decoct in 500ml of water until 200ml of liquid remains. Take half of the decoction warm, twice daily.

【Formula Analysis】

The function of this formula is to restore normal menstruation by transforming and resolving phlegm-damp which has stagnated in the penetrating and conception vessels.

Cāng zhú (Rhizoma Atractylodis), *fǎ bàn xià* (Rhizoma Pinelliae Praeparatum) and *dǎn nán xīng* (Arisaema cum Bile) act together to resolve dampness and phlegm. However, *zào jiǎo cì* (Spina Gleditsiae) has a particularly strong phlegm-transforming effect, while *fú líng* (Poria) fortifies the Spleen and drains dampness. *Zhǐ qiào* (Fructus Aurantii), *chén pí* (Pericarpium Citri Reticulatae) and *xiāng fù* (Rhizoma Cyperi) activate the movement of qi and blood, while *shén qū* (Massa Medicata Fermentata) and *shēng jiāng* (Rhizoma Zingiberis Recens) invigorate both the Spleen and Stomach and regulate the middle jiao. Finally, *tù sī zǐ* (Semen Cuscutae) acts to regulate and tonify the penetrating and conception vessels.

【Modifications】

➢ With vomiting or fullness and oppression of the chest and hypochondrium, remove *tù sī zǐ* (Semen Cuscutae) and *shén qū* (Massa Medicata Fermentata), and add *guā lóu pí* (Pericarpium Trichosanthis) 10g, *hòu pò* (Cortex Magnoliae Officinalis) 12g, *zhú rú* (Caulis Bambusae in Taenia) 12g, and *tíng lì zǐ* (Semen Lepidii Semen Descurainiae) 10g.

➢ With damp-heat, a yellow and greasy tongue coating may be present. Add *huáng lián* (Rhizoma Coptidis) 10g, and *huáng qín* (Radix Scutellariae) 12g.

➢ With heat signs due to phlegm stagnation, add *huáng qín* (Radix Scutellariae) 12g, *yú xīng cǎo* (Herba Houttuyniae) 20g and *xià kū cǎo* (Spica Prunellae) 20g.

> For particularly tenacious phlegm conditions, add *kūn bù* (Thallus Laminariae) 12g, *zhè bèi mǔ* (Bulbus Fritillariae Thunbergii) 20g and *shān cí gū* (Pseudobulbus Cremastrae seu Pleiones) 20g.

> With Kidney deficiency, add *gǒu qǐ zǐ* (Fructus Lycii) 10g, *shān zhū yú* (Fructus Corni) 12g, *yín yáng huò* (Herba Epimedii) 12g, and *ròu cōng róng* (Herba Cistanches) 12g.

(3) Blood Stasis due to Congealing Cold

【Syndrome Characteristics】

This pattern is characterized by persistent amenorrhea lasting for over 6 months. Typical symptoms include coldness of the trunk and limbs, and lower abdominal pain that is relieved by warmth, yet aggravated by pressure. Complexion may be pale, and tongue appears dusky purple with white coating. Pulses are deep and tight in quality.

【Treatment Principle】

Warm the channels to dispel cold, invigorate blood and promote menstruation.

【Commonly Used Medicinals】

Medicinals include *dāng guī* (Radix Angelicae Sinensis), *chuān xiōng* (Rhizoma Chuanxiong), *pào jiāng* (Rhizoma Zingiberis Praeparata), *ròu guì* (Cortex Cinnamomi), *é zhú* (Rhizoma Curcumae), *mǔ dān pí* (Cortex Moutan), *wū yào* (Radix Linderae), *chuān niú xī* (Radix Cyathulae), *guì zhī* (Ramulus Cinnamomi), *zǐ sū yè* (Folium Perillae), and *xiāng fù* (Rhizoma Cyperi).

【Representative Formula】

Wēn Jīng Tāng (温经汤)

【Ingredients】

人参	rén shēn	12g	Radix Ginseng
当归	dāng guī	12g	Radix Angelicae Sinensis
川芎	chuān xiōng	9g	Rhizoma Chuanxiong

白芍	bái sháo	12g	Radix Paeoniae Alba
莪术	é zhú	10g	Rhizoma Curcumae
肉桂	ròu guì	10g	Cortex Cinnamomi
牡丹皮	dān pí	12g	Cortex Moutan
牛膝	chuān niú xī	12g	Radix Cyathulae
甘草	gān cǎo	6g	Radix et Rhizoma Glycyrrhizae

Decoct in 500ml of water until 200ml of liquid remains. Take half of the decoction warm, twice daily.

【Formula Analysis】

This combination of medicinals warms the channels to dispel cold, as well as functioning to invigorate blood and promoting menstruation. *Ròu guì* (Cortex Cinnamomi) warms the channels and dispels cold, while *dāng guī* (Radix Angelicae Sinensis) and *chuān xiōng* (Rhizoma Chuanxiong) together nourish and invigorate blood. The warm nature and sweet flavor of *rén shēn* (Radix et Rhizoma Ginseng) determines its function to both tonify qi and, in combination with *ròu guì* (Cortex Cinnamomi), to warm the channels to dispel cold. *É zhú* (Rhizoma Curcumae), *mǔ dān pí* (Cortex Moutan) and *chuān niú xī* (Radix Cyathulae) function to invigorate blood and remove stasis. These medicines assist the functions of *dāng guī* (Radix Angelicae Sinensis) and *chuān xiōng* (Rhizoma Chuanxiong). In addition, *bái sháo* (Radix Paeoniae Alba) and *gān cǎo* (Radix et Rhizoma Glycyrrhizae) are useful in relieving urgent abdominal pain and spasms.

【Modifications】

If the patient displays a dark yellow complexion, a dusky purple tongue, and severe cold pain of the lower abdomen, add *ài yè* (Folium Artemisiae Argyi) 10g, *fù piàn* (Prepared Radix Aconiti Lateralis Praeparata) 10g and *xiān líng pí* (Herba Epimedii) 12g.

Additional Treatment Modalities

1. Chinese patent medicine

(1) Promote Menstruation by Dispelling Blood Stasis

1) *Dà Huáng Zhè Chóng Wán* (大黄蛰虫丸)

This patent medicine treats amenorrhea of stasis type by breaking up stagnated blood to dispel stasis. Dosage: Large honeyed pills, take 1 or 2 pills, up to 3 times daily. Small honeyed pills, take 3-6g per dose, or 3g for water-honeyed pill. Take with warm water. Contraindicated in pregnant women. Discontinue use immediately if any signs of allergic skin reaction appear.

2) *Fù Kē Tōng Jīng Wán* (妇科通经丸)

Promotes menstruation in conditions due to blood stasis. Take 30 pills with foxtail millet water or yellow rice wine before the morning meal. Contraindicated in pregnancy, or in patients with loose stools or signs of qi and blood deficiency.

3) *Shào Fù Zhú Yū Wán* (少腹逐瘀丸)

Treats amenorrhea due to congealing cold and blood stasis. This patent medicine warms the channels and dispels cold, regulates menstruation and relieves pain. Take 1 pill, twice daily.

4) *Xuè Fǔ Zhú Yū Wán* (血府逐瘀丸)

This patent medicine activates both qi and blood to relieve pain and regulate menstruation. Indicated for patients with stagnation of both qi and blood due to Liver depression. Take 1 pill, twice daily.

(2) Induce Menstruation by Enriching Insufficiency

1) *Kūn Líng Wán* (坤灵丸)

The pill is selected for deficiency of both the Liver and Kidney. It strengthens the Liver and Kidney while regulating the penetrating and conception vessels. Take 15 pills, twice daily.

2) *Bā Zhēn Yì Mǔ Wán* (八珍益母丸)

Indicated for cases of qi and blood deficiency. It nourishes both qi and blood while regulating the penetrating and conception vessels. Take 1 pill, three times daily.

3) *Wū Jī Bái Fèng Wán* (乌鸡白凤丸)

For patterns of yin and blood insufficiency. This formula nourishes both yin and blood, while regulating the penetrating and conception vessels. Take 1 pill, twice daily.

4) *Ài Fù Nuǎn Gōng Wán* (艾附暖宫丸)

Treats congealing cold and blood stasis. This formula promotes menstruation by warming the channels and invigorating blood. Take 1 pill, twice daily.

(3) Promote Menstruation by Nourishing Deficiency and Dispelling Blood Stasis

Fù Kē Huí Shēng Dān (妇科回生丹)

This formula both tonifies qi and invigorates blood. Indicated for amenorrhea due to qi deficiency and blood stasis. Take 1 pill, twice daily.

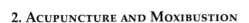
2. Acupuncture and Moxibustion

(1) Deficiency Patterns

1) Deficiency of Kidney Qi

【Treatment Principle】

Tonify the Kidney and replenish the essence.

【Point Selection】

BL 23	shèn shù	肾俞
RN 6	qì hǎi	气海
SP 6	sān yīn jiāo	三阴交
KI 3	tài xī	太溪

【Manipulation】

Puncture BL 23 (*shèn shù*) perpendicularly to a depth of 1-1.5*cun*. Manipulate with lifting, thrusting and rotating until a sore, distending sensation appears. For SP 6 (*sān yīn jiāo*) and KI 3 (tài xī), insert the needle 0.5-1*cun* perpendicularly, and manipulate with with supplementation after arrival of qi. Insert RN 6 (*qì hǎi*) perpendicularly to 0.5*cun*, manipulate gently and slowly with lifting, thrusting and rotating methods until a distending and downbearing sensation is obtained. Retain the needles for 20 minutes. Treatment is given once every two days.

2) Deficiency of Both the Liver and Kidney

【Treatment Principle】

Tonify and regulate the Liver and Kidney.

【Point Selection】

RN 4	guān yuán	关元
BL 23	shèn shù	肾俞

BL 18	gān shù	肝俞
SP 6	sān yīn jiāo	三阴交
KI 3	tài xī	太溪
LV 3	tài chōng	太冲

【Manipulation】

Puncture RN 4 (*guān yuán*) perpendicularly to a depth of 0.5-1*cun*. Supplement with lifting, thrusting and rotating until a distending and downbearing sensation is obtained. For BL 23 (*shèn shù*), insert the needle perpendicularly 1.5-2*cun* and manipulate until a sore, distending sensation appears. Puncture BL 18 (*gān shù*) with oblique insertion to 1*cun*. After the arrival of qi, supplement with rotation. Puncture SP 6 (*sān yīn jiāo*), to a depth of 0.5-1*cun*, then supplement until a sensation is propagated toward the foot. Needle KI 3 0.5-1*cun* perpendicularly and supplement with rotation. Insert LV 3 (*tài chōng*) to 0.5*cun*, supplement after the arrival of qi by lifting and thrusting. Retain the needles for 20 minutes. Treatment is given once every two days.

3) Deficiency of Qi and Blood

【Treatment Principle】

Nourish both qi and blood.

【Point Selection】

ST 36	zú sān lǐ	足三里
SP 6	sān yīn jiāo	三阴交
RN 6	qì hǎi	气海
ST 29	guī lái	归来
BL 20	pí shù	脾俞
BL 21	wèi shù	胃俞

【Manipulation】

Needle with gentle manipulation. Puncture ST 36 (*zú sān lǐ*) perpendicularly to 0.5-1*cun*. Supplement with lifting and thrusting or rotation after arrival of qi. Needle SP 6 perpendicularly to 0.5-1*cun*, and supplement until a sore, distending sensation appears. For RN 6 (*qì hǎi*) and ST 29 (*guī lái*), insert perpendicularly 0.5*cun*, manipulate gently and slowly with lifting, thrusting and rotating methods until a distending and downbearing sensation is obtained. BL 20 (*pí shù*) and BL 21 (*wèi shù*) are inserted obliquely to 0.5-1*cun*. After the arrival of qi, supplement with rotation. Retain the needles for 20 minutes. Treatment is given once every two days.

(2) Excess Patterns

1) Qi Stagnation and Blood Stasis

【Treatment Principle】
Invigorate blood and dispel blood stasis.

【Point Selection】

LI 4	hé gǔ	合谷
SP 6	sān yīn jiāo	三阴交
SP 8	dì jī	地机
SP 10	xuè hǎi	血海
ST 30	qì chōng	气冲

【Manipulation】
Insert LI 4 (*hé gǔ*) perpendicularly to 0.5-1*cun*. Supplement with lifting and thrusting until a local distending sensation appears which may be transmitted to the tip of the index finger.Puncture SP 6 (*sān yīn jiāo*) directed upwardly into to a depth of 1-1.5*cun*. Drain with lifting and thrusting until a sensation is propagated upwardly along the leg. For SP 8 (*dì jī*), puncture perpendicularly to 0.5-1*cun*. Drain with lifting and thrusting, until the needling sensation transmits upward. Needle SP 10 (*xuè hǎi*) perpendicularly to 1*cun*, drain with lifting and thrusting,

or rotation. Finally, ST 30 (*qì chōng*) is needled 1*cun* perpendicularly. Manipulate with the even method until a distending and downbearing sensation is obtained. Retain the needles for 20 minutes, manipulating periodically.

2) Stagnation of Phlegm-damp

【Treatment Principle】

Eliminate dampness and transform phlegm.

【Point Selection】

BL 20	pí shù	脾俞
BL 22	sān jiāo shù	三焦俞
RN 3	zhōng jí	中极
RN 12	zhōng wǎn	中脘
SP 6	sān yīn jiāo	三阴交
ST 40	fēng lóng	丰隆

【Manipulation】

Puncture BL 20 (*pí shù*) and BL 22 (*sān jiāo shù*) obliquely to 1-1.5*cun* with the even method, rotating until a distending sensation is obtained. For RN 3 (*zhōng jí*), insert perpendicularly to 1 *cun* with drainage. Perform lifting and thrusting until a distending sensation appears in the lower abdomen. Needle RN 12 (*zhōng wǎn*) to 1-1.5*cun*, using the even method. Use lifting and thrusting to produce a sensation of distention and numbness in the upper abdomen. ST 40 (*fēng lóng*) is needled perpendicularly to 1-1.5*cun*. Drain with lifting and thrusting until the needling sensation is transmitted to the foot. Insert SP 6 (*sān yīn jiāo*) perpendicularly to 1*cun* using the even method. Perform lifting and thrusting until a sore, distending sensation is obtained which may be transmitted upward or downward. Retain the needles for 20 minutes, manipulating periodically.

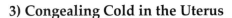

3) Congealing Cold in the Uterus

【Treatment Principle】

Warm the channels and dispel cold.

【Point Selection】

RN 4	guān yuán	关元
ST 25	tiān shū	天枢
ST 29	guī lái	归来
SP 6	sān yīn jiāo	三阴交
DU 3	yāo yáng guān	腰阳关
BL 26	guān yuán shù	关元俞

【Manipulation】

Puncture RN 4 and ST 25 (*tiān shū*) to 1-1.5*cun* perpendicularly. Supplement with rotation to produce a distending sensation in the abdomen. The burning mountain warming method can also be applied to these two points, producing a sensation of heat in the abdomen. Insert ST 29 (*guī lái*) perpendicularly to 0.5-1*cun* and BL 26 (*guān yuán shù*) to 1.5-2*cun*. Supplement both until a downbearing sensation is obtained. Puncture SP 6 (*sān yīn jiāo*) perpendicularly to 1-1.5*cun*. Perform lifting and thrusting until the needling sensation appears which may be transmitted upward or downward. Puncture DU 3 (*yāo yáng guān*) to 0.5-1*cun* perpendicularly until the needling sensation appears. Retain the needles for 20 minutes, manipulating periodically.

(3) Electroacupuncture

【Point Selection】

ST 25	tiān shū	天枢
SP 10	xuè hǎi	血海
ST 29	guī lái	归来

SP 6	sān yīn jiāo	三阴交
ST 30	qì chōng	气冲
SP 8	dì jī	地机

【Manipulation】

Select points in pairs, choosing one point from the abdomen and one point from the lower limbs. Apply electroacupuncture to one pair of points for each treatment. Set to dense wave, moderate intensity, for 10-15 minutes.

(4) Cutaneous needling

【Point Selection】

Select points along the first lateral line of bladder channel in lumbosacral area as well as from below the umbilicus along the penetrating and conception channels. Other applicable points include:

ST 29	guī lái	归来
SP 10	xuè hǎi	血海
ST 36	zú sān lǐ	足三里

【Manipulation】

Apply tapping with a plum blossom needle along the channels, three times each. Treat BL 18 (*gān shù*) and BL 23 (*shèn shù*) in particular, and then treat the remaining points. Treat with moderate intensity. Treatment is given once every two days, ten days constitute one course of treatment. Allow 3-5 days between each course.

(5) Auricular Acupuncture

【Point Selection】

endocrine	CO 18	nèi fēn mì	内分泌
ovary		luǎn cháo	卵巢

subcortex	AT 4	pí zhì xià	皮质下
Liver	CO 12	gān	肝
Kidney	CO 10	shèn	肾
shenmen	TF 4	shén mén	神门

【Manipulation】

3-4 points are selected for each treatment. If treating with filiform needles, use moderate stimulation, retaining the needles for 20 minutes. Treat once every two days. If embedding ear seeds, 2-3 times per week is sufficient.

3. Simple prescriptions and empirical formulas

(1) Yǎng Xuè Tōng Jīng Tāng (养血通经汤)

胎盘粉	tāi pán fěn	30g	Placenta Hominis Powder
生水蛭	shēng shuǐ zhì	10g	Hirudo (raw)
鸡内金	jī nèi jīn	15g	Endothelium Corneum Gigeriae Galli
生山楂	shēng shān zhā	20g	Fructus Crataegi (raw)
熟地黄	shú dì huáng	20g	Radix Rehmanniae Praeparata
当归	dāng guī	15g	Radix Angelicae Sinensis
白芍	bái sháo	15g	Radix Paeoniae Alba
甘草	gān cǎo	15g	Radix et Rhizoma Glycyrrhizae
川芎	chuān xiōng	15g	Rhizoma Chuanxiong

Indicated for Kidney deficiency and blood stasis. This prescription acts to tonify the Kidney, invigorate blood and promote menstruation.

Powder the first three and decoct with the remaining medicinals. Take half, twice daily. 10 days constitute one course.

(2) Huà Tán Tōng Jīng Tāng (化痰通经汤)

半夏	bàn xià	10g	Rhizoma Pinelliae
胆南星	dǎn nán xīng	10g	Arisaema cum Bile
浙贝母	zhè bèi mǔ	10g	Bulbus Fritillariae Thunbergii

当归	dāng guī	10g	Radix Angelicae Sinensis
红花	hóng huā	10g	Flos Carthami
三棱	sān léng	10g	Rhizoma Sparganii
莪术	é zhú	10g	Rhizoma Curcumae
香附	xiāng fù	10g	Rhizoma Cyperi
茯苓	fú líng	15g	Poria
益母草	yì mǔ cǎo	20g	Herba Leonuri
川牛膝	chuān niú xī	30g	Radix Cyathulae

Indicated for blood stasis and phlegm stagnation in patients who have not yet become sexually active. This prescription acts to transform phlegm, invigorate blood and promote menstruation.

Take half as one dose twice daily, 5 days per week. 20 doses constitute one course of treatment. If menstruation is not restored, wait five days and begin a second course.

PROGNOSIS

Long-term amenorrhea and anovulation increase the risk of endometrial cancer. This condition is detrimental to both bone metabolism and reproductive function. Associated conditions include premature menopause, infertility, reduced bone density and sexual dysfunction. Recent studies also have shown an association with hypoestrogenism, hyperinsulinism and hyperlipidemia, and an increased chance of developing arteriosclerosis, hypertension and heart disease. Amenorrhea is a significant factor in the development of these conditions.

PREVENTIVE HEALTHCARE

Health counseling has clearly been shown to benefit women's reproductive health. There are a variety of lifestyle issues that must be addressed to assist in the prevention of amenorrhea.

During the menstrual period, women should not eat too many raw or cold-natured foods. Excessive exposure to cold weather or cold water is to be avoided. Personal hygiene is also particularly important during the menstrual or post-partum periods. Effective contraception can help avoid unwanted abortions. Breastfeeding should not be continued beyond the normal period. Excessive dieting and weight loss should be avoided. Women should be aware of conditions that lead to amenorrhea, such as late periods, scant menstrual flow, inflammation of the genitals, tuberculosis, diabetes, and diseases of the adrenal and thyroid glands. Prompt treatment should be sought for any of the above conditions. For patients with amenorrhea related to contraceptive agents, other methods are to be advised.

Lifestyle Modification

Recommend that the patient create a reasonable schedule that balances both work and rest. Regular exercise and a balanced diet are both extremely beneficial in supporting body constitution.

Dietary Recommendation

Chinese dietary therapy is based on pattern differentiation. For patients with deficiency conditions, the following medicinals may be added to the daily diet.

Bái zhú (Rhizoma Atractylodis Macrocephalae), *shān yào* (Rhizoma Dioscoreae), *gǒu qǐ zǐ* (Fructus Lycii), *tāi pán* (placenta), *biē* (turtle) and *sāng jì shēng* (Herba Taxilli). For patients with excess conditions, add *jī xuè téng* (Caulis Spatholobi), *hóng huā* (Flos Carthami), *yì mǔ cǎo* (Herba Leonuri), *chuān xiōng* (Rhizoma Chuanxiong) and *táo rén* (Semen Persicae).

(1) *Dùn Bái Gē* (炖白鸽)

白鸽	bái gē	1	White Pigeon
鳖甲	biē jiǎ	50g	Carapax Amydae

Rinse the bird well. Add yellow rice wine and equal amount of water to a earthen pot. After the bird is cooked thoroughly, consume the broth and meat. Prepare 4-5 times per month, and take every other day. Another recipe is to stuff the bird with small pieces of *biē jiǎ* (Carapax Trionycis) 50g before cooking. Benefits patients with deficiency of both Liver and Kidney yin.

(2) *Shòu Ròu Biē Tāng* (瘦肉鳖汤)

鳖	biē	1	turtle
瘦肉	shòu ròu	100g	lean pork

Braise the turtle with 100g of lean pork, season to taste. Consume the broth and meat once per day for several days each month. Benefits patients with deficiency of both Liver and Kidney yin.

(3) *Tāi Pán Mò* (胎盘末)

Put a thoroughly cleaned fresh placenta onto a baking sheet or pan and bake on low heat till dry. Pestle into a powder and mix with yellow rice wine. Take 15g, twice daily, consuming one placenta per month. This preparation benefits patients with deficiency of essence and blood, and regulates the penetrating and conception vessels.

(4) *Yì Mǐ Biǎn Dòu Shān Zhā Zhǔ Hóng Táng* (薏米扁豆山楂煮红糖)

薏苡仁	yì yǐ rén	60g	Coicis Semen
炒扁豆	chǎo bǎi biǎn dòu	15g	Semen Lablab Alba (dry-fried)
山楂	shān zhā	15g	Fructus Crataegi
红糖	hóng táng		Brown Sugar

Make porridge with the above ingredients. Take once per day, 7-8 times per month. Benefits patients with Spleen deficiency, blood stasis, and phlegm stagnation.

(5) *Jī Xuè Téng Yào Dàn* (鸡血藤药蛋)

| 鸡血藤 | jī xuè téng | 30g | Caulis Spatholobi |
| 鸡蛋 | jī dàn | 2 | eggs |

Boil both ingredients with water, remove the eggshells and filter out the dregs. Dissolve up to 20g white sugar into the decoction. Drink once per day for several days.

Regulation of Emotional and Mental Health

A balanced emotional state is very beneficial to reproductive health. Avoid stressful and depressive conditions. Consciously cultivating a generous and tolerant attitude towards others can create an easygoing personality that promotes good health.

CLINICAL EXPERIENCE OF RENOWNED PHYSICIANS

Empirical Formulas

1. *Sì Èr Wǔ Hé Fāng* (四二五合方) FROM LIU FENG-WU

【Ingredients】

Sì Wù Tāng (四物汤), *Èr Xiān Tāng* (二仙汤) with *Wǔ Zǐ Yǎn Zōng Wán* (五子衍宗丸).

当归	dāng guī	Radix Angelicae Sinensis
生地	shēng dì huáng	Radix Rehmanniae
白芍	bái sháo	Radix Paeoniae Alba
川芎	chuān xiōng	Rhizoma Chuanxiong
仙茅	xiān máo	Rhizoma Curculiginis
仙灵脾	xiān líng pí	Herba Epimedii
菟丝子	tù sī zǐ	Semen Cuscutae
覆盆子	fù pén zǐ	Fructus Rubi

枸杞子	gǒu qǐ zǐ	Fructus Lycii
五味子	wǔ wèi zǐ	Fructus Schisandrae Chinensis
车前子	chē qián zǐ	Semen Plantaginis

【Indications】

Amenorrhea associated with Kidney and blood deficiency.

【Formula Analysis】

Wǔ Zǐ Yǎn Zōng Wán tonifies Kidney qi. The medicinal *tù sī zǐ* (Semen Cuscutae) has a bitter flavor and is neutral. It tonifies the Kidney and nourishes both essence and marrow. *Fù pén zǐ* (Fructus Rubi), is sweet and sour with a mildly warm nature, and strengthens the Kidney to secure the essence. *Gǒu qǐ zǐ* (Fructus Lycii), with its sweet and sour flavor, is used to nourish Kidney yin. *Wǔ wèi zǐ* (Fructus Schisandrae Chinensis) is named the "five-flavored seed" because it reaches all five viscera. However, it is particularly effective in tonifying the Kidney. The cold and downbearing nature of *chē qián zǐ* (Semen Plantaginis) enable it to disinhibit the urogenital canal and promote urination. Its function here is to dispel turbid-damp while nourishing Kidney yin. Using the combination of *xiān máo* (Rhizoma Curculiginis) and *xiān líng pí* (Herba Epimedii) from *Èr Xiān Tāng*, this formula also tonifies Kidney yang. Yang activates Kidney qi, while yin produces Kidney essence. This explains the combination of *Wǔ Zǐ Yǎn Zōng Wán* and *Èr Xiān Tāng*. When the qi and essence of the Kidney become sufficient, hair growth is stimulated, vaginal fluids will increase, sexual desire will be improved, and menstruation will resume. The presence of *Sì Wù Tāng* as part of this formula strengthens its blood and yin nourishing effect. The addition of *chuān niú xī* (Radix Cyathulae), adds to the formula's Kidney tonifying effect. The formula clearly focuses on tonification rather than purging. After both the Kidney qi and essence are replenished, the source of the menses becomes sufficient, thereby restoring menstruation.

(Beijing Chinese Medicine Hospital, Beijing Chinese Medical College. *Gynecological Experiences of Liu Feng-wu* 刘奉五妇科经验 . Beijing: People's Medical Publishing House, 1982. 281-282)

2. *Huà Tán Pò Yū Tōng Jīng Tāng* (化痰破瘀通经汤) FROM LI CHUN-HUA
【Ingredients】

当归	dāng guī	15g	Radix Angelicae Sinensis
柴胡	chái hú	15g	Radix Bupleuri
白芍	bái sháo	15g	Radix Paeoniae Alba
茯苓	fú líng	15g	Poria
白术	bái zhú	15g	Rhizoma Atractylodis Macrocephalae
益母草	yì mǔ cǎo	15g	Herba Leonuri; Leonuri
鸡血藤	jī xuè téng	15g	Caulis Spatholobi
川芎	chuān xiōng	10g	Rhizoma Chuanxiong
陈皮	chén pí	10g	Pericarpium Citri Reticulatae
法半夏	fǎ bàn xià	10g	Rhizoma Pinelliae Praeparatum

【Indications】
Amenorrhea due to blood stasis and phlegm stagnation.
【Formula Analysis】
In this formula, *fú líng* (Poria) and *bái zhú* (Rhizoma Atractylodis Macrocephalae) both fortify the Spleen to transform phlegm and eliminate dampness. They act together with *chén pí* (Pericarpium Citri Reticulatae) and *fǎ bàn xià* (Rhizoma Pinelliae Praeparatum) to this effect. *Dāng guī* (Radix Angelicae Sinensis), *chuān xiōng* (Rhizoma Chuanxiong), *yì mǔ cǎo* (Herba Leonuri) and *jī xuè téng* (Caulis Spatholobi) all invigorate blood and dispel stasis, while *chái hú* (Radix Bupleuri) and *bái sháo* (Radix Paeoniae Alba) relieve constraint by both nourishing and emolliating the Liver.
【Modifications】
➢ With severe blood stasis, add *táo rén* (Semen Persicae) 10g, and *hóng huā* (Flos Carthami) 10g.

➢ With excessive phlegm-damp, add *dǎn nán xīng* (Arisaema cum Bile) 10g and *bái jiè zǐ* (Sinapis Semen) 15g.

➢ With obvious signs of qi stagnation, add *xiāng fù* (Rhizoma Cyperi) 15g, and *yù jīn* (Radix Curcumae) 15g.

➢ With predominant Kidney yang deficiency, add *xiān máo* (Rhizoma Curculiginis) and *xiān líng pí* (Herba Epimedii).

(Chen Jin-rong, Li Chun-hua. Experience Treating Phlegm Stagnation and Blood Stasis in Stubborn Gynecological Diseases 运用痰瘀学说治疗妇科疑难病的经验 . *New Journal of Traditional Chinese Medicine* 新中医 , 1995. (6)：5)

Selected Case Studies

1. MEDICAL RECORDS OF SHI JIN-MO: AMENORRHEA DUE TO QI AND BLOOD DEFICIENCY WITH BLOOD STASIS OF THE PENETRATING AND CONCEPTION VESSELS

【Initial Visit】

Miss Xie, age 22.

Chief complaint: Absent menstruation for 1 year.

Cessation of menstruation for 1 year, accompanied by symptoms such as emaciation, lassitude, poor memory, scant leucorrhea, lower back soreness, and a downbearing pain of the lower abdomen. Her complexion appeared darkish, and the tongue body dark red. Pulses were deep and rough in quality

【Pattern Differentiation】

Qi and blood deficiency with blood stasis.

【Treatment Principle】

Invigorate blood and promote menstruation. Follow up with tonification and regulation of qi and blood.

【Prescription】

| 两头尖 | liǎng tóu jiān | 10g | Rhizoma Anemones Raddeanae |
| 凌霄花 | líng xiāo huā | 6g | Flos Campsis |

茜草根	qiàn cǎo gēn	6g	Radix et Rhizoma Rubiae
茺蔚子(酒炒)	chōng wèi zǐ	6g	Fructus Leonuri (fried with wine)
酒玄胡索	jiǔ yán hú suǒ	6g	Rhizoma Corydalis (fried with wine)
酒当归	jiǔ dāng guī	6g	Radix Angelicae Sinensis (fried with wine)
酒川芎	jiǔ chuān xiōng	5g	Rhizoma Chuanxiong (fried with wine)
酒丹参	jiǔ dān shēn	15g	Radix Salviae Miltiorrhizae (fried with wine)
祈艾叶	ài yè	5g	Folium Artemisiae Argyi
炙甘草	zhì gān cǎo	3g	Radix et Rhizoma Glycyrrhizae Praeparata cum Melle

4 doses were prescribed.

【Second Visit】

Menstruation was slightly restored after the second dose, followed by the appearance of dark purple menses with clotting. Her lower back and abdominal pain was also relieved. The patient was prescribed *Bā Bǎo Kūn Shùn Wán* (八宝坤顺丸) for one month, 1 pill twice daily.

Comments:

Despite the symptom of emaciation, which is considered to be a sign of qi and blood deficiency, the deep, rough pulses and dark red tongue color suggested the existence of blood stasis. Simple tonification is insufficient to restore menstruation without first dispelling static blood, while in conditions of deficiency the use of strong purgatives is contraindicated. The primary treatment principle here is to invigorate blood and dispel stasis. Qi and blood nourishing formulas like *Bā Bǎo Kūn Shùn Wán* (八宝坤顺丸) should only be given later. Once the stasis condition is resolved, qi and blood must be supplemented to promote menstruation. Only then can regular menstrual function be restored. Because *Liǎng tóu jiān* (Rhizoma Anemones Raddeanae) treats the blood aspect and also has an affinity to the Liver channel, it effectively invigorates blood and dispels stasis. It can also be used to treat both carbuncles and swellings. *Líng xiāo huā* (Flos Campsis) also promotes menstruation by removing masses and dispelling static blood.

(Zhu Shen-yu, Zhai Ji-sheng, Shi Ru-yu, etal. *Collection of Shi Jin-mo's Clinical Experience* 施今墨临床经验集. Beijing: Peoples Medical Publishing House, 1982. 184-187)

2. MEDICAL RECORDS OF SHI JIN-MO: AMENORRHEA DUE TO LIVER CONSTRAINT AND BLOOD STASIS

【Initial Visit】

Miss Zhang, 23 years old.

Chief complaint: Absent menstruation for 5 months.

This patient reported a long history of late periods. She had been suffering with symptoms of mental depression for several months, related to a domestic dispute. She also complained of lumbar and back pain, poor appetite, dizziness and weight loss. Sleep habits and excretion were normal. Tongue appeared darkish with a thin white coating. All six pulses were deep, rough and thready.

【Pattern Differentiation】

Constraint of Liver qi and blood stasis.

【Treatment Principle】

Course the Liver and invigorate blood.

【Prescription】

柴胡	chái hú	5g	Radix Bupleuri
砂仁	shā rén	6g	Fructus Amomi
玫瑰花	méi guī huā	5g	Flos Rosae Rugosae
赤芍	chì sháo	6g	Radix Paeoniae Rubra
白芍	bái sháo	6g	Radix Paeoniae Alba
生地黄	shēng dì huáng	6g	Radix Rehmanniae
熟地黄	shú dì huáng	6g	Radix Rehmanniae Praeparata
厚朴花	hòu pò huā	5g	Flos Magnoliae Officinalis
益母草	yì mǔ cǎo	12g	Herba Leonuri

酒川芎	jiǔ chuān xiōng	5g	Rhizoma Chuanxiong (fried with wine)
酒当归	jiǔ dāng guī	10g	Radix Angelicae Sinensis (fried with wine)
佛手花	fó shǒu huā	6g	Flos Fructus Citri Sarcodactylis
佩兰叶	pèi lán	10g	Herba Eupatorii
炒丹皮	chǎo mǔ dān pí	6g	Cortex Moutan (dry-fried)
月季花	yuè jì huā	6g	Flos Rosae Chinensis
泽兰叶	zé lán yè	10g	Herba Lycopi
炒丹参	chǎo dān shēn	6g	Radix Salviae Miltiorrhizae (dry-fried)
白蒺藜	bái jí lí	10g	Fructus Tribuli
沙蒺藜	shā jí lí	10g	Semen Astragali Complanati
炙甘草	zhì gān cǎo	3g	Radix et Rhizoma Glycyrrhizae Praeparata cum Melle

4 doses.

【Second Visit】

After 4 doses, the lumbar and back pain was relieved and her appetite improved. *Guì zhī* (Ramulus Cinnamomi) 3g and *xì xīn* (Radix et Rhizoma Asari) 1.5g were added to the formula, and another 4 doses prescribed.

【Third Visit】

Her menstruation was slightly restored. Dark colored menses were accompanied by a downbearing abdominal pain. The decoction was discontinued and the prescription was changed to *Bā Bǎo Kūn Shùn Wán* (八宝坤顺丸), 1 pill each morning, with *Yù Yè Jīn Dān* (玉液金丹), 1 pill each evening.

Comments:

There are a number of etiologies associated with amenorrhea, and we must clearly distinguish them to avoid taking the common approach of simply prescribing drastic purgatives and strong stasis dispelling medicinals. This case shows clear signs of blood stasis and Liver constraint, so the primary approach is to course the Liver and dispel static blood. The formula is based on *Chái Hú Sì Wù Tāng* (柴胡四物汤),

with the addition *méi guī huā* (Flos Rosae Rugosae), *yuè jì huā* (Flos Rosae Chinensis), *zé lán* (Herba Lycopi) and *yì mǔ cǎo* (Herba Leonuri). These medicinals both invigorate and nourish blood. Menstruation was restored after 8 doses of the decoction, and tonic pills were then prescribed to stabilize the therapeutic effect.

(Zhu Shen-yu, Zhu Shen-yu, Zhai Ji-sheng, Shi Ru-yu, etal. *Collection of Shi Jin-mo's Clinical Experience* 施今墨临床经验集 . Beijing: People's Medical Publishing House, 1982. 184-187)

3. MEDICAL RECORDS OF WANG WEI-CHUAN: AMENORRHEA DUE TO QI AND BLOOD DEFICIENCY WITH BLOOD STASIS

【Initial Visit】

Ms. Yu, age 35, laborer. Initial visit on May 21ˢᵗ, 1979.

Chief complaint: Absent menstruation for 7 months.

Menstruation ceased following an argument with her partner regarding a previous abortion. The primary symptoms were palpitations, lassitude, poor appetite, oppression of the chest, and abdominal pain that was aggravated by pressure. In addition, she complained of fishy smelling leucorrhea, and her face appeared swollen. Her tongue body was pale with a thin coating. Pulses were both rapid and wiry.

【Pattern Differentiation】

Deficiency of both qi and blood with blood stasis.

【Treatment Principle】

Nourish qi and blood, dispel stasis and eliminate dampness.

【Prescription】

The formula is a modification of *Hé Jiān Dì Huáng Yǐn Zǐ* (河间地黄饮子), *Tōng Qiào Huó Xuè Tāng* (通窍活血汤) and *Yín Jiǎ Jiān Jì* (银甲煎剂).

党参	dǎng shēn	30g	Radix Codonopsis
鸡血藤	jī xuè téng	18g	Caulis Spatholobi

生黄芪	shēng huáng qí	60g	Radix Astragali Cruda
黑故纸	hēi gù zhǐ	12g	Fructus Psoraleae
蛰虫	zhè chóng	10g	Eupolyphaga seu Steleophaga
水蛭	shuǐ zhì	6g	Hirudo
炒蒲黄	chǎo pú huáng	10g	Pollen Typhae (dry-fried)
泽兰	zé lán	12g	Herba Lycopi
益母草	yì mǔ cǎo	24g	Herba Leonuri
当归	dāng guī	10g	Radix Angelicae Sinensis
川芎	chuān xiōng	6g	Rhizoma Chuanxiong
红藤	hóng téng	24g	Sargentgloryvine Stem
蒲公英	pú gōng yīng	24g	Herba Taraxaci
槟榔	bīng láng	10g	Semen Arecae
琥珀末(冲服或布包煎)	hǔ pò mò	6g	Succinum Powder (infused or wrap-boiled)

12 doses were prescribed. (6 doses per week)

【Second Visit】

By the second visit the patient's energy level and appetite had improved, and her pain relieved. The leucorrhea was greatly reduced, with no foul odor. However, she was experiencing anxiety with severe pain of the chest and hypochondrium. Her tongue appeared red, with no coating. Pulses were wiry and rapid in quality. Further modifications were made to the formula.

党参	dǎng shēn	30g	Radix Codonopsis
鸡血藤	jī xuè téng	18g	Caulis Spatholobi
生黄芪	shēng huáng qí	60g	Radix Astragali Cruda
水蛭	shuǐ zhì	6g	Hirudo
生蒲黄	shēng pú huáng	10g	Pollen Typhae Crudum
红泽兰	hóng zé lán	12g	Herba Lycopi
益母草	yì mǔ cǎo	24g	Herba Leonuri
当归	dāng guī	10g	Radix Angelicae Sinensis
川芎	chuān xiōng	6g	Rhizoma Chuanxiong
女贞子	nǚ zhēn zǐ	24g	Fructus Ligustri Lucidi

旱莲草	hàn lián cǎo	15g	Ecliptae Herba
夏枯草	xià kū cǎo	15g	Spica Prunellae
薤白	xiè bái	12g	Bulbus Allii Macrostemonis
炒川楝	chǎo chuān liàn	10g	Fructus Toosendan (dry-fried)
生白芍	shēng bái sháo	12g	Radix Paeoniae Alba (raw)
覆盆子	fù pén zǐ	24g	Fructus Rubi
广木香	guǎng mù xiāng	10g	Radix Aucklandiae
沙参	shā shēn	20g	Radix Adenophorae seu Glehniae

12 doses were prescribed at 6 doses per week, with *Yín Jiǎ Wán* (银甲 丸), three times daily.

【Third Visit】

Her condition greatly improved with all previous symptoms resolved. However, she began menstruating profusely with an amount equivalent to 3 packs of sanitary napkins. She was subsequently diagnosed with pelvic inflammation. The tongue appeared light red with a thin white coating, and her pulse moderate. Several modifications were made to the previous formula.

党参	dǎng shēn	30g	Radix Codonopsis
鸡血藤	jī xuè téng	18g	Caulis Spatholobi
生黄芪	shēng huáng qí	60g	Radix Astragali (raw)
红泽兰	hóng zé lán	12g	Herba Lycopi
益母草	yì mǔ cǎo	24g	Herba Leonuri
覆盆子	fù pén zǐ	24g	Fructus Rubi
太子参	tài zǐ shēn	20g	Radix Pseudostellariae
仙鹤草	xiān hè cǎo	60g	Herba Agrimoniae
鸡内金	jī nèi jīn	9g	Endothelium Corneum Gigeriae Galli
何首乌	hé shǒu wū	30g	Radix Polygoni Multiflori
槟榔	bīng láng	6g	Semen Arecae
砂仁	shā rén	6g	Fructus Amomi
广藿香	guǎng huò xiāng	6g	Herba Pogostemonis

12 doses were prescribed at 6 doses per week, with *Yín Jiǎ Wán* (银甲

丸), three times daily.

【Fourth Visit】

All symptoms were resolved and treatments were discontinued. The patient later reported that menses remained regular, with no further appearance of leucorrhea.

Comments:

In this case, the etiology is associated with an emotional disturbance leading to a pattern of blood stasis coupled with qi and blood deficiency. Treatment focuses on nourishing qi and blood, eliminating pathogenic dampness, and dispelling static blood. *Dì Huáng Yǐn Zǐ* (地黄饮子) and *Tōng Qiào Huó Xuè Tāng* (通窍活血汤) combine effectively as *dǎng shēn* (Radix Codonopsis) and *huáng qí* (Radix Astragali) tonify qi, while the insect-based medicinals specifically dredge the meridians, promote the movement of blood and remove blood stasis. In addition, *Yín Jiǎ Wán* (银甲丸) eliminates excessive dampness. In these cases we must clearly distinguish the etiologies and progression of the disorder. Again, if we take the more common approach of simply prescribing drastic purgatives or stasis dispelling medicinals such as *Táo Hóng Sì Wù Tāng* (桃红四物汤), treatment will not be effective.

4. MEDICAL RECORDS OF WANG WEI-CHUAN: AMENORRHEA RESULTING FROM DEPLETION OF THE SEA OF BLOOD DUE TO EXUBERANT HEAT IN THE HEART AND STOMACH

【Initial Visit】

Miss Yang, age 20, laborer. Initial visit on June 7th, 1977.

Chief complaints: Absence of menstruation for about 3 months.

The patient appeared agitated and restless. She complained of lower back and upper abdominal pain as well as feverish sensations. Her upper abdominal discomfort was found to be aggravated by pressure. Other symptoms included poor appetite, poor sleep, and frequent episodes of syncope. Her stools were black, and the tongue body dusky purple with a yellow coating. Pulses were moderate.

【Pattern Differentiation】

Depletion of the Sea of Blood due to accumulated heat of the Heart and Stomach.

【Treatment Principle】

Purge pathogenic heat and preserve yin, stop bleeding and dispel stasis.

【Prescription】

Modifications of *Yín Jiǎ Jiān Jì* (银甲煎剂) and *Dà Huáng Zhè Chóng Wán* (大黄蛰虫丸). The medicinals include:

泡参	pào shēn	24g	Radix Adenophorae
生黄芪	shēng huáng qí	60g	Radix Astragali (raw)
鸡血藤	jī xuè téng	18g	Caulis Spatholobi
生地黄	shēng dì huáng	12g	Radix Rehmanniae
女贞子	nǚ zhēn zǐ	24g	Fructus Ligustri Lucidi
旱莲草	hàn lián cǎo	24g	Ecliptae Herba
红藤	hóng téng	24g	Caulis Sargentodoxae
蒲公英	pú gōng yīng	24g	Herba Taraxaci
地榆	dì yú	10g	Radix Sanguisorbae
槐花	huái huā	10g	Flos Sophorae
白芨	bái jí	15g	Rhizoma Bletillae
生蒲黄	shēng pú huáng	10g	Pollen Typhae Crudum
蛰虫	zhè chóng	10g	Eupolyphaga seu Steleophaga
九香虫	jiǔ xiāng chóng	9g	Aspongopus
仙鹤草	xiān hè cǎo	60g	Herba Agrimoniae
益母草	yì mǔ cǎo	30g	Herba Leonuri
当归	dāng guī	10g	Radix Angelicae Sinensis
琥珀末(冲服 或布包煎)	hǔ pò mò	6g	Succinum Powder (infused or wrap-boiled)

12 doses were prescribed at 6 doses per week.

【Second Visit】

After the third dose, menstruation was restored. After finishing 12 doses, her appetite and sleep condition had improved, and her stool appeared yellow in color. However, her abdominal complaint was persistent to some degree. The tongue coating was thick and yellow, and her pulse moderate.

Nǔ zhēn zǐ (Fructus Ligustri Lucidi), *hàn lián cǎo* (Ecliptae Herba), *dì yú* (Radix Sanguisorbae) and *huái huā* (Flos Sophorae) were removed from the formula. Added were *bài jiàng cǎo* (Herba Patriniae) 24g, *yán hú suǒ* (Rhizoma Corydalis) 9g, and *hóng zé lán* (Herba Lycopi) 12g. *Zhè chóng* (Eupolyphaga seu Steleophaga) was reduced to 9g.

【Third Visit】

After 12 doses of this formula, all symptoms were relieved. Menstruation was reported to be normal one year later.

Comments:

In this case, the condition is caused by a depletion of the sea of blood, associated with the presence of exuberant heat in the Heart and Stomach. The excess internal heat not only depletes yin and blood, but may also cause hemafecia due to an accumulation of heat in the large intestine. Based on pattern differentiation, the treatment principle is to purge the pathogenic heat while preserving yin, stop bleeding and dispel static blood.

In this formula, *shēng dì huáng* (Radix Rehmanniae), *hóng téng* (Sargentgloryvine Stem), *pú gōng yīng* (Herba Taraxaci), *nǔ zhēn zǐ* (Fructus Ligustri Lucidi) and *hàn lián cǎo* (Ecliptae Herba) purge pathogenic heat and preserve yin, while *dì yú* (Radix Sanguisorbae), *huái huā* (Flos Sophorae), *xiān hè cǎo* (Herba Agrimoniae), *bái jí* (Rhizoma Bletillae), *zhè chóng* (Eupolyphaga seu Steleophaga) and *pú huáng* (Pollen Typhae) are indicated to stop bleeding and dispel blood stasis. In addition, *jiǔ xiāng chóng* (Aspongopus) regulates Stomach qi. This formula combines a great variety of medicinals in order to acheive its therapeutic effect.

5. Medical Records of Wang Wei-chuan: Amenorrhea due to Blood Stasis

【Initial Visit】

Miss Yang, age 34. Initial visit on September 6th, 1975.

Chief complaint: Absence of menstruation for 4 years, infertility.

The patient was previously diagnosed as infertile due to an obstruction of the fallopian tube. Menstruation had ceased for 4 years. Her complexion appeared darkish green in color, and she reported frequent gas pains in the chest, hypochondrium, and lower abdomen. Other symptoms included mental depression, lassitude, giddiness and vertigo, insomnia, and fishy smelling yellow leucorrhea. Her tongue body appeared dusky purple with red spots near the edges. Pulses were both deep and wiry.

【Pattern Differentiation】

Amenorrhea due to blood stasis.

【Treatment Principle】

Invigorate blood and dispel stasis, course and regulate the Liver, dispel dampness.

【Prescription】

Modifications of *Xuè Fǔ Zhú Yū Tāng* (血府逐瘀汤) and *Zī Shuǐ Qīng Gān Yǐn* (滋水清肝饮).

钩藤	gōu téng	10g	Ramulus Uncariae cum Uncis
刺蒺藜	cì jí lí	18g	Fructus Tribuli
蚕蛹(焙干研末, 吞服)	cán yǒng	20pieces	Bombyx Mori (baked and powdered for swollowing)
当归	dāng guī	10g	Radix Angelicae Sinensis
川芎	chuān xiōng	6g	Rhizoma Chuanxiong

生白芍	shēng bái sháo	12g	Radix Paeoniae Alba (raw)
桃仁	táo rén	10g	Semen Persicae
红泽兰	hóng zé lán	12g	Strobilanthes Japonicus
蟅虫	zhè chóng	10g	Eupolyphaga seu Steleophaga
水蛭	shuǐ zhì	6g	Hirudo
红藤	hóng téng	24g	Caulis Sargentodoxae
蒲公英	pú gōng yīng	24g	Herba Taraxaci
熟枣仁	shú zǎo rén	12g	Semen Ziziphi Spinosae (dry-fried)
夜交藤	yè jiāo téng	60g	Caulis Polygoni Multiflori
槟榔	bīng láng	10g	Semen Arecae
琥珀末(冲服或布包煎)	hǔ pò mò	6g	Succinum Powder (infused or wrap-boiled)

12 doses were prescribed at 6 doses per week.

【Second Visit】

Scant and dark menses appeared with clots following dose 10, with an amount equivalent to one-half package of sanitary napkins. Her energy level, appetite and sleep quality returned to normal. The leucorrhea had improved and her pains in the chest and hypochondrium alleviated to some degree, with no further episodes of giddiness or vertigo. However, she expressed an aversion to cold with some persisting discomfort of the lower abdomen. Modifications were then made to the formula.

蚕蛹(焙干，研末吞服)	cán yǒng	20pieces	Bombyx Mori (baked and powdered for swollowing)
当归	dāng guī	10g	Radix Angelicae Sinensis
川芎	chuān xiōng	6g	Rhizoma Chuanxiong
红泽兰	hóng zé lán	12g	Strobilanthes Japonicus
蟅虫	zhè chóng	9g	Eupolyphaga seu Steleophaga
水蛭	shuǐ zhì	6g	Hirudo
槟榔	bīng láng	10g	Semen Arecae

琥珀末(冲服或布包煎)	hǔ pò mò	6g	Succinum Powder (infused or wrap-boiled)
穿山甲	chuān shān jiǎ	10g	Squama Manis
鲜生地渣(姜汁炒焦)	xiān shēng dì zhā	20g	Radix Rehmanniae dregs (scorch-fried with Rhizoma Zingiberis juice)
生姜渣(鲜生地汁炒焦)	shēng jiāng zhā	15g	Rhizoma Zingiberis Recens dregs (scorch-fried with Radix Rehmanniae juice)

12 doses, 6 doses per week.

【Third Visit】

After 18 doses, menses appeared red in color with no clotting. Her abdominal discomfort and aversion to cold were relieved. Although some leucorrhea persisted, it was now normal in color. The prescription was again modified.

穿山甲	chuān shān jiǎ	10g	Squama Manis
琥珀末(冲服或布包煎)	hǔ pò mò	6g	Succinum Powder (infused or wrap-boiled)
沙参	shā shēn	20g	Radix Adenophorae seu Glehniae
鸡血藤	jī xuè téng	18g	Caulis Spatholobi
生黄芪	shēng huáng qí	30g	Radix Astragali Cruda
女贞子	nǚ zhēn zǐ	15g	Fructus Ligustri Lucidi
旱莲草	hàn lián cǎo	15g	Ecliptae Herba
枸杞子	gǒu qǐ zǐ	12g	Fructus Lycii
益母草	yì mǔ cǎo	24g	Herba Leonuri
覆盆子	fù pén zǐ	24g	Fructus Rubi
制香附	zhì xiāng fù	12g	Rhizoma Cyperi Praeparata
炒川楝	chǎo chuān liàn	10g	Fructus Toosendan (dry-fried)

16 doses, 4 doses per week.

【Fourth Visit】

At dose 6, a gynecological examination was performed to find a recanalized fallopian tube. The following formula was prescribed.

穿山甲	chuān shān jiǎ	10g	Squama Manis
琥珀末(冲服或布包煎)	hǔ pò mò	6g	Succinum Powder (infused or wrap-boiled)
沙参	shā shēn	20g	Radix Adenophorae seu Glehniae
鸡血藤	jī xuè téng	18g	Caulis Spatholobi
生黄芪	shēng huáng qí	30g	Radix Astragali Cruda
女贞子	nǔ zhēn zǐ	15g	Fructus Ligustri Lucidi
旱莲草	hàn lián cǎo	15g	Ecliptae Herba
枸杞子	gǒu qǐ zǐ	12g	Fructus Lycii
益母草	yì mǔ cǎo	24g	Herba Leonuri
覆盆子	fù pén zǐ	24g	Fructus Rubi
制香附	zhì xiāng fù	12g	Rhizoma Cyperi Praeparata
炒川楝	chǎo chuān liàn	10g	Fructus Toosendan (dry-fried)
新鲜胎盘	xiān tāi pán	1	Placenta Hominis (unwashed, baked and powdered)

【Fifth Visit】

The patient continued on this formula till December 18th, 1975, and was eventually able to achieve a successful pregnancy.

Comments:

Amenorrhea can occur as a result of an invasion of the six pernicious influences, or due to internal disorders caused by the seven affects. There are many illustrative examples of this condition in relation to mental-emotional states. For instance, when a flood attacked Wuhan, the capital of Hubei province, amenorrhea emerged in more than half of the women residents. All of the symptoms in the population disappeared promptly after the flood, without any medical intervention.

In this case of amenorrhea, although blood stasis is clearly the primary pathomechanism, emotional depression due to her previous diagnosis of infertility was certainly a factor. For patterns of blood stasis accompanied by Liver constraint, the guiding principles here are to dispel static blood while coursing the Liver, as well as regulating the penetrating and conception vessels.

In the above formula, *gōu téng* (Ramulus Uncariae cum Uncis) and *cì jí lí* (Fructus Tribuli) aid the function of *cán yǒng* (Bombyx Mori), which is to regulate Liver qi and soothe spasms. The combination of *táo rén* (Semen Persicae), *hóng zé lán* (Strobilanthes Japonicus), *zhè chóng* (Eupolyphaga seu Steleophaga), *shuǐ zhì* (Hirudo) and *pú huáng* (Pollen Typhae) has a strong ability to invigorate blood and transform stasis. Its effect is considered to be no less than that of *Táo Hóng Sì Wù Tāng* (桃红四物汤). In addition, *hóng téng* (Caulis Sargentodoxae), *pú gōng yīng* (Herba Taraxaci) and *hǔ pò mò* (Succinum Powder) can dispel the damp-heat in the lower jiao, and are so regarded as effective medicinals for gynecological inflammation and morbid leucorrhea.

The preparation method of frying fresh *shēng dì huáng* (Radix Rehmanniae) and *shēng jiāng* (Rhizoma Zingiberis Recens) together with their juices is called *Jiāo Jiā Sǎn* (交加散) by doctor Wang Xu-gao. It is said to have the function of both promoting blood circulation and regulating the movement of qi. It is indicated for conditions associated with an imbalance of nutritive and defensive qi, especially for thoses with signs such as an aversion to cold.

Additionally, *bīng láng* (Semen Arecae) can activate the movement of qi without depleting it, while stir-fried *chuān liàn zǐ* (Fructus Toosendan) and *chuān shān jiǎ* (Squama Manis) are among the primary medicinals for the treatment of infertility and fallopian tube obstruction. When such medicinals are effectively combined and coordinated, infertility patients may effectively recover and become pregnant within 4 months of treatment.

(Wang Wei-chuan. *Wang Wei-chuan's Selected Experience of Stubborn Diseases* 王渭川疑难病症治验选. Chengdu: Sichuan Science and

Technology Publishing House, 1984. 218-220)

6. MEDICAL RECORDS OF LUO YUAN-KAI: AMENORRHEA DUE TO KIDNEY DEFICIENCY

【Initial Visit】

Ms. Huang, age 28, married. Initial visit on April 5th, 1978.

Chief complaints: Absent menstruation for 2 years.

Patient had been diagnosed with secondary amenorrhea of unknown origin for 2 years. Her last menstrual period was on April 14th, 1976. On her first visit, she complained of dizziness, tinnitus, lassitude, and palpitation, as well as soreness and weakness of the lower back and knees. Other symptoms included insomnia, frequent urination at night, a lack of libido, and dryness of the vagina. Her complexion appeared darkish, particularly below the eyes. Her tongue body was also darkish with a thin white coating. Pulses were both weak and thready.

GYN examination revealed normal development of secondary sexual characteristics consistent with a non childbearing vagina. Smooth vaginal tract, with a normal capacity. Slender cervix and infantile uterus were present with normal annexa on both sides.

【Pattern Differentiation】

Deficient Kidney, qi and blood deficiency.

【Treatment Principle】

Tonify Kidney, nourish qi and blood.

【Prescription】

菟丝子	tù sī zǐ	25g	Semen Cuscutae
怀牛膝	huái niú xī	15g	Radix Achyranthis Bidentatae
枸杞子	gǒu qǐ zǐ	15g	Fructus Lycii
当归	dāng guī	15g	Radix Angelicae Sinensis
川芎	chuān xiōng	10g	Rhizoma Chuanxiong
党参	dǎng shēn	15g	Radix Codonopsis

| 香附 | xiāng fù | 10g | Rhizoma Cyperi |
| 熟地黄 | shú dì huáng | 20g | Radix Rehmanniae Praeparata |

At a later date, *bǔ gǔ zhī* (Fructus Psoraleae), *xiān líng pí* (Herba Epimedii), *sāng jì shēng* (Herba Taxilli), *yì mǔ cǎo* (Herba Leonuri) and *wū yào* (Radix Linderae) were added to the formula. Given the relatively long history of the disorder, biomedicines were prescribed initially. After 3 months they were discontinued and treatment continued with Chinese medicinals alone. Eventually, menstruation was restored for an 8 month period. There was a 2 month recurrence following a contraction of the common cold with fever, which occurred in January, 1979. The same formula was prescribed, and menstruation was again restored. At a two-year follow-up visit, the patient reported that normal menstrual cycles had been maintained.

(Luo Yuan-kai. Discussion on Kidney Qi, Tian Gui, Penetrating and Conception Vessels, and Their Relationship with Gynecology 肾气、天癸、冲任的探讨及其与妇科的关系 . *Shanghai Journal of Traditional Chinese Medicine* 上海中医药杂志 . 1983, (1)：11-13)

7. Medical Records of Li Chun-hua: Amenorrhea due to Stagnation of Phlegm and Blood Stasis in the Penetrating and Conception Vessels

【Initial Visit】

Ms. Mo, age 23, married, laborer. Hospitalization on January 7th, 1987.

Chief complaint: Absent menstruation, intermittent for 3 years.

Patient reported a 3 year history of menstrual problems. Menses appeared only once every few months, appearing dark in color with clots and accompanied by stabbing pains of the lower abdomen. She also complained of dream-disturbed sleep.

GYN examination revealed a curd-like vaginal discharge. Abnormalities of the uterus were also found, including a forward displacement and abnormal size.

Lab tests showed lowered hormone levels, and bacteria present in the vaginal discharge.

【Pattern Differentiation】

Stagnation of phlegm and blood stasis in the penetrating and conception vessels.

【Treatment Principle】

Transform phlegm, dispel stasis, and promote menstruation.

【Prescription】

Modification of *Huà Tán Pò Yū Tōng Jīng Tāng* (化痰破瘀通经汤加减).

柴胡	chái hú	15g	Radix Bupleuri
当归	dāng guī	15g	Radix Angelicae Sinensis
白芍	bái sháo	15g	Radix Paeoniae Alba
白术	bái zhú	15g	Rhizoma Atractylodis Macrocephalae
茯苓	fú líng	15g	Poria
益母草	yì mǔ cǎo	15g	Herba Leonuri
鸡血藤	jī xuè téng	15g	Caulis Spatholobi
白芥子	bái jiè zǐ	15g	Semen Sinapis
川芎	chuān xiōng	10g	Rhizoma Chuanxiong
法半夏	fǎ bàn xià	10g	Rhizoma Pinelliae Praeparatum
陈皮	chén pí	10g	Pericarpium Citri Reticulatae
红花	hóng huā	10g	Flos Carthami

Decoct with water. One divided dose three times per a day. 32 days constitute one course of treatment.

【Second Visit】

In one month menstruation was restored for 4 days, with normal flow but accompanied by some aching pain in the lower back. As a long history of amenorrhea typically requires continued treatment, the patient was transferred to family practice.

The prescription was modified with the addition of *xiān máo* (Rhizoma Curculiginis), *bā jǐ tiān* (Radix Morindae Officinalis) and *tù sī zǐ* (Semen Cuscutae) 15g. Menstruation resumed the following month with normal flow and little clotting. The leucorrhea was resolved and all other symptoms disappeared.

(Chen Jin-rong, Li Chun-hua. Experience Treating Phlegm Stagnation and Blood Stasis in Stubborn Gynecological Diseases 李春华运用痰瘀学说治疗妇科疑难病的经验. *New Journal of Traditional Chinese Medicine* 新中医. 1995, (6)∶5)

Discussions

1. Luo Yuan-kai's Theories on Amenorrhea

Patients with primary amenorrhea often have underdeveloped secondary sexual characteristics and a generally weak constitution, even in the absence of an infantile uterus. For these patients, proper nutrition is essential, and tonification of both Kidney yin and Kidney yang is indicated. *Tian Gui* must be present along with a free flowing abundance of the penetrating and conception vessels. Only then can normal ovarian development and function occur. Patients with primary amenorrhea should seek treatment as early as possible. Clinical results are best in patients under the age of 22. Before tonification, the specific pattern should be accurately differentiated. Although the predominating pattern in amenorrhea cases is Kidney yin deficiency, patients also may present signs of deficient Kidney yang. Menses and ovum are both considered to be vital substances in the human body. These substances are both nourished by and coordinate with other essential substances, and in this way they are supported by the yang of the Kidney as well. This not only illustrates how yin and yang are interrelated, but also points to the treatment principle for primary amenorrhea. The primary approach is to nourish the yin of the Kidney, and the second, tonification of Kidney yang.

Most clinical cases of secondary amenorrhea are associated with patterns of deficiency, or more commonly, a combination of both deficiency and excess. Absolute excess is rarely seen, so the general treatment approach is to first tonify, then drain. The purging method is found to be more effective when applied after tonification. The supply of qi, blood, yin, and yang must be adequate, as well as the condition of the penetrating and conception vessels. Zhang Jing-yue's formula *Guī Shèn Wán* (归肾丸), modified with *Sì Wù Tāng* (四物汤) is selected to both tonify the Kidney and nourish nutrient-blood.

菟丝子	tù sī zǐ	Semen Cuscutae
枸杞子	gǒu qǐ zǐ	Fructus Lycii
山茱萸	shān zhū yú	Fructus Corni
杜仲	dù zhòng	Cortex Eucommiae
山药	shān yào	Rhizoma Dioscoreae
茯苓	fú líng	Poria
当归	dāng guī	Radix Angelicae Sinensis
川芎	chuān xiōng	Rhizoma Chuanxiong
熟地黄	shú dì huáng	Radix Rehmanniae Praeparata
白芍	bái sháo	Radix Paeoniae Alba

When the Kidney qi and nutrient-blood have become sufficient, apply the purging method with empirical formula, *Tiáo Jīng Tāng* (调经汤).

丹参	dān shēn	Radix Salviae Miltiorrhizae
川牛膝	chuān niú xī	Radix Cyathulae
当归	dāng guī	Radix Angelicae Sinensis
桃仁	táo rén	Semen Persicae

茺蔚子	chōng wèi zǐ	Fructus Leonuri
乌药	wū yào	Radix Linderae
山楂	shān zhā	Fructus Crataegi
川芎	chuān xiōng	Rhizoma Chuanxiong

If the patient presents deficiency of both yin and yang, *Fù Dì Tāng* (附地汤) is indicated.

| 熟地黄 | shú dì huáng | Radix Rehmanniae Praeparata |
| 熟附子 | shú fù zǐ | Radix Aconiti Lateralis Praeparata |

According to the theories of Dr. Luo Yuan-kai, *fù zǐ* (Radix Aconiti Lateralis Praeparata) and *shú dì huáng* (Radix Rehmanniae Praeparata) together provide nourishment to both yang and yin respectively. This combination promotes menstruation and benefits ovarian functioning.

Where a more severe yang deficiency is coupled with congealing cold, add *guì zhī* (Ramulus Cinnamomi), *gān jiāng* (Rhizoma Zingiberis) and *zhì gān cǎo* (Radix et Rhizoma Glycyrrhizae) to warm and course the channels.

Amenorrhea with blood stasis can be divided into three major categories: blood stasis with heat, blood stasis with qi stagnation and blood stasis with congealing cold. Modifications of *Xuè Fǔ Zhú Yū Tāng* (血府逐瘀汤)[1], *Gé Xià Zhú Yū Tāng* (膈下逐瘀汤)[2] and *Shào Fù Zhú Yū Tāng* (少腹逐瘀汤)[3] can be selected for these three patterns respectively.

For patients with signs of phlegm-damp stagnation, prescribe *Dāng Guī Bǔ Xuè Tāng* (当归补血汤) modified with *Cāng Fù Dǎo Tán Wán* (苍附导痰丸)[4].

For amenorrhea due to postpartum hemorrhage, modify *Èr Xiān Wēn Bǔ Tāng* (二仙温补汤). This formula nourishes qi and blood and warms Kidney yang. This condition should be treated for 1 to 2 months.

仙灵脾	xiān líng pí	Herba Epimedii
仙茅	xiān máo	Rhizoma Curculiginis
熟附子	shú fù zǐ	Radix Aconiti Lateralis Praeparata
炙甘草	zhì gān cǎo	Radix et Rhizoma Glycyrrhizae Praeparata cum Melle
人参	rén shēn	Radix et Rhizoma Ginseng
熟地黄	shú dì huáng	Radix Rehmanniae Praeparata
当归	dāng guī	Radix Angelicae Sinensis
川芎	chuān xiōng	Rhizoma Chuanxiong

For amenorrhea associated with uterine tuberculosis, modified *Huáng Jīng Tiě Pò Tāng* (黄精铁破汤) is recommended.

黄精	huáng jīng	Rhizoma Polygonati
穿破石	chuān pò shí	Radix Cudraniae
铁包金	tiě bāo jīn	Lineate Supplejack Root
百部	bǎi bù	Radix Stemonae
玉竹	yù zhú	Rhizoma Polygonati Odorati
山药	shān yào	Rhizoma Dioscoreae
丹参	dān shēn	Radix Salviae Miltiorrhizae
鸡血藤	jī xuè téng	Caulis Spatholobi
怀牛膝	huái niú xī	Radix Achyranthis Bidentatae

(Luo Yuan-kai. The Essentials of Gynecology 女科述要. *New Journal of Traditional Chinese Medicine* 新中医. 1992, (4)：14-15)

[1] [2] [3] Recorded in *Correction of Professional Errors* (医林改错, *Yī Lín Gǎi Cuò*).

[4] Recorded in *Ye Tian-shi's Ttheories of Gynecology* (叶天士女科, *Yè Tiān-shì Nǚ kē*).

2. Tang Ji-fu's Theories on Amenorrhea

Doctor Tang also holds that amenorrhea cases can be divided into two general treatment groups. In deficiency cases, medicinals that promote menstruation must be combined with those that are sufficiently tonifying.

We may select *dǎng shēn* (Radix Codonopsis), *huáng qí* (Radix Astragali), *dāng guī* (Radix Angelicae Sinensis), *shú dì huáng* (Radix Rehmanniae Praeparata), *qiàn cǎo* (Radix et Rhizoma Rubiae), *wū zéi gǔ* (Endoconcha Sepiae), *chuān xiōng* (Rhizoma Chuanxiong) and *xiāng fù* (Rhizoma Cyperi).

For patients in the excess group, the primary treatment principle is to transform phlegm-damp and dispel static blood. Modifications of *Qǐ Gōng Wán* (启宫丸) and *Cāng Shā Dǎo Tán Wán* (苍莎导痰丸) may be prescribed.

(Tang Ji-fu. Pattern Differentiation and Treatment of Amenorrhea 闭经证治 . *Journal of Traditional Chinese Medicine* 中医杂志. 1985, 26(8)：9-13)

3. Liu Feng-wu's Theories on Amenorrhea

Doctor Liu Feng-wu has distingished eight complex patterns in cases of amenorrhea.

(1) Constraint of Liver Qi and Blood Stasis

Medicinals include *chái hú* (Radix Bupleuri), *chuān xiōng* (Rhizoma Chuanxiong), *dāng guī* (Radix Angelicae Sinensis), *yì mǔ cǎo* (Herba Leonuri), *bái sháo* (Radix Paeoniae Alba) and *xiāng fù* (Rhizoma Cyperi).

(2) Blood Stasis due to Liver Heat

This pattern develops as a result of the flaring up of Liver heat which leads to counterflow of the blood.

Medicinals include *lú huì* (Aloe), *lóng dǎn cǎo* (Radix et Rhizoma Gentianae), *chuān niú xī* (Radix Cyathulae), *shēng dì huáng* (Radix Rehmanniae), *yì mǔ cǎo* (Herba Leonuri) and *zé lán* (Herba Lycopi).

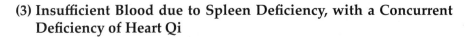

(3) Insufficient Blood due to Spleen Deficiency, with a Concurrent Deficiency of Heart Qi

Modified *Guī Pí Tāng* (归脾汤) is indicated for this pattern.

(4) Yin Deficiency and Stomach Dryness, with Dysfunction of the Penetrating Vessel

Medicinals include *guā lóu* (Fructus Trichosanthis), *shí hú* (Caulis Dendrobii), *shēng dì huáng* (Radix Rehmanniae), *xuán shēn* (Radix Scrophulariae), *mài dōng* (Radix Ophiopogonis), *huáng qín* (Radix Scutellariae), *qú mài* (Herba Dianthi), *chē qián zǐ* (Semen Plantaginis), *yì mǔ cǎo* (Herba Leonuri) and *chuān niú xī* (Radix Cyathulae).

(5) Deficiency of Both Blood and Kidney Essence

Medicinals include *dāng guī* (Radix Angelicae Sinensis), *chuān xiōng* (Rhizoma Chuanxiong), *shú dì huáng* (Radix Rehmanniae Praeparata), *chē qián zǐ* (Semen Plantaginis), *bái sháo* (Radix Paeoniae Alba), *fù pén zǐ* (Fructus Rubi), *gǒu qǐ zǐ* (Fructus Lycii), *wǔ wèi zǐ* (Fructus Schisandrae Chinensis), *xiān máo* (Rhizoma Curculiginis) and *xiān líng pí* (Herba Epimedii).

(6) Insufficiency of Both Yin and Blood, Leading to Malnourishment of the Penetrating and Conception Vessels

Modifications of *Sì Wù Tāng* (四物汤), *Zēng Yè Tāng* (增液汤) and *Èr Zhì Wán* (二至丸) may be selected.

(7) Congealing Cold and Blood Stasis in the Penetrating and Conception Vessels

Medicinals include *dāng guī* (Radix Angelicae Sinensis), *chuān xiōng* (Rhizoma Chuanxiong), *táo rén* (Semen Persicae), *hóng huā* (Flos Carthami), *wú zhū yú* (Fructus Evodiae), *xiǎo huí xiāng* (Fructus Foeniculi), *ròu guì* (Cortex Cinnamomi) and *chuān niú xī* (Radix Cyathulae).

(8) Blood Stasis Resulting in Obstruction of the Channels

Medicinals include *dāng guī* (Radix Angelicae Sinensis), *chuān xiōng* (Rhizoma Chuanxiong), *táo rén* (Semen Persicae), *hóng huā* (Flos Carthami), *xiāng fù* (Rhizoma Cyperi), *zé lán* (Herba Lycopi), *chì sháo* (Radix Paeoniae Rubra), *bái sháo* (Radix Paeoniae Alba) and *chuān niú xī* (Radix Cyathulae).

(Gao Yi-min. Doctor Liu Feng-wu's Theories on the Pattern Differentiation and Treatment of Amenorrhea 刘奉五老中医对闭经分型辨治的介绍 . *Journal of Traditional Chinese Medicine* 中医杂志 . 1985, 26(9)：34)

4. Xu Run-san's Treatment of Amenorrhea due to Kidney Deficiency

Doctor Xu Run-san regards Kidney deficiency as the essential etiology in most cases of amenorrhea. Therefore, his general approach to treatment focuses primarily on restoring Kidney function. By nourishing Kidney yin, warming Kidney yang, nourishing Liver blood and regulating the penetrating and conception vessels, essence will be replenished and the penetrating and conception vessels will become abundant. Although treatments that activate qi and blood and transform phlegm may in fact lead to menstruation, regular menstrual cycles can only be established by treatments that focus on the Kidney.

The following medicinals should be selected to supplement the Kidney and Liver, course the Liver and regulate the penetrating vessel.

女贞子	nǚ zhēn zǐ	Fructus Ligustri Lucidi
菟丝子	tù sī zǐ	Semen Cuscutae
当归	dāng guī	Radix Angelicae Sinensis
白芍	bái sháo	Radix Paeoniae Alba

紫河车	zǐ hé chē	Placenta Hominis
山茱萸	shān zhū yú	Fructus Corni
仙茅	xiān máo	Rhizoma Curculiginis
仙灵脾	xiān líng pí	Herba Epimedii
柴胡	chái hú	Radix Bupleuri
制香附	zhì xiāng fù	Rhizoma Cyperi Praeparata

With yang deficiency of both spleen and Kidney, warm the Kidney and fortify the Spleen, dispel the phlegm and invigorate blood. The following medicinals may be selected.

鹿角霜	lù jiǎo shuāng	Cornu Cervi Degelatinatum
白术	bái zhú	Rhizoma Atractylodis Macrocephalae
当归	dāng guī	Radix Angelicae Sinensis
生黄芪	shēng huáng qí	Radix Astragali
枳壳	zhǐ qiào	Fructus Aurantii
法半夏	fǎ bàn xià	Rhizoma Pinelliae Praeparatum
昆布	kūn bù	Thallus Laminariae
益母草	yì mǔ cǎo	Herba Leonuri
川芎	chuān xiōng	Rhizoma Chuanxiong
香附	xiāng fù	Rhizoma Cyperi

(Xu Run-san. Treatment of Amenorrhea Associated with the Kidney 从肾论治闭经. *Chinese Journal of Medicine* 中国医刊. 1992, (12)：38)

5. SUN NING-QUAN'S SIMULATED CYCLE THERAPY

Simulated cycle therapy emphasizes the regulation of the menstrual cycle through the following method.

During the time period following menstruation, the main treatment principles are to nourish yin and regulate the movement of qi and blood.

Medicinals include *shēng dì huáng* (Radix Rehmanniae), *shú dì huáng* (Radix Rehmanniae Praeparata), *nǚ zhēn zǐ* (Fructus Ligustri Lucidi), *hàn lián cǎo* (Ecliptae Herba), *dāng guī* (Radix Angelicae Sinensis), *dān shēn* (Radix Salviae Miltiorrhizae), *jī xuè téng* (Caulis Spatholobi), *zhì xiāng fù* (Rhizoma Cyperi Praeparata), *guǎng mù xiāng* (Radix Aucklandiae), *zé xiè* (Rhizoma Alismatis) and *shā rén* (Fructus Amomi).

During ovulation, select medicinals to warm the channels, free the collaterals, and invigorate qi and blood.

Medicinals include *guì zhī* (Ramulus Cinnamomi), *wú zhū yú* (Fructus Evodiae), *hóng huā* (Flos Carthami), *dān shēn* (Radix Salviae Miltiorrhizae), *gě gēn* (Radix Puerariae Lobatae), *dāng guī* (Radix Angelicae Sinensis), *zhì xiāng fù* (Rhizoma Cyperi Praeparata), *guǎng mù xiāng* (Radix Aucklandiae), *wū yào* (Radix Linderae), *chuān niú xī* (Radix Cyathulae) and *zé xiè* (Rhizoma Alismatis).

Preceding menstruation, the treatment includes equal tonification of both yin and yang, and also the regulation of qi and blood.

Medicinals include *shēng dì huáng* (Radix Rehmanniae), *shú dì huáng* (Radix Rehmanniae Praeparata), *xiān máo* (Rhizoma Curculiginis), *xiān líng pí* (Herba Epimedii), *nǔ zhēn zǐ* (Fructus Ligustri Lucidi), *hàn lián cǎo* (Ecliptae Herba), *dāng guī* (Radix Angelicae Sinensis), *dān shēn* (Radix Salviae Miltiorrhizae), *zhì xiāng fù* (Rhizoma Cyperi Praeparata), *wū yào* (Radix Linderae), *mù xiāng* (Radix Aucklandiae), *zhǐ qiào* (Fructus Aurantii), *fú líng* (Poria) and *yán hú suǒ* (Rhizoma Corydalis).

Finally, during the menstrual cycle one should select medicinals that primarily invigorate qi and blood and regulate the menses.

Medicines include *hóng huā* (Flos Carthami), *dān shēn* (Radix Salviae Miltiorrhizae), *dāng guī* (Radix Angelicae Sinensis), *zhì xiāng fù* (Rhizoma Cyperi Praeparata), *wū yào* (Radix Linderae), *mù xiāng* (Radix Aucklandiae), *zǐ sū gěng* (Caulis Perillae), *zhǐ qiào* (Fructus Aurantii), *chén pí* (Pericarpium Citri Reticulatae), *chuān niú xī* (Radix Cyathulae) and *zé xiè* (Rhizoma Alismatis).

(Sun Ning-quan. Chinese Medicine Treatment Principles to Regulate

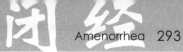

Menstruation 调整月经周期的中医治则. *Shanghai Journal of Traditional Chinese Medicine* 上海中医药杂志. 1983, (3)：22)

6. XIA GUI-CHENG'S THEORIES ON AMENORRHEA DUE TO PHLEGM-DAMP

Dr. Xia holds that amenorrhea associated with phlegm-damp is primarily caused by a deficiency of the Kidney. Of course, patterns of blood stasis and qi constraint are usually involved as well.

Amenorrhea due to phlegm-damp accumulation can be divided into three associated categories; Kidney yang deficiency, Kidney yin deficiency with Liver constraint, and blood stasis with masses. Therefore, specific objectives have been established for these patterns, that is, losing weight, promoting menstruation, and regulating periods.

(1) For patients with Kidney yang deficiency, both the root and branch should be treated simultaneously. In these cases, both tonify the Kidney and transform the phlegm-damp. A combination of medicinals from *Èr Xiān Tāng* (二仙汤), *Rén Shēn Lù Róng Wán* (人参鹿茸丸) and *Cāng Pò Èr Chén Tāng* (苍朴二陈汤) are recommended. The medicinals to include in the formula are listed below.

仙灵脾	xiān líng pí	Herba Epimedii
仙茅	xiān máo	Rhizoma Curculiginis
巴戟天	bā jǐ tiān	Radix Morindae Officinalis
鹿角片	lù jiǎo piàn	Cornu Cervi slices
续断	xù duàn	Radix Dipsaci
菟丝子	tù sī zǐ	Semen Cuscutae
苍术	cāng zhú	Rhizoma Atractylodis
厚朴	hòu pò	Cortex Magnoliae Officinalis
陈皮	chén pí	Pericarpium Citri Reticulatae
茯苓	fú líng	Poria
法半夏	fǎ bàn xià	Rhizoma Pinelliae Praeparatum
丹参	dān shēn	Radix Salviae Miltiorrhizae

In cases with severe symptoms, priority may be given to transforming phlegm-damp. A combination of *Cāng Pò Èr Chén Tāng* (苍朴二陈汤) and *Xiōng Guī Píng Wèi Wán* (芎归平胃丸) may be prescribed for the first two weeks. After this, a Kidney tonifying formula should also be prescribed. Combining of the formulas may be accomplished in several ways. The patient may either alternate between the two or take them together. A combination of decoctions and pills is also effective.

Tonifying the Kidney and warming the yang may require a relatively long-term treatment. During the tonification process it is appropriate to add blood nourishing medicinals to the prescription.

If the patient presents additional signs of Liver constraint, the formula may be modified to include medicinals from the formulas *Yòu Guī Wán* (右归丸), *Cāng Fù Dǎo Tán Tāng* (苍附导痰汤) and *Yuè Jū Wán* (越鞠丸).

For patients with signs both Kidney yang and Spleen qi deficiency, the treatment principles are to fortify the Spleen, warm yang, and disinhibit water. Combine medicinals from the formulas *Rén Shēn Lù Róng Wán* (人参鹿茸丸) and *Jiàn Gù Tāng* (健固汤) into basic formulas such as *Fáng Jǐ Huáng Qí Tāng* (防己黄芪汤) or *Wǔ Pí Yǐn* (五皮饮). If both Kidney and Spleen yang are deficient, add *Zhēn Wǔ Tāng* (真武汤) to the basic formulas mentioned above.

For patients with yin deficiency and concurrent Liver constraint, the treatment principles are to regulate qi and resolve constraint, transform phlegm-damp, and nourish yin and blood. Combine medicinals from formulas such as *Cāng Fù Dǎo Tán Tāng* (苍附导痰汤), *Yuè Jū Èr Chén Tāng* (越鞠二陈汤) and *Guī Sháo Dì Huáng Wán* (归芍地黄丸). The medicinals are listed below.

制苍术	zhì cāng zhú	Rhizoma Atractylodis (prepared)
制香附	zhì xiāng fù	Rhizoma Cyperi Praeparata
制南星	zhì nán xīng	Arisaema cum Bile (prepared)
制半夏	zhì bàn xià	Rhizoma Pinelliae Praeparatum

陈皮	chén pí	Pericarpium Citri Reticulatae
茯苓	fú líng	Poria
广郁金	guǎng yù jīn	Radix Curcumae
炒枳壳	zhǐ qiào	Fructus Aurantii (dry-fried)
丹参	dān shēn	Radix Salviae Miltiorrhizae
全瓜蒌	quán guā lóu	Fructus Trichosanthis
泽泻	zé xiè	Rhizoma Alismatis

For excessive phlegm-damp conditions with constipation, *Fáng Fēng Tōng Shèng Wán* (防风通圣丸) may be taken alone or combined with *Guī Sháo Dì Huáng Wán* (归芍地黄丸). For concurrent damp-heat in the Liver channel, combine *Lóng Dǎn Xiè Gān Tāng* (龙胆泻肝汤) with *Liù Wèi Dì Huáng Wán* (六味地黄丸).

With masses due to blood stasis, dispel static blood while transforming phlegm-damp. Combine medicinals from the formulas *Guì Zhī Fú Líng Wán* (桂枝茯苓丸) with *Cāng Fù Dǎo Tán Tāng* (苍附导痰汤).

苍术	cāng zhú	Rhizoma Atractylodis
香附	xiāng fù	Rhizoma Cyperi
茯苓	fú líng	Poria
瓜蒌	guā lóu	Fructus Trichosanthis
海藻	hǎi zǎo	Sargassum
穿山甲	chuān shān jiǎ	Squama Manis
莪术	é zhú	Rhizoma Curcumae
三棱	sān léng	Rhizoma Sparganii
桂枝	guì zhī	Ramulus Cinnamomi
桃仁	táo rén	Semen Persicae
丹皮	dān pí	Cortex Moutan
枳壳	zhǐ qiào	Fructus Aurantii

Alternatively, the formulas *Fáng Fēng Tōng Shèng Sǎn* (防风通圣散) and *Dà Huáng Zhè Chóng Wán* (大黄蛰虫丸) may also be prescribed.

(2) To free the channels, *Bǎi Zǐ Rén Wán* (柏子仁丸) is recommended.

柏子仁	bǎi zǐ rén	Semen Platycladi
卷柏	juǎn bǎi	Herba Selaginellae
牛膝	niú xī	Radix Achyranthis Bidentatae
泽兰	zé lán	Herba Lycopi
当归	dāng guī	Radix Angelicae Sinensis
赤芍	chì sháo	Radix Paeoniae Rubra
茺蔚子	chōng wèi zǐ	Fructus Leonuri
丹参	dān shēn	Radix Salviae Miltiorrhizae

(3) The theory of mutual growth and decline of yin and yang is the guiding principle behind the following method. Although regulating menstruation is generally based on the cyclic ebb and flow of both yin and yang, here the primary principle is to nourish yin. This approach promotes the creation of the fundamental substances that are essential to the menstruation process.

A combination of medicinals from *Guī Sháo Dì Huáng Tāng* (归芍地黄 汤) and *Yuè Jū Wán* (越鞠丸) may be prescribed to benefit yin.

In this modification, *shú dì huáng* (Radix Rehmanniae Praeparata) is replaced by *shēng dì huáng* (Radix Rehmanniae), *shān zhū yú* (Fructus Corni) is replaced by *nǚ zhēn zǐ* (Fructus Ligustri Lucidi), and *xù duàn* (Radix Dipsaci), *tù sī zǐ* (Semen Cuscutae) are added.

For patients with Spleen and Kidney yang deficiency, use *Jiàn Gù Tāng* (健 固 汤) added with *huái shān yào* (Rhizoma Dioscoreae), *gān dì huáng* (Radix Rehmanniae) and *huáng jīng* (Rhizoma Polygonati).

In the period preceding menstruation, we may warm yang with the addition of *Yù Lín Zhū* (毓麟珠). The medicinals are listed below.

川续断	chuān xù duàn	Radix Dipsaci
菟丝子	tù sī zǐ	Semen Cuscutae
紫河车	zǐ hé chē	Placenta Hominis

| 鹿角片 | lù jiǎo piàn | Cornu Cervi slices |
| 紫石英 | zǐ shí yīng | Fluoritum |

(Xia Gui-cheng. The Pattern Differentiation and Treatment of Amenorrhea due to Phlegm-Damp 痰湿闭经证治. *Jilin Journal of Traditional Chinese Medicine* 吉林中医药. 1989, (3)：1-2)

7. WU XI'S THEORIES ON AMENORRHEA

Doctor Wu Xi holds that there are two main etiologies for amenorrhea: deficiency of nutrient-blood, or obstruction of the channels. In the case of insufficient nutrient-blood, ammenoreah results because the essential substances needed to create menses can not be supplied. In cases of obstruction, the presence of stagnation or stasis in the channels prevents the free flow of menses. According to clinical experience, doctor Wu Xi points out that amenorrhea is most commonly associated with a deficiency. Even in clearly differentiated cases of excess, there is almost always some degree of deficiency present as well. When amenorrhea has persisted for 3 to 6 months, it is seldom a case of blood stasis alone.

Proper treatments for amenorrhea emphasize two main principles. The first is to nourish the nutrient-blood by fortifying the Spleen and Stomach, and the second is to relieve constraint and eliminate stagnation.

The theoretical basis of the first method is found in *The Yellow Emperor's Inner Classic* (黄帝内经 , *Huáng Dì Nèi Jīng*), which recorded, *"The essential qi derived from food is absorbed by the middle jiao. After a series of transformations it turns red and becomes blood."*

From this, we can see that the nutrient-blood originates from the refined nutritive substances that are absorbed by the middle jiao. Therefore, the penetrating vessel is subordinate to the Stomach. The condition of the Spleen and Stomach is then considered paramount in the effective treatment of amenorrhea. If an impairment of the Spleen's transforming and transporting function causes an insufficiency of nutrient-blood, combine *Sì Wù Tāng* (四物汤) with medicinals that fortify the Spleen, such as *rén shēn* (Radix et Rhizoma Ginseng), *bái zhú* (Rhizoma Atractylodis Macrocephalae), *shān yào* (Rhizoma Dioscoreae), *shēng gǔ yá* (Fructus Setariae Germinatus) and *shú gǔ yá* (prepared Fructus Setariae Germinatus).

Stagnation patterns can be divided into two subcategories. It may present either as a severe blockage due to blood stasis, or as a relatively milder condition resulting from qi stagnation.

Blood stasis may be caused by deficiency and cold of the lower origin, or by blood depletion in the vessels due to exuberant heat. Treatments may then be formulated based on the presence of cold or heat signs.

Qi is the commander of the blood. Therefore disorders of qi, such as stagnation, may certainly lead to a dysfunction in the movement of blood, the primary symptom in amenorrhea. For patients presenting this pattern, eliminating the qi stagnation should be given priority. Medicinals that nourish nutrient-blood and promote menstruation should be prescribed later in the treatment process.

Formulas such as *Wēn Jīng Tāng* (温经汤), *Jiāo Ài Sì Wù Tāng* (胶艾四物汤), *Dāng Guī Sì Nì Tāng* (当归四逆汤), *Rén Shēn Yǎng Róng Tāng* (人参养荣汤), *Shí Quán Dà Bǔ Tāng* (十全大补汤) and *Guī Pí Tāng* (归脾汤) are appropriate for patients presenting deficiency due to cold.

For deficiency due to heat, select from *Dān Zhī Xiao Yáo Sǎn* (丹栀逍遥散), *Guī Sháo Dì Huáng Tāng* (归芍地黄汤) or *Sì Wù Tāng* (四物汤). *Huáng qín* (Radix Scutellariae), *huáng lián* (Rhizoma Coptidis), *huáng bǎi* (Cortex Phellodendri Chinensis) and *zhī mǔ* (Rhizoma Anemarrhenae) may also be added.

Medicinals created from animals have a special ability to course the channels and nourish yin. Therefore *guī bǎn* (Carapax et Plastrum Testudinis) and *biē jiǎ* (Carapax Trionycis) may be added.

The formulas *Liù Wèi Dì Huáng Wán* (六味地黄丸) and *Zhī Bǎi Bā Wèi Wán* (知柏八味丸) can be used to both tonify the Kidney and replenish the source of menses. This approach treats the fundamental conditions associated with amenorrhea.

Furthermore, for excess conditions due to heat we may use formulas such as *Dà Huáng Zhè Chóng Wán* (大黄蛰虫丸) and *Táo Rén Chéng Qì Tāng* (桃仁承气汤), while in excess cold patterns, *Guì Zhī Fú Líng Wán* (桂枝茯苓丸) is indicated.

(Wu Xi. *A Review of Wu Xi's Gynecology* (*Volume Two*) 吴熙妇科朔洄第二集 . Xiamen University Publishing House, 1996. 38-41)

8. Ma Bao-zhang's Theories on Amenorrhea

(1) Pattern Differentiation

After a literature review of amenorrhea treatment throughout Chinese history, Dr. Ma Bao-zhang compiled the following twelve primary patterns associated with amenorrhea.

Heart and Lung yin deficiency, Heart and Spleen deficiency, Spleen deficiency, Stomach fire, Kidney qi deficiency, Kidney yang deficiency, Kidney yin deficiency, Liver blood deficiency, Liver yin deficiency, exhaustion of yin and blood, qi stagnation and blood stasis, congealing cold and blood stasis, and stagnation of phlegm-damp.

He determined nine major patterns of disharmony by combining the yin deficient patterns into one category.

Deficiency patterns include:
➢ Kidney qi deficiency
➢ Kidney yang deficiency
➢ Spleen deficiency
➢ Spleen and Heart deficiency
➢ Depletion of yin and blood

Excess patterns include:
➢ Stomach fire

➤ Qi stagnation and blood stasis

➤ Congealing cold and blood stasis

➤ Stagnation of phlegm-damp

(2) Treatment Principles

Dr. Ma regards Kidney tonification as the primary treatment approach in most cases of amenorrhea. Normal menstruation requires a sufficiency of Kidney qi, an abundant sea of blood, and the free flow of qi and blood. Based on these facts, he established a three week course of therapy called: "Nourish Kidney yin, Warm Kidney yang, and invigorate blood to promote menstruation".

Week one: Tonify the Kidney and nourish essence and blood.

Week two: Tonify Kidney yang (medicinals that nourish yin are also involved) and gently invigorate blood.

Week three: Warm Kidney yang, and strongly invigorate blood to promote menstruation.

(Ma Bao-zhang, Han Feng, Liu Ya-chao. A Discussion on Kidney Tonifying Therapy and the Pattern Differentiation of Amenorrhea 关于闭经的辨证分型与补肾疗法的探讨 . *Information on Traditional Chinese Medicine* 中医药信息 . 1989, (6)：14-16)

9. YAO YU-CHEN'S TREATMENT OF AMENORRHEA RELATED TO THE HEART

Doctor Yao Yu-chen observes that female patients are more likely to suffer from depressive conditions. Stressful circumstances may lead to affect damage, often causing a stagnation of Heart qi and a depletion of Heart yin. Patterns related to disorders of the seven affects are often associated with the development of menstrual dysfunction.

In addition to their chief complaint, patients presenting this pattern often report emotionally labile states such as depression or anxiety. Menstrual cycles may occur infrequently, or become completely absent.

The tongue may appear dark red, with pulses both thready and rough. The correct treatment is to tonify the Heart and free the collaterals.

Bǎi Zǐ Rén Wán (柏子仁丸) is recommended. For this pattern, generally avoid acrid medicinals with drying qualities. Sweet and moist medicinals are indicated, as well as those which clear heat and purge fire. Nourishing the Heart in this way both promotes the free flow of qi and clears heat from the collaterals, regulating blood and vessels.

For longstanding amenorrhea, the "three purples" (San Zi) may also be prescribed. They function together to tonify the heart, course the collaterals, and calm the spirit. Add *zǐ shí yīng* (Fluoritum), *zǐ dān shēn* (Radix et Rhizoma Salviae Miltiorrhizae) and *zǐ shēn* (Rhizoma Bistortae).

(Yao Shi-an: Yao Yu-chen's Experiences of Regulating the Heart in Gynecological Diseases 姚寓晨运用调心法治疗妇科病的经验. *Liaoning Journal of Traditional Chinese Medicine* 辽宁中医杂志. 1990, (6)：9-10)

PERSPECTIVES OF INTEGRATIVE MEDICINE

Challenges and Solutions

In Chinese medicine theory, menstruation requires a harmonious condition of the Kidney qi and *Tian Gui*, as well as the penetrating and conception vessels and uterus. The regular production of menses requires coordinated functioning of these elements. Qi and blood is the fundamental substance. The penetrating and conception vessels must be abundant in this substance to ensure the normal functioning of the uterus. Kidney qi also plays a primary and essential role in the physiology of menstruation. Therefore, disorders associated with any of these elements will have a negative impact on the production of menstruation. Re-establishing regular and predictable menstrual cycles and restoring normal ovulatory function is a difficult process in both primary and secondary conditions. However, there are a variety of potential solutions when approaching this challenging condition.

Challenge #1: Inducing Menstruation

Menstruation is generally regarded as a sign of healthy of reproductive function. During pubescence, the onset of menarche is considered to indicate a stage of maturation that includes the development of reproductive function. There are often patient concerns regarding reproductive health following a delay of menarche or after the cessation of a previously established cycle. For women of reproductive age, and those nearing menopause, menstruation is also considered to be a sign related to general well-being. Since absent periods may indicate pregnancy, or disease, most individuals seek medical attention within six months of onset. As a result, most patients in the clinic have received biomedical treatment before a differential diagnosis has been made. Some seek treatment after attempting to resolve the condition themselves, while others find their condition to persist in spite of biomedical treatment. Amenorrhea is considered to be an often tenacious condition, where rapid clinical effects are usually not obtained by either Chinese medicine or modern biomedicine.

The primary goal of treatment is to promote menstruation. However that process includes the establishment of regular cycles which are necessary for the restoration of reproductive health. The clinical effects of treatment and the prognosis of the disorder are case-specific. For example, cases associated with infertility are treated differently than when a premature decline of reproductive function is encountered. Other issues related to fertility and future reproductive health may arise after the re-establishment of menstruation. Furthermore, lowered estrogen levels will eventually lead to endometrial thickening. Although hormone replacement therapy may induce menstruation, the result may be only temporary. Amenorrhea often recurs after 1-3 menstrual cycles.

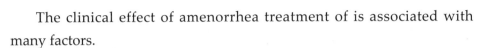

The clinical effect of amenorrhea treatment of is associated with many factors.

(1) Age of the patient

(2) Patient history

(3) Type of amenorrhea

(4) Progression of the disorder

(5) The ovarian primordial follicle in reserve and the functional condition of the hypothalamic-pituitary-ovarian axis

(6) The effect of previous treatment

(7) Patient compliance

In consideration of these factors, we should perform a thorough case history, complete the relevant exams, and integrate biomedical treatment as well as psychological and lifestyle counseling. The patients should be fully informed to help ensure compliance with treatment. An integration of Chinese medicine with modern biomedical treatment may be the most effective approach.

CHALLENGE #2: INFERTILITY DURING THE REPRODUCTIVE PERIOD

For amenorrhea associated with a general decline of reproductive function, especially for those approaching menopause, there are several objectives. While promoting menstruation and improving the constitutional symptoms we must, if possible, delay the natural decline of reproductive function. For those seek childbirth, regular and predictable ovulatory cycles must also be established. This remains another difficulty in the treatment of amenorrhea.

Therapy which aims to promote ovarian function requires a clear strategy. Treatment must proceed in several phases, with clearly defined principles and objectives for each phase. These objectives include:

(1) Improvement of the constitutional symptoms. In cases of premature menopause, the restoration of regular cycles is especially

difficult, so the improvement of constitutional symptoms becomes the primary objective.

(2) Establishment of anovular menstrual cycles. This phase may help address the associated psychological issues.

(3) Establishment or restoration of normal ovulation. For patients who seek childbirth, this may be the final objective of treatment.

The effective treatment of amenorrhea is a difficult process, so an emphasis on preventative measures that promote reproductive health is essential.

Insight from Empirical Wisdom

There are two approaches to the prescription of medicinals in the clinic. One is to choose a single formula that has been shown to be effective in the treatment of the patient's disorder. The other approach is to carefully combine formulas based on pattern differentiation. To treat amenorrhea we may choose from formulas to nourish blood and regulate qi, fortify the Spleen and course the Liver, course the Liver and drain heat, invigorate blood and dispel stasis, or to transform phlegm-damp. Another empirically effective method of treatment is to take a two-step approach. First, promote menstruation while relieving symptoms, and second, regulate the menstruation and support ovulation. Treatment should proceed in light of the inevitable natural decline of reproductive function, and then focus on both short-term and long-term therapeutic effects.

1. Pathogenesis: Deficiency Conditions Predominate with Blood Stasis

The diagnosis of amenorrhea requires an absence of menstruation for over 6 months. If treatment begins during this period, the patient is likely to obtain relief from the uncomfortable symptoms usually associated with excess conditions. However, longstanding untreated conditions usually result in some degree of deficiency. What was previously an excess pattern may have been transformed into a predominately deficient condition. Therefore we rarely see cases of pure excess as most patients seeking treatment will present either deficient or mixed patterns.

Furthermore, the diagnosis of local symptoms must be seen as separate from the overall constitutional condition. Patients may show signs of deficient qi and blood in the penetrating and conception vessels where no general deficiency pattern is observed. Therefore when prescribing medicinals, we must consider their effects on both. For example, in the treatment of localized deficiency, we may prescribe tonifying medicinals which over time may cause weight gain. Monitoring the patient's weight is indicated, especially in cases associated with obesity. During the course of treatment, appropriate modifications must be made, and the correct therapeutic approach should be determined.

In Chinese medicine, the Kidney governs reproduction. Because amenorrhea is essentially an impairment or decline of reproductive function, its pathogenesis can be directly associated with Kidney deficiency. However, almost all cases eventually present some degree of blood stasis, regardless of the initial etiology and pathogenesis. Kidney deficiency and blood stasis are the most common patterns associated with amenorrhea, therefore the general treatment principles here are to tonify the Kidney and dispel static blood.

2. TREATMENT BASED ON UTERINE STORAGE AND RELEASE

A dysfunction of uterine storage and release manifests itself as a deficiency of essence and blood, with blood stasis in the uterine vessels. The general treatment principle is to tonify deficiency and dispel static blood. However, it is difficult to make an objective evaluation regarding the storage and release function of the uterus. It is also unlikely that we can accurately predict the appearance or timing of the menses. Because of this, there is always some difficulty in determining the correct treatment approach for this particular condition. Clinical experience has determined two methods for making a proper evaluation.

The first is direct examination and testing. We must examine the size of the uterus, the thickness of the endometria, and the condition of the ovarian follicle. Also measure uterine and ovarian blood circulation by performing type-B ultrasonic and color Doppler exams.

The other method is an indirect evaluation. This requires the measurement of basal body temperature, vaginal discharges, cervical mucus, blood hormones, and an index of hemorheology. Typically the patient may show slight discharge, a small uterus, and endometrial thickness of less than 0.5cm, with no mature ovarian follicle present.

Other possibilities are single-phase BBT, low estrogen level, slight cervical mucus with little or no crystallization, and insufficient uterine and ovarian blood. In this case the treatment should focus on tonification of the Liver and Kidney as well as and the nourishment qi and blood.

For other patients, effective treatment emphasizes the purging method. If the index of hemorheology points to blood stasis, add medicinals to invigorate blood and dispel stasis. However, if the endometrial thickness exceeds that of late proliferation, and qi and blood moving medicinals are not sufficient to restore menstruation, administer progestin. Follow up with Chinese medicinals to regulate menstruation.

Summary

Amenorrhea is a symptom that may occur as a result of many existing medical conditions. It has many causes and widespread physical effects, and the prognosis is also not clear. In clinic, a biomedical diagnosis is primary. Cases associated with uterine disease, hypothalamic-pituitary-ovarian disorders, and other non-gonadal pathologies should be clearly distinguished from each other. Evaluate the prognosis and create an integrated medical treatment plan based on reasonable treatment goals.

In the course of amenorrhea treatment there are two primary goals. First we must establish menstruation, and secondly we aim to re-establish reproductive health. This requires regulation of the menstrual cycles over a sufficient period of time. In promoting the maturity and discharge of the ovarian follicle, Chinese medicine, biomedicine, and integrative approaches may all be effective. To benefit the uterus, select Chinese medicinals to both tonify the Kidney and regulate qi and blood. Estrogen therapy may be indicated. To promote circulation in the uterus, select Chinese medicinals that invigorate qi and blood and dispel blood stasis. We may also prescribe progestin if needed. Evaluation of uterine storage and release is the diagnostic foundation for selecting the proper treatment method, whether in Chinese medicine or modern biomedicine.

For conditions associated with the hypothalamic-pituitary-ovarian axis, a relatively long course of therapy is indicated, including both Chinese medicinals and hormone therapy. Hormone replacement alone often resolves this condition and its associated symptoms. However, it is important to note that ovarian function may be compromised over time when prescribing hormones. Degeneration of the ovary may occur in severe cases, which are marked by the cessation of menstruation soon after the discontinuation of hormone therapy. Although hormone therapy has no adverse effect in patients who do not desire childbirth, after 3 months of treatment it may become harmful to those who do. For these cases, Chinese medicine may be a better choice.

SELECTED QUOTES FROM CLASSICAL TEXTS

Yellow Emperor's Inner Classic, Plain Questions-Chapter 7, Discussions on the Differences between Yin and Yang (素问 · 阴阳别论篇第七 , *Sù Wèn · Yīn Yáng Bié Lùn Piān Dì Qī*):

"二阳之病发心脾，有不得隐曲，女子不月。"

"Disorders of the Heart or Spleen due to disease in the yang brightness channels can cause disturbances of urination and defecation, and also amenorrhea in women."

Yellow Emperor's Inner Classic, Plain Questions-Chapter 40, Discussions on Abdominal Diseases (素问 • 腹中论篇第四十 , *Sù Wèn • Fù Zhōng Lùn Piān Dì Sì Shí*):

"有病胸胁支满者，妨于食，病至则先闻腥臊臭，出清液，先唾血，四支清，目眩，时时前后血……病名血枯，此得之年少时，有所大脱血，若醉入房，中气竭，肝伤，故月事不来也。"

"Fullness of the chest and hypochondrium, poor appetite, a fishy odor before fluid regurgitation, spitting blood, coldness in the limbs, dizziness, and the intermittent presence of blood in the urine and stools are all symptoms of blood exhaustion. Amenorrhea often develops after profuse bleeding, especially in young people. Sexual intercourse following alcohol abuse will also damage the Liver and exhaust qi of the middle jiao, which leads to a sudden or gradual cessation of menses."

Yellow Emperor's Inner Classic, Plain Question- Chapter 33, Discussions on Heat Diseases (素问 • 评热病论篇第三十三 , *Sù Wèn • Píng Rè Bìng Lùn Piān Dì Sān Shí Sān*):

"月事不来者，胞脉闭也。胞脉者属心而络于胞中，今气上迫肺，心气不得下通，故月事不来也。"

"The absence of menstruation results from obstruction of the uterine vessels. The uterine vessel homes to the Heart and nets to the uterus. If the Lung is oppressed by counterflow qi, Heart qi will not be able to descend, causing amenorrhea."

Classified Canon-Category of Diseases-Section 63, Blood Exhaustion (类经·疾病类·六十三血枯, *Lèi Jīng · Jí Bìng Lèi · Liù Shí Sān Xuè Kū*):

"血枯一证，与血隔相似，皆经闭不通之候。然枯之与隔，则相反有如冰炭。夫枯者，枯竭之谓，血虚之极也。隔者，阻隔之谓，血本不虚，而或气或寒或积有所逆也。"

"Even though amenorrhea is associated with blood exhaustion and blood obstruction, their etiologies are quite opposite, like ice and burning embers. Blood exhaustion refers to an extreme blood deficiency, whereas blood obstruction is not associated with deficiency. Blood obstruction is due to counterflow as a result of qi disorders, congealing cold, or accumulation."

Essentials from the Golden Cabinet-Chapter 22, Pulse, Symptoms and Treatment of Miscellaneous Diseases of Gynecology (金匮要略 · 妇人杂病脉证并治第二十二 , *Jīn Guì Yào Luè · Fù Rén Zá Bìng Mài Zhèng Bìng Zhì Dì Èr Shí Èr*):

"妇人经水不利下，抵挡汤主之。"

"For absent or inhibited menstruation, *Dǐ Dǎng Tāng* (抵 挡 汤) is indicated."

Origin and Indicators of Disease-Miscellaneous Diseases of Gynecology, Section 1, Menstrual Block (诸病源候论 · 妇人杂病一 · 月水不通候, *Zhū Bìng Yuán Hòu Lùn · Fù Rén Zá Bìng Yī · Yuè Shuǐ Bù Tōng Hòu*):

"醉以入房，则内气竭绝，伤肝，使月事衰少不来也。所以尔者，肝藏於血，劳伤过度，血气枯竭於内也。"

"又，先经唾血，及吐血、下血，谓之脱血，使血枯，亦月事不来也。"

"Sexual intercourse following alcohol abuse exhausts qi and damages the Liver, causing a sudden or gradual cessation of menses. When the blood-storing function of the Liver is taxed, an exhaustion of qi and blood may result."

"Initial symptoms of blood collapse include the spitting or vomiting of blood, with blood in the urine or stool. This exhausts blood further, resulting in amenorrhea."

"妇人月水不通者，由劳损血气，致令体虚受风冷。风冷邪气客于胞内，伤损冲任之脉，并手太阳少阴经，致胞络内绝，血气不通，故也。"

"A taxation of qi and blood weakens the body's resistance to wind and cold, which if contracted can lead to amenorrhea. Pathogenic wind-cold that settles in the uterus can cause depletion and obstruction in the penetrating vessel, conception vessel, hand greater yang small intestine channel and hand lesser yin heart channel. This damage may lead to obstruction of the uterine vessel while blocking the free flow of qi and blood."

Orthodox Treatise of Medicine-Gynecology (医学正传 · 妇人科 , *Yī Xué Zhèng Zhuàn · Fù Rén Kē*):

"况月经全赖肾水施化，肾水既乏，则经血日以干涸，以致或先或后，淋漓无时。若不早治，渐而致于闭塞不通，甚则为症瘕血隔劳极之证，不易治也。"

"Kidney water is the source of menses. An insufficiency of Kidney water leads to the gradual drying up of the menstrual blood. Menstruation becomes unpredictably advanced or delayed, with sporadic spotting. Without proper treatment, other difficult patterns may appear including masses and conglomerations, blood obstruction, and taxation-damage of the Kidney."

Complete Works of Jingyue-Gynecology-Section 1, Chapter 16, Menstrual Block due to Blood Exhaustion (景岳全书 · 妇人规上 · 血枯经闭十六 , *Jǐng Yuè Quán Shū · Fù Rén Guī Shàng · Xuè Kū Jīng Bì Shí Liù*):

"血枯之与血隔，本自不同……凡妇女病损至旬月半载之后，则未有不闭经者。正因阴竭，所以血枯。枯之为义，无血而然。故或以羸弱，或以困倦，或以咳嗽，或以夜热，或以食饮减少，或以亡血失血，及一切无胀无痛，无阻无隔，而经有久不至者，即无非血枯经闭之候。欲其不枯，无如养营，欲以通之，无如充之，但使雪消则春水自来，血盈则经脉自止，源泉混混，又孰有能阻之者。奈何今之为治者，不论有滞无滞，多兼开导之药，其有甚者，则专以桃仁、红花之类，通利为事。岂知血滞者可通，血枯者不可通也。血既枯矣，而复通之，则枯者愈枯，其与榨干汁者何异，为不知枯字之义耳，为害不小，无或蹈此弊也。"

"The root causes of blood exhaustion and blood obstruction are quite different. Amenorrhea will be present in almost all women who have been ill for several months. Such blood exhaustion is due to yin depletion. As exhaustion suggests a severe blood deficiency, we may find many associated symptoms. Weakness and emaciation, debilitation, cough, fever at night, poor appetite, bleeding or blood loss, or an absence of menstruation without signs of fullness, pain, blockage or obstruction. For blood exhaustion patterns focus on nourishing blood rather than removing obstruction. As the melting snow fills the river in springtime, the blood will flow smoothly in the vessels and channels from an abundant source. However, regardless of the presence of obstruction, most contemporary treatments focus on dredging methods. Some even use medicinals such as *táo rén* (Semen Persicae) and *hóng huā* (Flos Carthami) for all amenorrhea patterns. They have not recognized that such medicinals are indicated for blood obstruction, rather than blood exhaustion. To be unaware of exhaustion, and to only dredge the deficient blood, will only exacerbate the depletion. Learn from this harmful method and never repeat such a mistake."

Secrets from the Orchid Chamber-Gynecology-Three Etiologies of Menstrual Block (兰室秘藏 · 妇人门 · 经闭不行有三论 , *Lán Shì Mì Cáng · Fù Rén Mén · Jīng Bì Bù Xíng Yǒu Sān Lùn*):

"妇人脾胃久虚，或形羸气血俱衰，而致经水断绝不行。或病中消胃热，善食渐瘦，津液不生。夫经者血脉津液所化，津液既绝，为热所灼，肌肉消瘦，时见渴燥，血海枯竭，病名曰血枯经绝。宜泻胃之燥热，补益气血，经自行矣……或因劳心，心火上行，月事不来，安心和血、泻火，经自行矣。"

"Amenorrhea may result from a longstanding Spleen and Stomach deficiency, or occur as a result of emaciation due to qi and blood exhaustion. Amenorrhea can also be caused by central consumption (middle xiao) and Stomach heat. As heat burns the fluids that are the source of menstruation, an exhaustion of the sea of blood may result. As the fluids and blood in the vessels are consumed, symptoms such as excessive eating with weight loss, emaciation, and a dry mouth may be present. This pattern is called blood exhaustion amenorrhea, and its treatment principles are to purge the dryness-heat while nourishing qi and blood. In addition, amenorrhea may be associated with taxation of the Heart leading to Heart fire flaming upward. For this pattern, menstruation can be restored by calming the Heart, regulating blood and purging fire."

Dan-xi's Experience-Chapter 93, Procreation (丹溪心法 · 子嗣九十三， *Dān Xī Xīn Fǎ · Zǐ Sì Jiǔ Shí Sān*):

"若是肥盛妇人，禀受甚浓，恣于酒食之人，经水不调，不能成胎，谓之躯脂满溢，闭塞子宫。"

"Amenorrhea is often associated with infertility in obese women. They are born with abundant constitutions, and consume too much food and wine. This leads to excessive fat congesting the uterus."

Necessities for Women's Diseases-Regulating Menstruation (女科切要·调经门, *Nǚ Kē Qiè Yào · Tiáo Jīng Mén*):
"其肥白妇人，经闭而不通者，必是湿痰与脂膜壅塞之故也。"

"Amenorrhea in obese women may result from a congestion of phlegm-damp and an accumulation of fat in the uterine membranes."

Wan's Gynecology-Chapter of Regulating Menstruation, Section of Menstrual Block (万氏妇人科 · 调经章 · 经闭不行 , *Wàn Shì Fù Rén Kē · Tiáo JīngZhāng · Jīng Bì Bù Xíng*):
"有忧思怨怒、气郁血滞，而经不行者。"

"Anxiety, over-thinking, anger and hatred can all lead to amenorrhea by causing qi constraint and blood stasis."

Basic Introduction to Medicine-Outer Volume-Chapter 4, Internal Impairment-Category of Deficiency-Section on Miscellaneous Worms (医学入门 · 外集 · 卷四 · 内伤类 · 虚类 · 诸虫, *Yī Xué Rù Mén · Wài Jí · Juàn Sì · Nèi Shāng Lèi · Xū Lèi · Zhū Chóng*):
"妇人经闭，腹大仅一月间便能动作，乃至过期不产，或有腹痛，此必虫证。"

"Some women who are not pregnant present symptoms such as cessation of menstruation with abdominal distention, and a feeling of movement in the abdomen after one month. This is caused by parasites. Abdominal pain may also be present."

Fu Qing-zhu's Obstetrics and Gynecology-Regulating Menstruation-Section 17, Menstruation at Irregular Intervals (傅青主女科 · 调经 · 经水先后无定期十七, *Fù Qīng-zhǔ Nǚ Kē · Tiáo Jīng · Jīng Shuǐ Xiān Hòu Wú Dìng Qī Shí Qī*):

"经水出诸肾。"

"Menses originate from the Kidney."

Fu Qing-zhu's Obstetrics and Gynecology-Regulating Menstruation-Section 28, Advanced Cessation of Menstruation (傅青主女科 · 调经 · 年未老经水断二十八, *Fù Qīng-zhǔ Nǚ Kē · Tiáo Jīng · Nián Wèi Lǎo Jīng Shuǐ Duàn Èr Shí Bā*):

"经原非血，乃天一之水，出自肾中。"

"经水早断，似乎肾水衰涸。"

"矧肾气本虚，又何能盈满而化经水外泄耶。"

"Menses is not in the form of blood initially. It is the Water of Tian-yi coming from the Kidney."

"Premature menopause is similar to the exhaustion of Kidney water."

"If Kidney qi is deficient instead of abundant, qi fails to become transformed and menses can not be discharged."

MODERN RESEARCH

Clinical Research

1. PATTERN DIFFERENTIATION AND CORRESPONDING TREATMENT

(1) Doctor Yang Ying divides tuberculosis-related amenorrhea into three patterns according to their etiology, pathogenesis and

manifestations.

The primary patterns are Lung and Kidney yin deficiency with hyperactive Heart and Liver fire, hyperactivity of fire due to yin deficiency with blood stasis, and qi and blood deficiency affecting the Lung and Spleen.

Tuberculosis depletes Lung yin, and the Lung fails to transport fluids to the Kidney. This condition manifests as a Lung and Kidney yin deficiency with hyperactive fire. If the Lung cannot nourish the Kidney, yin will gradually become deficient and fail to nourish the Liver and Heart. Pathogenic fire in the Heart and Liver may then affect the Lung as well. This vicious cycle in the four viscera exhausts the essence and blood causing further deficiencies of the Lung and Kidney yin. These complex conditions often result in amenorrhea.

Other symptoms of this pattern include cough, shortness of breath, blood-streaked sputum, steaming bone disorder, tidal fever, night sweats, vexing heat in the in the chest, palms and soles, anxiety and irascibility, and dream-disturbed sleep. The tongue body is often red or crimson, with little coating. Pulses are thready and rapid. The treatment principles are to nourish yin and clear heat, moisten the Lung and relieve cough, and to replenish blood while regulating menstruation. *Băi Hé Gù Jīn Tāng* (百合固金 汤) is recommended.

For excessive heat, add *huáng lián* (Rhizoma Coptidis), *huáng băi* (Cortex Phellodendri Chinensis) and *zhī mŭ* (Rhizoma Anemarrhenae) which, due to their bitter flavor and cold nature, act to purge pathogenic fire and preserve yin.

For cough with the expectoration of turbid yellow phlegm, add *sāng bái pí* (Cortex Mori), *huáng qín* (Radix Scutellariae) and *yú xīng căo* (Herba Houttuyniae) to clear heat and transform phlegm.

For severe spitting of blood, add *hēi zhī zĭ* (Fructus Gardeniae Praeparatus), *dà huáng tàn* (Carbonized Radix et Rhizoma Rhei) and *dì yú tàn*

(Carbonized Radix Sanguisorbae) to cool blood and stop bleeding.

Hyperactive fire with blood stasis may result from a Kidney and Lung yin deficiency. As tuberculosis depletes the Lung yin, so the Lung metal fails to promote Kidney water. Deficient fire may also consume yin and blood, leading to blood stasis in the sea of blood. When the penetrating and conception vessels are obstructed, amenorrhea may result.

For this pattern, clinical manifestations include scanty menses with dark color and clots, anxiety and insomnia, emaciation, scaly skin, steaming bone disorder, tidal fever, night sweats, cough, wheezing and blood-streaked sputum. The tongue and lips may appear deep-red and dry, with dark spots indicating stasis. Pulses are deficient and rapid. The treatment principle is to nourish yin and clear heat, dispel blood stasis and replenish blood. A modified combination of *Dà Bǔ Yīn Wán* (大补阴丸) and *Dà Huáng Zhè Chóng Wán* (大黄蛰虫丸) is recommended.

Tuberculosis may affect the Lung yin and also the Spleen. Due to the mother-son relationship in this case, the Lung may deplete the Spleen in order to nourish itself, leading to a deficiency of qi and blood. The Spleen is the source of engendering and transformation. When the source is insufficient, there will be a deficiency of blood in the penetrating and conception vessels. The empty sea of blood fails to be filled and discharged on time, resulting in amenorrhea.

This pattern is often marked by late periods with scanty menses that gradually decrease to none. Other symptoms include cough, blood-streaked sputum, tidal fever, night sweats or spontaneous sweating, a pale or greenish-yellow complexion, dizziness, shortness of breath and weak voice, palpitations of various degree, lassitude, and poor appetite. The tongue color is often pale, and the pulses thready and weak. Treatment principles are to fortify the Spleen and benefit the Lung, nourish blood and regulate menstruation. Modified *Bā Zhēn Tāng* (八珍汤)

is recommended. [1]

(2) Doctor Yan Wen-fei, a student of professor Zhu Nan-sun, established a cyclic method of therapy.

The therapy consists of four cyclic phases of treatment: postmenstrual, inter-menstrual, premenstrual, and menstrual treatment periods.

Following the menstrual cycle, tonify the Kidney and nourish blood with medicinals such as *zhì hé shŏu wū* (Radix Polygoni Multiflori Praeparata cum Succo Glycines Sotae), *gŏu qĭ zĭ* (Fructus Lycii), *tù sī zĭ* (Semen Cuscutae), *shān zhū yú* (Fructus Corni), *lù jiăo piàn* (Cornu Cervi), *xù duàn* (Radix Dipsaci), *ròu cōng róng* (Herba Cistanches), *xiān máo* (Rhizoma Curculiginis), *xiān líng pí* (Herba Epimedii), *dāng guī* (Radix Angelicae Sinensis) and *bái sháo* (Radix Paeoniae Alba).

The next phase of treatment aims to course the Liver and to nourish and invigorate blood. Select medicinals such as *zhì xiāng fù* (Rhizoma Cyperi Praeparata), *guăng yù jīn* (Radix Curcumae), *bā yuè zhá* (Fructus Akebiae), *jī xuè téng* (Caulis Spatholobi), *chōng wèi zĭ* (Fructus Leonuri), *chuān niú xī* (Radix Cyathulae), *chì sháo* (Radix Paeoniae Rubra), *yì mŭ căo* (Herba Leonuri) and *sān léng* (Rhizoma Sparganii).

During the premenstrual phase, warm yang and tonify qi with medicinals such as *xiān líng pí* (Herba Epimedii), *xiān máo* (Rhizoma Curculiginis), *suŏ yáng* (Herba Cynomorii), *bā jĭ tiān* (Radix Morindae Officinalis), *lù jiăo piàn* (Cornu Cervi), *gŏu qĭ zĭ* (Fructus Lycii), *guī băn* (Carapax et Plastrum Testudinis), *shān yào* (Rhizoma Dioscoreae), *dăng shēn* (Radix Codonopsis), *huáng qí* (Radix Astragali) and *huáng jīng* (Rhizoma Polygonati).

During the menstrual period the treatment approach is to course the Liver, invigorate blood and regulate menstruation.

Select from *dāng guī* (Radix Angelicae Sinensis), *chuān xiōng* (Rhizoma Chuanxiong), *chì sháo* (Radix Paeoniae Rubra), *dān shēn* (Radix Salviae Miltiorrhizae), *yì mŭ căo* (Herba Leonuri), *dăng shēn* (Radix Codonopsis), *huáng qí* (Radix Astragali), *bái zhú* (Rhizoma Atractylodis Macrocephalae), *bā jǐ tiān* (Radix Morindae Officinalis), *guì zhī* (Ramulus Cinnamomi) and *jī xuè téng* (Caulis Spatholobi).

For abdominal pain during menstruation, add *pú huáng* (Pollen Typhae), *wǔ líng zhī* (Faeces Togopteri) and *yán hú suǒ* (Rhizoma Corydalis).

For scant menses, add *sān léng* (Rhizoma Sparganii) and *é zhú* (Rhizoma Curcumae). For breast distention and pain, add *zhì xiāng fù* (Rhizoma Cyperi Praeparata), *chuān liàn zǐ* (Fructus Toosendan) and *bā yuè zhá* (Fructus Akebiae).

Three months constitutes one course of treatment. This effective rate was 89.47% after one course of treatment. [2]

(3) Doctor Zhang Gui-zhen distinguishes five main patterns associated with amenorrhea. They are Liver and Kidney deficiency, yin deficiency with blood dryness, qi and blood deficiency, phlegm-damp obstruction, and qi stagnation with blood stasis.

For Liver and Kidney deficiency, treatment tonifies the Liver and Kidney while regulating menstruation. Select *hé shǒu wū* (Radix Polygoni Multiflori) 30g, *shān yào* (Rhizoma Dioscoreae) 30g, *fú líng* (Poria) 30g, *dù zhòng* (Cortex Eucommiae) 15g, *dāng guī* (Radix Angelicae Sinensis) 10g, *gǒu qǐ zǐ* (Fructus Lycii) 10g, *shān zhū yú* (Fructus Corni) 10g, *lù jiǎo shuāng* (Cornu Cervi Degelatinatum) 10g, *fù pén zǐ* (Fructus Rubi) 20g, *shú dì huáng* (Radix Rehmanniae Praeparata) 20g, *jī xuè téng* (Caulis Spatholobi) 20g and *tù sī zǐ* (Semen Cuscutae) 20g.

For yin deficiency and blood dryness, treatment should nourish blood, dispel wind and regulate menstruation. Select *quán guā lóu* (Fructus Trichosanthis) 20g, *shēng dì huáng* (Radix Rehmanniae) 20g, *chuān niú xī* (Radix Cyathulae) 20g, *huáng jīng* (Rhizoma Polygonati) 20g, *yì mǔ cǎo* (Herba Leonuri) 20g, *dān shēn* (Radix Salviae Miltiorrhizae) 20g, *hàn lián cǎo* (Ecliptae Herba) 20g, *huáng lián* (Rhizoma Coptidis) 5g, *shí hú* (Caulis Dendrobii) 12g, *xuán shēn* (Radix Scrophulariae) 15g, *mài dōng* (Radix

Ophiopogonis) 15g and *qú mài* (Herba Dianthi) 15g.

For qi and blood deficiency, select *rén shēn* (Radix et Rhizoma Ginseng) 12g, *bái zhú* (Rhizoma Atractylodis Macrocephalae) 10g, *yuǎn zhì* (Radix Polygalae) 10g, *wǔ wèi zǐ* (Fructus Schisandrae Chinensis) 10g, *dāng guī* (Radix Angelicae Sinensis) 10g, *jī xuè téng* (Caulis Spatholobi) 30g, *dān shēn* (Radix Salviae Miltiorrhizae) 20g, *fú líng* (Poria) 20g, *bái sháo* (Radix Paeoniae Alba) 20g, *huáng qí* (Radix Astragali) 20g, *shú dì huáng* (Radix Rehmanniae Praeparata) 20g, *yì mǔ cǎo* (Herba Leonuri) 20g and *chuān niú xī* (Radix Cyathulae) 20g.

For obstruction of phlegm-damp, select from *cāng zhú* (Rhizoma Atractylodis) 10g, *bái zhú* (Rhizoma Atractylodis Macrocephalae) 10g, *dāng guī* (Radix Angelicae Sinensis) 10g, *dǎn nán xīng* (Arisaema cum Bile) 10g, *zhǐ shí* (Fructus Aurantii Immaturus) 15g, *xiāng fù* (Rhizoma Cyperi) 12g, *fǎ bàn xià* (Rhizoma Pinelliae Praeparatum) 12g, *fú líng* (Poria) 30g, *chuān niú xī* (Radix Cyathulae) 20g, *quán guā lóu* (Fructus Trichosanthis) 20g, *chuān xiōng* (Rhizoma Chuanxiong) 5g and *gān cǎo* (Radix et Rhizoma Glycyrrhizae) 5g.

For qi stagnation and blood stasis, select from *táo rén* (Semen Persicae) 12g, *jié gěng* (Radix Platycodonis) 12g, *chì sháo* (Radix Paeoniae Rubra) 20g, *chuān niú xī* (Radix Cyathulae) 20g, *dān shēn* (Radix Salviae Miltiorrhizae) 20g, *shēng dì huáng* (Radix Rehmanniae) 20g, *chuān xiōng* (Rhizoma Chuanxiong) 10g, *hóng huā* (Flos Carthami) 10g, *dāng guī* (Radix Angelicae Sinensis) 10g, *chái hú* (Radix Bupleuri) 10g, *zhǐ shí* (Fructus Aurantii Immaturus) 10g, *zé lán* (Herba Lycopi) 10g and *yì mǔ cǎo* (Herba Leonuri) 30g.

For blood stasis symptoms such as a lower abdominal pain that is aggravated by pressure, add *jiāng huáng* (Rhizoma Curcumae Longae) and *sān léng* (Rhizoma Sparganii).

In clinical testing, each patient was prescribed one dose per day, decocted. Standards for efficacy were as follows.

Recovery: Regular menstrual cycles are restored and maintained for

3-6 months after treatment. Double phase BBT is present or pregnancy has occurred.

Improved: Menstruation is restored, yet with scanty flow and irregular cycles. Condition may worsen after discontinuation of treatment. Unstable double phase BBT present.

No response: Symptoms improved after 2-4 months, yet menstruation is absent. Monophase BBT present.

Clinical trials show an effective rate of 81.69%. [3]

2. SPECIFIC FORMULAS

(1) Bǔ Shèn Yǎng Xuè Tāng (补肾养血汤)

The medicinals include *huáng qí* (Radix Astragali) 30g, *shú dì huáng* (Radix Rehmanniae Praeparata) 30g, *dāng guī* (Radix Angelicae Sinensis) 15g, *hé shǒu wū* (Radix Polygoni Multiflori) 20g, *nǚ zhēn zǐ* (Fructus Ligustri Lucidi) 15g, *hàn lián cǎo* (Ecliptae Herba) 15g, *dān shēn* (Radix Salviae Miltiorrhizae) 15g, *jī xuè téng* (Caulis Spatholobi) 30g, *tù sī zǐ* (Semen Cuscutae) 10g. This formula was studied in 52 cases of deficient amenorrhea. The standards of efficacy were as follows.

Clinical recovery: Regular menstrual cycles restored, with normal menstrual flow.

Improved: Menstruation restored, yet can be maintained only through the administration of the formula.

No response: Menstruation absent after 2 months of treatment.

Clinical trials showed 42 cases achieving clinical recovery, 6 cases improved, and 4 cases with no response. The total effective rate reached 92.31%. [4]

(2) Shùn Qì Tāng (顺气汤)

The medicinals include *jiāo mài yá* (Scorch-fried Fructus Hordei

Germinatus) 60g, *xià kū cǎo* (Spica Prunellae) 30g, *bái sháo* (Radix Paeoniae Alba) 30g, *shān zhā* (Fructus Crataegi) 30g, *pú gōng yīng* (Herba Taraxaci) 30g, *mǔ lì* (Concha Ostreae) 30g, *biē jiǎ* (Carapax Trionycis) 10g, *xiāng fù* (Rhizoma Cyperi) 10g, *wū yào* (Radix Linderae) 10g, *chuān niú xī* (Radix Cyathulae) 10g, *chē qián zǐ* (Semen Plantaginis) 20g, *shēng dì huáng* (Radix Rehmanniae) 20g, *dāng guī* (Radix Angelicae Sinensis) 15g, *hóng huā* (Flos Carthami) 6g, and *gān cǎo* (Radix et Rhizoma Glycyrrhizae) 6g. This formula was studied in patients with amenorrhea due to hyperprolactinemia. One decocted dose per day, 3 months constituting one course.

Clinical trials showed an total effective rate of 80% after 1-2 courses. [5]

(3) *Tài Chōng Dān* (太冲丹)

The formula consists of *hǎi piāo xiāo* (Endoconcha Sepiae), *qiàn cǎo* (Radix et Rhizoma Rubiae), *lù jiǎo jiāo* (Colla Cornus Cervi), *huáng qí* (Radix Astragali), *dāng guī* (Radix Angelicae Sinensis), *shēng dì huáng* (Radix Rehmanniae), *shú dì huáng* (Radix Rehmanniae Praeparata), *bái sháo* (Radix Paeoniae Alba), and *xuè jié* (Sanguis Draconis). One pill of *Tài Chōng Dān* (太冲丹) contains 1g crude herbs. 34 patients were prescribed 8 pills per dose, twice a day, taken with warm water. 3 months constitutes one course.

The trial showed 21 cases recovered (menstruation maintained for over 3 cycles without the formula), 9 cases improved (menstruation restored, yet irregular and scanty, also not maintained for 3 months), 4 cases no response (symptoms and relevant laboratory examinations showed no improvement). The total effective rate reached 88.24% . [6]

(4) *Tiáo Chōng Fāng* (调冲方)

The medicinals include *dāng guī* (Radix Angelicae Sinensis) 12g, *shú dì huáng* (Radix Rehmanniae Praeparata) 12g, *chuān xiōng* (Rhizoma

Chuanxiong) 8g, *jī xuè téng* (Caulis Spatholobi) 15g, *gǒu qǐ zǐ* (Fructus Lycii) 15g, *shān yào* (Rhizoma Dioscoreae) 15g, *tù sī zǐ* (Semen Cuscutae) 15g, *yín yáng huò* (Herba Epimedii) 15g, *chuān niú xī* (Radix Cyathulae) 10g, *zhì xiāng fù* (Rhizoma Cyperi Praeparata) 10g, and *lù lù tōng* (Fructus Liquidambaris) 10g.

Zhang Li-xian studied the effect of *Tiáo Chōng Tāng* (调冲汤) on amenorrhea conditions associated with contraceptive drugs. Modifications are as follows.

With qi deficiency, remove *shú dì huáng* (Radix Rehmanniae Praeparata), and add *dǎng shēn* (Radix Codonopsis) 12g, *jiāo bái zhú* (Scorch-fried Rhizoma Atractylodis Macrocephalae) 12g, *shén qū* (Massa Medicata Fermentata) 12g.

With oppression of the chest and abdominal distention, add *chén pí* (Pericarpium Citri Reticulatae) 10g, *zhǐ qiào* (Fructus Aurantii) 10g.

With aversion to cold, coldness in the limbs and loose stools, remove *shú dì huáng* (Radix Rehmanniae Praeparata) and *gǒu qǐ zǐ* (Fructus Lycii) and add *bǔ gǔ zhī* (Fructus Psoraleae) 10g, *zhì fù piàn* (Prepared Radix Aconiti Lateralis Praeparata) 10g, *zhì huáng qí* (Fried with liquid Radix Astragali) 15g.

With dream-disturbed sleep, add *yè jiāo téng* (Caulis Polygoni Multiflori) 30g.

In 26 cases, 18 cases showed recovery (menstruation maintained for 3 cycles), and 8 cases improved (menstruation restored but with irregular cycles). [7]

(5) *Bǔ Shèn Tiáo Chōng Tāng* (补肾调冲汤)

The formula includes *tù sī zǐ* (Semen Cuscutae) 20g, *gǒu qǐ zǐ* (Fructus Lycii) 15g, *nǚ zhēn zǐ* (Fructus Ligustri Lucidi) 15g, *fù pén zǐ* (Fructus Rubi) 15g, *sāng jì shēng* (Herba Taxilli) 15g, *chōng wèi zǐ* (Fructus Leonuri) 12g, *zhì shǒu wū* (Radix Polygoni Multiflori Praeparata cum Succo Glycines

Sotae) 12g, *shú dì huáng* (Radix Rehmanniae Praeparata) 12g, *ròu cōng róng* (Herba Cistanches) 12g, *bái zhú* (Rhizoma Atractylodis Macrocephalae) 12g, *yù jīn* (Radix Curcumae) 12g, *xiāng fù* (Rhizoma Cyperi) 12g.

In a study of the effect of *Bǔ Shèn Tiáo Chōng Tāng* (补肾调冲汤) in 56 patients with amenorrhea, Chen Yi-chun simulated artificial cycles and tested BBT at random. He also modified the formula accordingly for different phases of the menstrual cycle. After one course of treatment the results showed 34 cases recovered, 13 cases effective, 7 cases improved and 2 cases with no effect. The total effective rate reached 95.42%.[8]

(6) *Yì Tōng Yǐn* (益通饮)

The medicinals include: *shú dì huáng* (Radix Rehmanniae Praeparata) 30g, *zǐ hé chē* (Placenta Hominis) 15g, *chuān xù duàn* (Radix Dipsaci) 15g, *chuān niú xī* (Radix Cyathulae) 15g, *bái sháo* (Radix Paeoniae Alba) 15g, *bǎi zǐ rén* (Semen Platycladi) 12g, *juǎn bǎi* (Herba Selaginellae) 12g, *zé lán* (Herba Lycopi) 12g.

The formula was studied in 32 cases of functional amenorrhea associated with artificial abortion. All patients reported amenorrhea persisting for over 3 months. They were prescribed a daily decoction of the formula, and treatment continued for 1-3 months after the establishment of menstruation. Another 31 cases undergoing estrogen and progestin therapy were chosen as a control group. The standards for efficacy were as follows.

Clinical recovery: Regular menstrual cycles maintained for over three months after treatment.

Improved: Restored but not maintained for 3 cycles. Irregular and scant menstruation.

Ineffective: Absent menstruation after three months of treatment.

20 cases showed clinical recovery in the Chinese medicine group and 11 in the control group. 7 cases were improved in the Chinese medicine

group, with 8 cases in the control group. 5 cases were shown ineffective in the Chinese medicine group and 12 cases in control group. The effective rate of Chinese medicine group was obviously higher than that of the control group with a statistical significance (P < 0.05). [9]

(7) *Yì Shèn Huà Yū Tāng* (益肾化瘀汤)

This formula includes *yín yáng huò* (Herba Epimedii) 20g, *dù zhòng* (Cortex Eucommiae) 15g, *tù sī zǐ* (Semen Cuscutae) 15g, *gǒu qǐ zǐ* (Fructus Lycii) 15g, *dāng guī* (Radix Angelicae Sinensis) 15g, *chuān niú xī* (Radix Cyathulae) 15g, *dān shēn* (Radix Salviae Miltiorrhizae) 15g, *hé shǒu wū* (Radix Polygoni Multiflori) 12g, *táo rén* (Semen Persicae) 12g, *hóng huā* (Flos Carthami) 10g, *gān cǎo* (Radix et Rhizoma Glycyrrhizae) 10g and *suān zǎo rén* (Semen Ziziphi Spinosae) 10g.

For qi deficiency and blood stasis, add *huáng qí* (Radix Astragali) 20g and *dǎng shēn* (Radix Codonopsis) 15g.

For congealing cold and blood stasis, add *ròu guì* (Cortex Cinnamomi) 10g and *fù zǐ* (Radix Aconiti Lateralis Praeparata) 5g.

For qi stagnation and blood stasis, add *wū yào* (Radix Linderae) 10g and *xiāng fù* (Rhizoma Cyperi) 15g.

30 patients ranged in age from 25 to 36 years old, and all reported amenorrhea persisting for 2-12 months. The results showed clinical recovery in 15 cases where menstruation maintained for one year. Improvement was shown in 12 cases, where symptoms were improved and menstruation maintained for 6 months. 3 cases showed no response after 30 days. Treatment courses ranged from 20-60 days, with an average of 15 days. The total effective rate reached 90%. [10]

(8) *Yù Lín Zhū* (毓麟珠)

The formula consists of *lù jiǎo shuāng* (Cornu Cervi Degelatinatum), *chuān xiōng* (Rhizoma Chuanxiong), *chì sháo* (Radix Paeoniae Rubra), *táo*

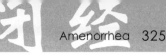

rén (Semen Persicae), *hóng huā* (Flos Carthami), *zhǐ qiào* (Fructus Aurantii), *yán hú suǒ* (Rhizoma Corydalis), *wǔ líng zhī* (Faeces Togopteri), *mǔ dān pí* (Cortex Moutan), *wū yào* (Radix Linderae), *zhì xiāng fù* (Rhizoma Cyperi Praeparata) and *gān cǎo* (Radix et Rhizoma Glycyrrhizae).This formula was prescribed with added *huáng qí* (Radix Astragali) and slices of placenta. Subjects were prescribed four doses per week for 3 up to 5 months, or until menstruation occurred.

22 subjects with secondary amenorrhea ranging in age from 17 to 36 years reported amenorrhea persisting for 6-24 months. After 2 to 4 months of treatment, 12 cases reported regular cycles, 6 cases reported delayed menstruation in a range of 35 to 57 days, and 4 cases showed no response. The total effective rate reached 81.82%. [11]

(9) *Guā Shí Liù Wèi Tāng* (瓜石六味汤)

The formula consists of *quán guā lóu* (Fructus Trichosanthis), *shí hú* (Caulis Dendrobii), *yì mǔ cǎo* (Herba Leonuri), *mǔ dān pí* (Cortex Moutan), *dān shēn* (Radix Salviae Miltiorrhizae) and *chuān niú xī* (Radix Cyathulae). This formula was studied in 65 cases of amenorrhea. Patients were aged from 16 to 46, and all reported amenorrhea persisting for 3 months up to 10 years.

For yin deficiency and blood-heat, add *shēng dì huáng* (Radix Rehmanniae), *xuán shēn* (Radix Scrophulariae), *mài dōng* (Radix Ophiopogonis) and *huáng lián* (Rhizoma Coptidis).

For qi stagnation and blood stasis, add *chái hú* (Radix Bupleuri), *zhǐ qiào* (Fructus Aurantii), *xiāng fù* (Rhizoma Cyperi), *bǎi zǐ rén* (Semen Platycladi), *zé lán* (Herba Lycopi), *wáng bù liú xíng* (Semen Vaccariae) and *juǎn bǎi* (Herba Selaginellae).

For disharmony between the Liver and Spleen, add *chái hú* (Radix Bupleuri), *bái zhú* (Rhizoma Atractylodis Macrocephalae), *fáng fēng* (Radix Saposhnikoviae), *xiāng fù* (Rhizoma Cyperi), *fú líng* (Poria) and *qīng pí*

(Pericarpium Citri Reticulatae Viride).

For Liver and Kidney deficiency, add *shēng dì huáng* (Radix Rehmanniae), *shú dì huáng* (Radix Rehmanniae Praeparata), *shān yào* (Rhizoma Dioscoreae), *shān zhū yú* (Fructus Corni), *chuān xù duàn* (Radix Dipsaci) and *gǒu qǐ zǐ* (Fructus Lycii).

For obstruction of phlegm-damp, add *fǎ bàn xià* (Rhizoma Pinelliae Praeparatum), *fú líng* (Poria), *dǎn nán xīng* (Arisaema cum Bile), *cāng zhú* (Rhizoma Atractylodis) and *zhú rú* (Caulis Bambusae in Taenia).

Subjects were prescribed one dose decocted, twice daily. The results showed normal menstruation restored and maintained for over 3 months in all 65 cases. Many of the patients continued therapy to maintain and regulate menstruation after the conclusion of the study. [12]

(10) *Tiáo Jīng Huí Rǔ Tāng* (调经回乳汤)

The formula includes *chái hú* (Radix Bupleuri) 10g, *zhǐ qiào* (Fructus Aurantii) 10g, *bái sháo* (Radix Paeoniae Alba) 10g, *chē qián zǐ* (Semen Plantaginis) 10g, *shēng mài yá* (Raw Fructus Hordei Germinatus) 60g, *chuān niú xī* (Radix Cyathulae) 15g and *gān cǎo* (Radix et Rhizoma Glycyrrhizae) 5g.

For Liver constraint and blood stasis, add *xiāng fù* (Rhizoma Cyperi) 10g, *yīn chén* (Herba Artemisiae Scopariae) 10g, *huáng qín* (Radix Scutellariae) 10g, *é zhú* (Rhizoma Curcumae) 10g, *mǔ dān pí* (Cortex Moutan) 10g and *yù jīn* (Radix Curcumae) 10g.

For Liver and Kidney deficiency, remove *chē qián zǐ* (Semen Plantaginis), and add *shú dì huáng* (Radix Rehmanniae Praeparata) 20g, *huái shān yào* (Rhizoma Dioscoreae) 20g, *jī xuè téng* (Caulis Spatholobi) 20g, *dāng guī* (Radix Angelicae Sinensis) 10g, *gǒu qǐ zǐ* (Fructus Lycii) 10g and *hé shǒu wū* (Radix Polygoni Multiflori) 10g.

For obstruction of phlegm-damp, remove *bái sháo* (Radix Paeoniae Alba) and add *cāng zhú* (Rhizoma Atractylodis) 10g, *xiāng fù*

(Rhizoma Cyperi) 10g, *fú líng* (Poria) 10g, *fǎ bàn xià* (Rhizoma Pinelliae Praeparatum) 10g, *shí chāng pú* (Rhizoma Acori Tatarinowii) 10g and *chén pí* (Pericarpium Citri Reticulatae) 5g.

The medicinals were decocted in 400ml of water until 200ml of liquid remained. The formula was prescribed twice daily and taken with warm water with one month constituting one course of treatment. After 1-3 courses the total effective rate reached 93.33%. [13]

(11) *Cù Pái Luǎn Tāng* (促排卵汤)

The medicinals include *tù sī zǐ* (Semen Cuscutae) 30g, *bā jǐ tiān* (Radix Morindae Officinalis) 30g, *yín yáng huò* (Herba Epimedii) 30g, *gǒu qǐ zǐ* (Fructus Lycii) 25g, *shú dì huáng* (Radix Rehmanniae Praeparata) 25g, *chuān xiōng* (Rhizoma Chuanxiong) 25g, *chuān niú xī* (Radix Cyathulae) 25g, *dān shēn* (Radix Salviae Miltiorrhizae) 25g, *dǎng shēn* (Radix Codonopsis) 10g, and *gān cǎo* (Radix et Rhizoma Glycyrrhizae) 10g.

For Kidney yin deficiency, add *shēng dì huáng* (Radix Rehmanniae) 25g, *nǚ zhēn zǐ* (Fructus Ligustri Lucidi) 25g and *sāng shèn* (Fructus Mori) 25g.

For Kidney yang deficiency, add *xiān máo* (Rhizoma Curculiginis) 20g, *bǔ gǔ zhī* (Fructus Psoraleae) 20g and *ài yè* (Folium Artemisiae Argyi) 20g.

For disorder of the penetrating and conception vessels, add *guī bǎn* (Carapax et Plastrum Testudinis) 15g, *lù róng* (Cornu Cervi Pantotrichum) 10g, *ròu cōng róng* (Herba Cistanches) 15g, *mài dōng* (Radix Ophiopogonis) 15g, *tiān dōng* (Radix Asparagi) 15g, and *ē jiāo* (Colla Corii Asini) 10g.

For Spleen qi deficiency, add *huáng qí* (Radix Astragali) 20g and *ròu guì* (Cortex Cinnamomi) 20g.

For Liver constraint, add *chái hú* (Radix Bupleuri) 15g and *bái sháo* (Radix Paeoniae Alba) 15g.

A decoction was prescribed twice daily, with 14 days as one course. The total effective rate reached 85.13% after 3 courses of treatment. [14]

(12) *Bǔ Shèn Huó Xuè Tāng* (补肾活血汤)

The formula includes *shú dì huáng* (Radix Rehmanniae Praeparata) 12g, *shān yào* (Rhizoma Dioscoreae) 12g, *shān zhū yú* (Fructus Corni) 6g, *bā jǐ tiān* (Radix Morindae Officinalis) 6g, *xiān líng pí* (Herba Epimedii) 15g, *huáng jīng* (Rhizoma Polygonati) 12g, *nǚ zhēn zǐ* (Fructus Ligustri Lucidi) 9g, *bǔ gǔ zhī* (Fructus Psoraleae) 12g, *dān shēn* (Radix Salviae Miltiorrhizae) 9g, *hóng huā* (Flos Carthami) 9g and *xiāng fù* (Rhizoma Cyperi) 6g.

For fear of cold, *fù zǐ* (Radix Aconiti Lateralis Praeparata) 9g and *ròu guì* (Cortex Cinnamomi) 3g was added.

In 16 cases of amenorrhea, ovulation was restored in 10 subjects, 5 cases showed positive effect and 1 case showed no response. The total effective rate reached 93.7% . [15]

(13) Modified *Sì Wù Tāng* (四物汤加减)

The medicinals include *dāng guī* (Radix Angelicae Sinensis), *chuān xiōng* (Rhizoma Chuanxiong), *shú dì huáng* (Radix Rehmanniae Praeparata), *bái sháo* (Radix Paeoniae Alba), *huáng qí* (Radix Astragali), *jī xuè téng* (Caulis Spatholobi) and *chuān niú xī* (Radix Cyathulae).

For qi and blood deficiency, increase the dosage of *huáng qí* (Radix Astragali).

For qi stagnation and blood stasis, replace *bái sháo* (Radix Paeoniae Alba) with *chì sháo* (Radix Paeoniae Rubra), and replace *shú dì huáng* (Radix Rehmanniae Praeparata) with *shēng dì huáng* (Radix Rehmanniae). *Táo rén* (Semen Persicae), *hóng huā* (Flos Carthami), *chái hú* (Radix Bupleuri) and *zhǐ qiào* (Fructus Aurantii) may be added as well.

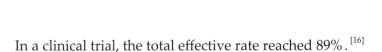

In a clinical trial, the total effective rate reached 89%.[16]

(14) *Tōng Dá Tāng* (通达汤)

The medicinals include *sān léng* (Rhizoma Sparganii) 6g, *é zhú* (Rhizoma Curcumae) 6g, *táo rén* (Semen Persicae) 10g, *zé lán* (Herba Lycopi) 10g, *jī xuè téng* (Caulis Spatholobi) 30g, *chuān xiōng* (Rhizoma Chuanxiong) 10g and *chuān niú xī* (Radix Cyathulae) 10g.

In the treatment of drug-induced galactorrhea-amenorrhea syndrome, the total effective rate reached 92.5%. The course of treatment ranged from 4-18 weeks. [17]

(15) Modified *Cāng Fù Dǎo Tán Wán* with *Shēng Huà Tāng* (苍附导痰丸加生化汤)

The formula consists of *chén pí* (Pericarpium Citri Reticulatae), *fú líng* (Poria), *fǎ bàn xià* (Rhizoma Pinelliae Praeparatum), *cāng zhú* (Rhizoma Atractylodis), *xiāng fù* (Rhizoma Cyperi), *dǎn nán xīng* (Arisaema cum Bile), *zhǐ qiào* (Fructus Aurantii), *dān shēn* (Radix Salviae Miltiorrhizae), *chuān xiōng* (Rhizoma Chuanxiong), *dāng guī* (Radix Angelicae Sinensis), *táo rén* (Semen Persicae) and *shēng jiāng* (Rhizoma Zingiberis Recens).

In a study of amenorrhea associated with antipsychotic medications, the total effective rate reached 91%. [18]

(16) *Huó Xuè Huà Yū Jīng Yàn Fāng* (活血化瘀经验方)

The medicinals include *táo rén* (Semen Persicae) 12g, *hóng huā* (Flos Carthami) 12g, *dāng guī* (Radix Angelicae Sinensis) 15g, *chuān xiōng* (Rhizoma Chuanxiong) 15g, *chì sháo* (Radix Paeoniae Rubra) 12g, *chuān niú xī* (Radix Cyathulae) 15g, *sān léng* (Rhizoma Sparganii) 12g, *é zhú* (Rhizoma Curcumae) 12g, *xiāng fù* (Rhizoma Cyperi) 20g and *gān cǎo* (Radix et Rhizoma Glycyrrhizae) 10g.

In a study of amenorrhea associated with antipsychotic medications, the decoction was prescribed twice per day. The total effective rate reached 85%. [19]

(17) *Xuè Fǔ Zhú Yū Jiāo Náng* (血府逐瘀胶囊)

In a study treating amenorrhea associated with neurosis with *Xuè Fǔ Zhú Yū Jiāo Náng,* the total effective rate reached 90.3%. [20] 6 tablets were prescribed twice per day. This formula is manufactured by the fifth Chinese medicinal factory of Tianjin. [20]

(18) *Féi Pàng Bì Jīng Fāng* (肥胖闭经方)

The formula consists of *jiāng bàn xià* (Rhizome Pinelliae Praeparata), *fú líng* (Poria), *yì yǐ rén* (Semen Coicis), *tiān huā fěn* (Radix Trichosanthis), *zhú rú* (Caulis Bambusae in Taenia), *chǎo zhǐ qiào* (Dry-fried Fructus Aurantii), *dāng guī* (Radix Angelicae Sinensis), *jiāo bái sháo* (Scorch-fried Radix Paeoniae Alba), *shā shēn* (Radix Adenophorae seu Glehniae), *nǚ zhēn zǐ* (Fructus Ligustri Lucidi), *dǎn nán xīng*(Arisaema cum Bile), *shēng shān zhā* (Raw Fructus Crataegi), *zé lán* (Herba Lycopi) and *zé xiè* (Rhizoma Alismatis). 43 cases of amenorrhea associated with obesity were treated.

The study showed 13 cases responding with excellent effect, 23 showing positive effect, and 7 cases with no response. The total effective rate reached 83.7% . [21]

3. ACUPUNCTURE AND MOXIBUSTION

(1) Lu Ping treated 32 cases of amenorrhea with acupuncture.

SP 6 *(sān yīn jiāo)* was selected as the primary point prescription. Acupuncture was performed once daily, with ten days constituting one course of treatment.

For deficiency, RN 4 (*guān yuán*), RN 6 (*qì hǎi*) and ST 36 (*zú sān lǐ*) were added, manipulating with even supplementation and drainage.

For excess patterns, ST 40 (*fēng lóng*), LV 3 (*tài chōng*) and SP 10 (*xuè hǎi*) were added, manipulating with drainage.

Neither Chinese medicinals nor biomedicines were prescribed during treatment. With treatment beginning 10 days before the normal menstrual date, 10 cases resumed menstruation within one course of treatment. After 1-3 courses of treatment, 18 subjects maintained normal menstruation for more than 3 months. 4 cases showed a positive effect, yet discontinued the therapy for other treatment methods. [22]

(2) Lou Yu-fang treated 60 cases of secondary amenorrhea associated with induced abortion.

The experimental group were treated with acupuncture and moxibustion, the control group with Chinese medicinals. The patients were aged from 20-40, with amenorrhea persisting for 4 to 7 months. Among the 60 cases, 12 presented Kidney deficiency, 18 with qi stagnation and blood stasis, 16 with qi and blood deficiency, and 14 showed congealing cold and blood stasis conditions.

The primary points chosen were RN 4 with ST 29, SP 6 and SP 10 (*xuè hǎi*) bilaterally.

For Kidney deficiency, KI 3 (*tài xī*) was added.

For qi stagnation and blood stasis, LV 3 and RN 6 was added.

For qi and blood deficiency, ST 36 was added.

For congealing cold and blood stasis, moxibustion was indicated.

The treatment was performed once per day, with ten days constituting one course. After 3 courses of treatment, 20 cases were recovered (regular menstruation maintained for 3 months), 8 cases showed obvious improvement, (menstruation restored, yet with irregular cycles and menses) and 2 cases without effect (menstruation absent with no response). [23]

In a study treating amenorrhea associated with drug abuse, Nie Hui-ming divided patients into two groups: an ear acupoint pressing therapy group, and a control group, each with 21 subjects.

The control group was given routine psychological treatment for 30 days. The other patients were treated with ear acupoint pressing therapy using *wáng bù liú xíng* (Semen Vaccariae). Subjects were treated 10 times, every third day, in addition to psychological treatment. During the 30-day period following detoxification, the patients' menstrual periods were recorded. The severities of withdrawal and abstinent symptoms were also evaluated before and after treatment.

In the ear acupoint pressing therapy group, 17 subjects established menstruation within 30 days, with 5 subjects in the control group. The restoration rate of ear acupoint pressing therapy group was significantly higher than that of the control group, while the average time needed to establish menstruation was significantly shorter in the ear acupoint group. The symptoms of abstinence and withdrawal such as craving, anxiety, muscular pain, and sleep disturbance scored lower in the ear acupoint group.

The trial showed that ear acupoint pressing therapy has excellent effect in treating secondary amenorrhea, and also in reducing the protracted abstinence and withdrawal abstinent symptoms in female drug addicts. [24]

(3) Han Yan studied the effect of abdominal acupuncture in the treatment of secondary amenorrhea.

The primary points chosen were RN 12 (*zhōng wǎn*), RN 10 (*xià wǎn*), RN 6 and RN 4 (these four points are called *Yǐn Qì Guī Yuán Fāng* (引气归元方) in abdominal acupuncture), along with KI 13 (*qì xué*) and ST 28 (*shuǐ dào*).

Method: Using 0.25mm×40mm filiform needles, insert slowly until a mild resistance appears, then retain the needles for 30 minutes without further manipulation. Treat three times per week, 10 times as one course, with a short break between courses.

Subjects received 2 courses of treatment and a 6 month follow-up. 7 patients established menstruation after 5 treatments, 14 subjects established menstruation after one course, 8 patients required 2 courses, and 4 subjects showed no response after 2 courses of treatment.

With abdominal acupuncture, 21 subjects established regular menstruation, with an total recovery rate of 63.63%. 8 subjects presented irregular menstruation, with an effective rate of 24.24%. 4 cases showed no response, with an ineffective rate of 12.13%. The total effective rate reached 87.87%. [25]

(4) Liu Bing-quan studied acupuncture in the treatment of 86 cases of secondary amenorrhea.

The primary points were DU 1 (*cháng qiáng*), RN 4 , RN 7 (*yīn jiāo*), SP 6 (*sān yīn jiāo*), *zǐ gōng* (EX-CA1), LI 4 (*hé gǔ*) and LV 3. Needles were inserted to a depth of 1.2-1.5*cun*.

For qi and blood deficiency, ST 36 was added.

For qi stagnation and blood stasis, SP 10 (*xuè hǎi*) was added.

For Liver and Kidney deficiency, BL 23 (*shèn shù*) was added.

With symptoms of congealing cold, warming needle acupuncture was applied to RN 4.

Treatment was performed once daily, 6 days per week, 12 treatments as one course.

Following 6 courses of treatment, the study showed 45 subjects achieving clinical recovery, 26 cases showed improvement, and 15 cases showed no effect. The total effective rate reached 82.6%. [26]

4. ADDITIONAL TREATMENT MODALITIES

(1) Electroacupuncture

Dr. Yu Peng treated 24 cases of galactorrhea-amenorrhea syndrome with electroacupuncture.

The primary points were RN 17 (*dàn zhōng*), ST 18 (*rǔ gēn*), ST 36 (*zú sān lǐ*), SP 6 (*sān yīn jiāo*) and BL 23 *(shèn shù)*, using 0.35mm × 40mm filiform needles.

RN 17 and ST 18 were inserted transversely at 15° to a depth of 20mm.

ST 36 and SP 6 were needled perpendicularly to a depth of 25mm.

BL 23 was inserted obliquely toward the spine at 45°, to a depth of 25mm.

A G68052 II electric acupuncture apparatus was then connected and set to continuous wave, 6V, 215mA, at 80Hz.

Treatment was given daily for 30 minutes, 10 days as one course. Subjects received 2 courses of treatment, with an interval of 7 days.

The total effective rate reached 75.10%. PRL approached normal after treatment. [27]

(2) Point Application

Dr. Qiu Min studied umbilical compress therapy using *Yì Shèn Tōng Jīng Sǎn* (益肾通经散).

The medicinals for this method include *lù róng* (Cornu Cervi Pantotrichum) 6g, *bā jǐ tiān* (Radix Morindae Officinalis) 30g, *ròu cōng róng* (Herba Cistanches) 30g, *zǐ hé chē* (Placenta Huminis) 30g, *shú dì huáng* (Radix Rehmanniae Praeparata) 30g, *yì mǔ cǎo* (Herba Leonuri) 30g, *huáng qí* (Radix Astragali) 40g, *dāng guī* (Radix Angelicae Sinensis) 30g, *rén shēn* (Radix et Rhizoma Ginseng) 30g, *shān zhā* (Fructus Crataegi) 30g and *jī nèi jīn* (Endothelium Corneum Gigeriae Galli) 30g.

All medicinals are pestled into a fine powder which can be stored in bottles. 10g of powder are mixed with wine and formed into a small round shape. Press the preparation into the navel, cover with gauze, and fix with adhesive plaster. Repeat every three days, 7 treatments as a course.

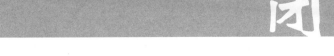

In a clinical study, the total effective rate reached 93.44%. [28]

Dr. Pang Bao-zhen studied umbilical compress therapy using *Xìn Tōng Dān* (信通丹) in 122 cases.

The formula consists of *lù róng* (Cornu Cervi Pantotrichum) 6g, *bā jǐ tiān* (Radix Morindae Officinalis) 30g, *ròu cōng róng* (Herba Cistanches) 30g, *zǐ hé chē* (Placenta Hominis) 30g, *shú dì huáng* (Radix Rehmanniae Praeparata) 30g, *yì mǔ cǎo* (Herba Leonuri) 30g, *huáng qí* (Radix Astragali) 40g, *dāng guī* (Radix Angelicae Sinensis) 30g, *rén shēn* (Radix et Rhizoma Ginseng) 30g, *shān zhā* (Fructus Crataegi) 30g, *jī nèi jīn* (Endothelium Corneum Gigeriae Galli) 30g and *xiāng fù* (Rhizoma Cyperi) 30g.

All medicinals are pestled into a fine powder and can be stored in bottles. 10g of powder is mixed with wine and formed into a small round shape. Press the preparation into the navel, cover with gauze, and fix with adhesive plaster. Repeat every three days, 10 treatments as a course.

After 10 courses of treatment, 74 cases reported recovered, 30 cases showed positive effect, 10 cases were improved, and 8 cases showed no response. The total effective rate reached 93.44%. [29]

Wang He-zhen studied ear acupoint pressing therapy in treating 65 cases of secondary amenorrhea.

The ear acupoints in this method include uterus (internal genital), ovary, central rim, endocrine, Liver, Kidney and Spleen. Press one seed of *wáng bù liú xíng* (Semen Vaccariae) or *bái jiè zǐ* (Sinapis Semen), *tù sī zǐ* (Semen Cuscutae), *cí shí* (Magnetitum) onto the selected point, and cover with a square 0.16cm × 0.16cm adhesive. Pinch and press with the thumb and index finger until a sensation of soreness, numbness, distention, or heat is produced. Press the points 4 to 5 times per day, for 5 to 10 minutes.

After treatment, all 65 cases established menstruation. Among them, 38 established menstruation with one course of treatment, 12 cases after two, and 15 cases required over 3 courses. [30]

Experimental Studies

1. Research on The Efficacy of Single Chinease Medicinals

Wei Mei-juan's study found that Chinese medicinals which tonify the Kidney can increase the mass of interstitial glands in the ovaries of anovular rats treated with androgen. Other effects were observed as well. A decrease of intracytoplasm lipid droplets in interstitial glands, activities of the estrogen and especially progestin receptors were increased, and the dissolution of mitochondria and autophagy of the adenopituicyte ceased. Chinese medicinals which tonify the Kidney have a marked effect on the anabolic hormone metabolism of ovaries and pituitary glands in rats.

The medicinals involved in the study included *shú fù zǐ* (Radix Aconiti Lateralis Praeparata), *ròu guì* (Cortex Cinnamomi), *bǔ gǔ zhī* (Fructus Psoraleae), *xiān líng pí* (Herba Epimedii), *tù sī zǐ* (Semen Cuscutae), *huáng jīng* (Rhizoma Polygonati) and *shú dì huáng* (Radix Rehmanniae Praeparata). [31]

2. Research on the Efficacy of Acupuncture

Dr. Yang Dan-hong studied the effects of acupuncture treatment on amenorrhea associated with excessive gonad stimulating hormone levels.

The primary points were RN 4 (*guān yuán*), RN 3 (*zhōng jí*), KI 12 (*dà hè*), *zǐ gōng* (EX-CA1), ST 29 (*guī lái*), BL 17 (*gé shù*), BL 18 (*gān shù*) and BL 23 (*shèn shù*). Other points such as ST 36 (*zú sān lǐ*), SP 6 (*sān yīn jiāo*), LV 3 (*tài chōng*) and SP 8 (*dì jī*) were added as clinically indicated.

Method: select 6 to 8 points for each treatment. Abdominal points require a relatively deep insertion. After the arrival of qi, manipulate with even supplementation and drainage until a strong needling sensation is produced in the lower abdomen. Retain the needles for 30 minutes. Treat once every two days.

The results showed markedly decreased FSH levels at the end of the treatment period, as well as when measured at 30 and 60 days. The FSH Levels after the treatment were obviously lower than that before the treatment with statistical significances ($P<0.001$). The LH levels were also decreased for 60 days, with no statistical significances. The E_2 levels after the treatment were obviously higher than that before the treatment with statistical significances ($P<0.001$). [32]

3. RESEARCH ON THE EFFICACY OF HERBAL PRESCRIPTIONS

(1) The Effect on Hypothalamic-Pituitary-Ovarian Axis

The water-soluble elements of *Bŭ Shèn Fāng* (补肾方) are found to increase uterine and ovarian mass and increase cellular substance in the interstitial glands of polycystic rat ovaries. This indicates that the water-soluble portion of Kidney tonics may play a particular role in the regulation of ovarian function.

The formula consists of *fù zĭ* (Radix Aconiti Lateralis Praeparata), *ròu guì* (Cortex Cinnamomi), *bŭ gŭ zhī* (Fructus Psoraleae), *xiān líng pí* (Herba Epimedii), *tù sī zĭ* (Semen Cuscutae), *huáng jīng* (Rhizoma Polygonati) and *shú dì huáng* (Radix Rehmanniae Praeparata). [33]

Dr. Xia Rong-xi randomly divided 40 immature female rats into four treatment groups. They were administered medicinals to tonify the Kidney, regulate the penetrating vessel, tonify the Kidney and regulate the penetrating vessel, and a normal saline group. A decoction was infused into the rats' stomach, and cells from the stratum granulosum of the ovarian follicle were later observed under an electron microscope.

In the Kidney tonification group, the cellular cytoplasm of the stratum granulosum displayed abundant rough endoplasmic reticulums, chondrosomes and lipid droplets, and few smooth endoplasmic reticulums.

In the regulating the penetrating vessel group, the Golgi complex was developed, chondrosomes abundant and the rough endoplasmic reticulum distended.

In the group both tonifying the Kidney and regulating the penetrating vessel, the Golgi complex was developed, chondrosomes and ribosomes were abundant, smooth endoplasmic reticulum increased, and lipid droplets were present.

No obvious changes were found in the normal saline group.

This indicates that Chinese medicinals which tonify the Kidney and regulate the penetrating vessel may also activate cellular function in the stratum granulosum of the ovarian follicle. [34]

Dr. Ma Zheng-li found that the formulas and medicinals which tonify Kidney and benefit essence can both decrease A-cells and increase B-cells in the PVN of the hypothalamus. Also found were increased GN and N cells of the pituitary gland, improved development and blood-supply of the ovarian follicle, increased interstitial cellular substance of the endometria, improved development of the endometrial glands, with a decrease of collagenous fibers.

This indicates that tonifying the Kidney and nourishing essence with Chinese medicinals may also regulate the function of hypothalamic-pituitary-ovarian axis to some extent. [35]

Dr. Wang Xuan researched how Chinese medicinals which tonify the Kidney and invigorate blood can affect serum hormone levels in cases of traumatic amenorrhea. The term traumatic amenorrhea refers to amenorrhea resulting from physical damage to the endometria. Such causes include abortion, hysteromyomectomy, intrauterine curettage after induced labor and diagnostic curettage. Subjects were treated with a self composed formula, *Bǔ Shèn Huó Xuè Tāng* (补肾活血汤), containing *lù jiǎo piàn* (Sliced Cornu Cervi).

The trial resulted in an effective rate of 93.55%.

Chinese medicinals which tonify the Kidney and invigorate blood may also markedly increase blood serum levels of E_2, P, FSH and LH. [36]

(2) The Effects on Development of the Ovarian Follicle

Dr. Li Gui-xian researched the effect of *Cù Pái Luǎn Tāng* (促排卵汤) on the ovaries and endometria of reproductive age Jimpy mice.

The formula contains medicinals such as *chái hú* (Radix Bupleuri), *chì sháo* (Radix Paeoniae Rubra), *bái sháo* (Radix Paeoniae Alba), *gǒu qǐ zǐ* (Fructus Lycii) and *tù sī zǐ* (Semen Cuscutae).

The results showed increased lipid and 3-β-HSDH activity in theca interna and stratum granulosum of the ovarian follicle, and also in the cytoplasm of luteal cells. Increased levels of glucoprotein and lipid were found in the endometrial epidermis and stroma. The above changes were observed in both preestrus and metestrus.

This indicates that *Cù Pái Luǎn Tāng* (促排卵汤) may promote the secretion of steroid hormone in the ovarian follicle and corpus luteum, nourish the endometria, and promote the implantation and development of the embryo. [37]

Dr. Li Wen-pei studied the effect of a Kidney tonifying and blood invigorating decoction on a group of mature rabbits. The dosage was infused directly into the stomach at a dose 20 times greater than that indicated for an adult woman.

The diameter and mass of the ovarian follicle was measured before and after the experiment. Greater ovarian follicle size was observed in the Chinese medicinal group compared with the normal saline group. The weights of the ovarian and uterus between the two groups had no statistical significances. [38]

(3) The Effect on the Internal Insulin Level

Dr. Zhang Yue-ping studied the effect of a Kidney yin tonifying decoction infused into the stomachs of androgen-sterilized rats.

The formula included *shēng dì huáng* (Radix Rehmanniae), *shān zhū yú* (Fructus Corni), *nǚ zhēn zǐ* (Fructus Ligustri Lucidi), *shān yào* (Rhizoma Dioscoreae), *zé xiè* (Rhizoma Alismatis), *fú líng* (Poria) and *zhī mǔ* (Rhizoma Anemarrhenae).

As a result, ovarian mass was increased, and follicles developed with a decrease of cystic follicles. Testosterone production in vitro had also decreased. Glucose tolerance increased, and blood insulin and bodyweight levels were both reduced.

This implies that Chinese medicinals may promote the development of the ovarian follicle. In androgen-sterilized rats, ovulation is promoted through the reduction of insulin and testosterone levels. [39]

4. Research on New Forms of Chinese Medicinals

Medicinal cakes such as *Bǎo Zhēn Yào Bǐng* (葆真药饼) both tonify the Kidney and Liver as well as nourishing essence and blood. It includes medicinals such as *hé shǒu wū* (Radix Polygoni Multiflori) and *nǚ zhēn zǐ* (Fructus Ligustri Lucidi).

Ma Zheng-li studied 21 month old female rats that had been consuming the medicinal cake for 7 months. It was observed that 1 to 6 developing ovarian follicles were present in all rats, up to 6 corpus luteum, few scattered interstitial glands, and healthy blood vessels in the medullary ovarian substance. However, ovarian follicles were not as well developed in the control group, where 5 degenerative follicles were found in 7 rats. In addition, agglomerated cells and sporadic interstitial glands were abundant, where corpus luteum and blood vessels in the medullary ovarian substance were few.

The results indicate that medicinals which tonify the Kidney and Liver while nourishing essence and blood may also promote the development of the ovarian follicle. [35]

REFERENCES

[1] Yang Ying, Cheng Xiao-xi. Pattern Differentiation and Treatment of Amenorrhea due to Deficiency (虚痨之闭经的辨证治疗). *Shanxi Journal of Traditional Chinese Medicine* (陕西中医). 2005, (2)：192.

[2] Yan Wen-Fei. Treatment in 223 Cases of Amenorrhea According to Staged Pattern Differentiation (辨证分期论治闭经 38 例). *Zhejiang Journal of Traditional Chinese Medicine.* (浙江中医杂志). 2001, (8)：344.

[3] Zhang Gui-zhen. Treatment in 60 Cases of Amenorrhea According to Pattern Differentiation (辨证分型治疗闭经 60 例). *Journal of Practical Traditional Chinese Medicine* (实用中医药杂志). 2004, 20(4)：176-177.

[4] Kang Cui-mei. Treatment in 52 Cases of Deficiency Pattern Amenorrhea with the Empirical Formula Bu Shen Yang Xue Tang (自拟补肾养血汤治疗虚证闭经 52 例). *Jilin Journal of Traditional Chinese Medicine* (吉林中医药). 2005, 25 (1)：27.

[5] Chen Xiao-xia. Treatment in 74 Cases of Hyperprolactinemia Amenorrhea with the Empirical Formula Shun Qi Tang (自拟顺气汤治疗高泌乳素血症 74 例). *Zhejiang Journal of Traditional Chinese Medicine* (浙江中医杂志). 2005, (2)：63.

[6] Cheng Yan. Clinical Observation of Tai Chong Dan Formula in Treatment of 34 Cases of Amenorrhea due to Blood Exhaustion (太冲丹治疗血枯经闭 34 例临床观察). *New Journal of Traditional Chinese Medicine* (新中医). 1998, 30(1)：31.

[7] Zhang Li-xian, Yu Shu-ren. Treatment in 26 Cases of Amenorrhea Associated with Contraceptive Drugs Using Tiao Chong Fang (调冲方治疗避孕药引起闭经 26 例). *Journal of Anhui Traditional Chinese Medical College* (安徽中医学院学报). 1994, 13(3)：16.

[8] Chen Yi-chun. Treatment in 56 Cases of Secondary Amenorrhea with Bu Shen Tiao Chong Tang (补肾调冲汤加减治疗继发性闭经 56 例). *Sichuan Journal of Traditional Chinese Medicine* (四川中医). 2001, 19(8)：52-53.

[9] Xi Jia. Treatment in 32 Cases of Amenorrhea Associated with Abortion with Yi Tong Yin (益通饮治疗人流术后闭经 32 例). *Jiangsu Journal of Traditional Chinese Medicine* (江苏中医). 1994, 15(12)：15.

[10] Ji Yun-hai. Treatment in 30 Cases of Amenorrhea Associated with Abortion Using Yi Shen Hua Yu Tang (益肾化瘀汤治疗人工流产闭经 30 例). *Jilin Journal of*

Traditional Chinese Medicine (吉林中医药). 1995, (5)：24.

[11] Deng Ke. Treatment in 22 Cases of Amenorrhea with Yu Lin Zhu (毓麟珠治疗闭经 22 例). *Jilin Journal of Traditional Chinese Medicine* (吉林中医药). 1994, (6)：25.

[12] Tang Kun-hua, Zhu Guang-hua. Treatment in 65 Cases of Amenorrhea with Gua Shi Liu Wei Tang (瓜石六味汤治疗闭经 65 例). *Jiangsu Journal of Traditional Chinese Medicine* (江苏中医). 1993, 14(11)：9.

[13] Ye Tian-zhen. Treatment in 15 Cases of Galactorrhea-Amenorrhea Syndrome with Tiao Jing Hui Ru Tang (调经回乳汤治疗闭经泌乳综合征 15 例). *Zhejiang Journal of Traditional Chinese Medicine* (浙江中医杂志). 2001, 7：296.

[14] Dong Jin-mei, Liu Wen-jiang, Yang Hong-fei. Clinical Observation of Treatment in 34 Cases of Amenorrhea with the Tonifying the Kidney and Coursing the Liver Method (补肾舒肝法治疗闭经 34 例临床观察). *Information on Traditional Chinese Medicine* (中医药信息). 2006, 23(1)：27.

[15] An Lian-ying. Observation of Inducing Ovulation in 58 Cases with Bu Shen Huo Xue Tang (补肾活血汤促排卵 58 例疗效观察). *Henan Journal of Traditional Chinese Medicine* (河南中医). 2001, 21(3)：49-50.

[16] Tang Gui-lan. Treatment in 28 Cases of Amenorrhea Associated with Abortion Using Modified Si Wu Tang (四物汤加减治疗人流术后闭经 28 例). *Beijing Journal of Traditional Chinese Medicine* (北京中医). 2000, 6：59.

[17] Ding Ying, Zhou Geng-sheng, Song Hai-dong. Treatment in 40 Cases of Drug-Induced Galactorrhea-Amenorrhea Syndrome with Tong Da Tang (通达汤治疗药源性闭经泌乳综合征 40 例·临床观察). *Journal of Snake* (蛇志). 2001, 13(3)：41-42.

[18] Zhang Mei-ru. Treatment of Amenorrhea Associated with Antipsychotic Medication Using Cang Fu Dao Tan Wan Modified with Sheng Hua Tang (苍附导痰丸合并生化汤治疗抗精神病药引起的闭经). *Tianjin Journal of Traditional Chinese Medicine* (天津中医). 2001, 18(1)：47-48.

[19] Xu Ai-min, Zhang Feng-xiang, Yang Jun. Treatment in 40 Cases of Amenorrhea Associated with Antipsychotic Medication Using the Invigorating Blood and Dispelling Stasis Method (活血化瘀法治疗抗精神病药物所致闭经 40 例). *Journal of Traditional Chinese Medicine* (光明中医). 17(102)：61-62.

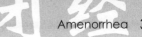

[20] Zhao Hong-tao, Long Jing, Luan Huo, et al. Study of Treatment in 60 Cases of Amenorrhea Associated with Neurosis Using Xue Fu Zhu Yu Jiao Nang (血府逐瘀胶囊治疗神经症伴发闭经60例对照研究). *Tianjin Journal of Traditional Chinese Medicine* (天津中医). 2002, 19(4)：50.

[21] Mi Weiyi, Zhang Lan. Treatment in 43 cases of Amenorrhea due to Obesity Using the Nourishing Yin and Dispelling Phlegm Method (运用养阴祛痰法治疗肥胖性闭经 43 例). *Chinese Journal of Traditional Medical Science and Technology* (中国中医药科技). 2002, 9(3)：185-186.

[22] Lu Ping. Treatment in 32 Cases of Amenorrhea with Acupuncture Using SP 6 (针刺三阴交为主治疗闭经 32 例). *Journal of Clinical Acupuncture and Moxibustion* (针灸临床杂志). 2000, 16(6)：44.

[23] Lou Yu-fang. Treatment in 30 Cases of Secondary Amenorrhea Associated with Abortion Using Acupuncture and Moxibustion (针刺结合艾灸治疗人工流产后继发性闭经 30 例). *Journal of Clinical Acupuncture and Moxibustion* (针灸临床杂志). 1999, 15(9)：17-18.

[24] Nie Hui-ming, Qiao Feng-ying, Sun Jia-fu, et al. Analysis of the Treatment of Secondary Amenorrhea and Protracted Abstinent Symptoms in Drug Addicts with Ear Acupoint Pressing Therapy (耳穴压迫法治疗吸毒者继发性闭经及稽延性戒断症状疗效分析). *Chinese Journal of Drug Dependence* (中国药物依赖性杂志). 2001, 10(3)：204-206.

[25] Han Yan. Treatment in 33 Cases of Secondary Amenorrhea by Regulating the Penetrating and Conception Vessels with Abdominal Acupuncture (腹针疗法调冲任治疗继发性闭经 33 例的临床报道). *Journal of Clinical Acupuncture and Moxibustion* (针灸临床杂志). 2002, 18(8)：3-4.

[26] Liu Bing-quan. Treatment in 88 Cases of Secondary Amenorrhea with Acupuncture and Moxibustion (针灸治疗继发性闭经86例). *Journal of Clinical Acupuncture and Moxibustion* (针灸临床杂志). 2003, 19(2)：16.

[27] Yu Peng, Yu Miao, Zhang Xiu-qi. Treament in 24 Cases of Galactorrhea-Amenorrhea Syndrome with Electroacupuncture (电针治疗泌乳闭经综合征 24 例). *Chinese Acupuncture & Moxibustion* (中国针灸). 2005, (9)：670.

[28] Qiu Min. Treament in 122 Cases of Amenorrhea with Umbilical Compress Therapy Using Yi Shen Tong Jing San (益肾通经散贴脐治疗闭经122 例). *Forum on*

Traditional Chinese Medicine (国医论坛). 2003, 18(5)：32.

[29] Pang Bao-zhen, Liu Xiang-ying, Hou Xian-liang, et al. Treament in 122 Cases of Amenorrhea with Umbilical Compress Therapy Using Xin Tong Dan (信通丹贴脐治疗闭经 122 例). *Journal of External Therapy of Traditional Chinese Medicine* (中医外治杂志). 2004, 13(4)：42-43.

[30] Wang He-zhen, Cao Zhi-ru. Observation of Treatment in 65 Cases of Secondary Amenorrhea with Ear Acupoint Pressing Therapy (耳压法治疗继发性闭经 65 例观察). *Chengdu Medical Journal* (成都医药). 2002, 28(3)：146.

[31] Wei Meijuan, Yu Jin. Observation of the Morphological Effect of Kidney-Tonifying Chinese Medicinals on Hypophysis Cerebri and Ovaries of Androgen-Sterilized Rats (补肾药对雄激素致无排卵大鼠垂体及卵巢的形态学变化观察). *Chinese Journal of Integrated Traditional and Western Medicine* (中国中西医结合杂志). 1993, 13(3)：164-166.

[32] Yang Dan-hong. Treatment in 31 Cases of Amenorrhea Associated with Excessive Gonad-Stimulating Hormone Levels with Acupuncture (针灸治疗高促性腺激素性闭经 31 例). *Journal of Zhejiang College of Traditional Chinese Medicine* (浙江中医学院学报学报). 2005, 29(5)：71-72.

[33] Yu Jin, Chen Hong-ying, Mao Qiu-zhi, et al. Experimental Study of the Kidney Governing Reproduction (肾主生殖的实验研究). *Chinese Journal of Integrated Traditional and Western Medicine* (中国中西医结合杂志). 1989, 9(9)：548-551.

[34] Xia Rong-xi, Cui Hong-ying. Experimental Study of the Effect of Tonifying the Kidney and Regulating the Penetrating Vessel Method on the Genitals of Immature Rats (补肾调冲法对幼鼠生殖系统作用的实验研究). *Tianjin Journal of Traditional Chinese Medicine* (天津中医). 1994, 11(3)：34-35.

[35] Ma Zheng-li, Shi Yu-hua, Wang Li-ya, et al. Study of the Morphological Effect of Essence-Replenishing and Kidney-Tonifying Chinese Medicinals on Hypothalmic-Pituitary-Adrenal Axis of Mature Rats (填精补肾中药对老年大鼠下丘脑 - 垂体 - 性腺 - 胸腺轴的形态学研究). *Journal of Traditional Chinese Medicine* (中医杂志). 1989, 30(8)：45.

[36] Wang Xuan, He Guo-pei, Wang Xian. The Effect of Kidney-Tonifying and Blood-Invigorating Chinese Medicinals on Serum Hormones in Patients with Traumatic Amenorrhea (补肾活血中药对创伤性闭经患者血清激素水平的影响). *The Practical Journal of*

Integrating Chinese with Mordern Medicine (中华实用中西医杂志). 2003, 3(16)：1690-1691.

[37] Li Gui-xian, Shi Xiao-lin, Zhang Ya-bin, et al. Histochemistry Research of the Effect of Cu Pai Luan Tang on the Ovaries and Endometria of Jimpy Mice (中草药促排卵汤对小鼠卵巢及子宫内膜作用的组织化学研究). *Reproduction & Contraception* (生殖与避孕). 1995, 15(6)：429-433.

[38] Li Wen-pei, Fu Shi-gui, Wu Guo-zhen, et al. Experimental Study of Kidney-Tonifying and Blood-Invigorating Chinese Medicinals on the Ovulation of Rabbits (Abstract) (补肾活血中药对家兔排卵的实验（摘要）). *Chinese Journal of Integrated Traditional and Western Medicine* (中国中西医结合杂志). 1986, 6(12)：745.

[39] Zhang Yue-ping, Yu Jin, Gui Sui-qi. Pathogenesis in Androgen-Sterilized Rats and the Ovulation-Inducing Effect of Chinese Medicinals that Nourish Kidney Yin (雄激素致不孕大鼠发病机制及滋肾阴药对其促排卵作用). *Chinese Journal of Endocrinology* (中华内分泌代谢杂志). 1994, 10(2)：98-101.

Index by Disease Names and Symptoms

Index by Chinese Medicinals and Formulas

General Index

Kidney deficiency with Liver qi stagnation, 011

Kidney deficiency, 009, 039, 048, 059, 086, 109, 110, 112, 150, 183, 184, 201, 204, 231, 233, 249, 281, 290, 305, 331

Kidney essence deficiency, 041

Kidney qi deficiency, 155, 299

Kidney yang and Spleen qi deficiency, 294

Kidney yang deficiency, 031, 041, 068, 116, 128, 154, 156, 161, 175, 179, 185, 186, 205, 266, 293, 299, 327

Kidney yin deficiency with Liver constraint, 293

Kidney yin deficiency, 040, 068, 092, 112, 116, 154, 158, 163, 175, 185, 186, 284, 299, 327

kòu rén, 098

kǔ dīng chá, 067

Kǔ Jiǔ Jiān, 053

kǔ shēn, 156

kūn bù, 249, 291

kūn cǎo, 052, 119, 120, 121, 122

L

lack of appetite, 243

lack of libido, 238, 281

lái fú yīng, 089, 090

lái fú zǐ, 044, 089, 090

lassitude with sleepiness, 018

lassitude, 013, 033, 037, 043, 063, 069, 081, 087, 090, 189, 234, 236, 246, 266, 270, 276, 281, 316

late menarche, 233

Latent heat in the sea of blood,

119

Leonuri, 265

leucopenia, 048

lián fáng tàn, 088, 108, 170

lián qiào, 021, 030, 102

lián ròu, 164

lián xū, 120, 121

lián zǐ xīn, 112, 154

Liǎng Dì Tāng, 173

liǎng tóu jiān, 266, 267

life gate fire, 010

Lignm Sappan, 117

Lignum Dalbergiae Odoriferae, 131

Limonitum, 070, 071, 072, 074, 096

Lineate Supplejack Root, 287

líng xiāo huā, 266, 267

Litchi Chinensis Sonn, 068, 175

Liù Jūn Zǐ Tāng, 101

Liù Wèi Dì Huáng Tāng, 152

Liù Wèi Dì Huáng Wán, 153, 178, 190, 295, 298

Liver and Kidney deficiency, 160, 188, 318, 326, 333

Liver and Kidney yin deficiency, 028, 064, 094, 127, 160

Liver and Stomach disharmony, 171

Liver blood deficiency, 090, 299

Liver constraint affecting the Spleen, 043

Liver constraint and blood stasis, 268, 326

Liver Constraint with Blood-heat, 022

Liver constraint, 294, 327

Liver depression, 251

Liver qi constraint, 008

Liver qi stagnation and excessive heat, 179

Liver qi stagnation, 011, 097, 101, 109, 178, 188, 194, 204

Liver yin deficiency, 299

lóng dǎn cǎo, 288

Lóng Dǎn Xiè Gān Tāng, 295

lóng gǔ, 034, 100, 131, 187, 197, 241

lóng yǎn ròu, 036, 099, 192

longstanding blood stasis transforming into heat, 025

Longstanding Qi Deficiency Impairing Yang, 105

loose stools, 033, 035, 037, 043, 085, 122, 172, 234, 251, 322

lower abdominal discomfort, 033

lower abdominal distention and pain, 024

lower abdominal pain, 027, 234, 249, 319

lower back and upper abdominal pain, 273

lower back soreness, 266

lower jiao, 280

lù dǎng shēn, 041, 076, 181

lú huì, 288

lù jiǎo jiāo, 026, 029, 038, 055, 065, 088, 094, 099, 108, 132, 157, 168, 201, 321

lù jiǎo piàn, 032, 037, 213, 240, 293, 297, 317, 338

lù jiǎo shuāng, 061, 086, 093, 095, 128, 155, 159, 162, 166, 167, 186, 198, 238, 291, 318, 324

Notes